A Suitable Case for Treatment

The NHS and Reform

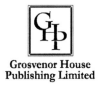

To Roger
Best wishes
Norman

by

Norman Warner

Grosvenor House
Publishing Limited

Norman Warner is hereby identified as author of this
work in accordance with Section 77 of the Copyright, Designs
and Patents Act 1988

The book cover picture is copyright to Inmagine Corp LLC

This book is published by
Grosvenor House Publishing Ltd
28-30 High Street, Guildford, Surrey, GU1 3HY.
www.grosvenorhousepublishing.co.uk

A CIP record for this book
is available from the British Library

ISBN 978-1-908105-32-5

Dedication

This book is dedicated to my children and grandchildren,
who deserve a better NHS inheritance.

About the Author

Norman Warner is a Labour member of the House of Lords and a member of the Lords Select Committee on Science and Technology. He is also a member of the independent Commission on Care and Support appointed by the Coalition Government. He was a Health Minister in the Blair Government and worked on NHS reform. He has been the senior policy adviser to the Home Secretary; and set up and chaired the Youth Justice Board for England and Wales to oversee reform of youth justice. As Kent's Director of Social Services in the 1980s he was heavily involved in reform of community care. He has chaired voluntary organisations and the National Council of Voluntary Organisations, as well as working as a management consultant and advising private companies.

Contents

Preface

Scene - setting

Personal and political context

One afternoon in June 2003 the telephone rang and No.10 asked me if I would speak to the Prime Minister. By 6pm that evening I was a Health Minister. For the next few years my life changed as I found myself back in the Department of Health, nearly twenty years after I had left it as a civil servant. This was the start of a chaotic, absorbing and often frustrating experience at a time of great change and turmoil for a national icon – the NHS. Suddenly riches beyond its wildest dreams had become available after years of penury. But the cash was accompanied by an avalanche of change driven by the Prime Minister, special advisers and a small cadre of Ministers and civil servants. The NHS liked the idea of the money but was less keen on the 'change' bit of the deal.

My time as a Minister was one of political controversy. The events of 9/11 had led to a war in Iraq driven from the other side of the Atlantic. A British Prime Minister had decided to support an unpopular US President and in doing so used up a lot of his domestic political capital within his own party, the public and the public services. The Labour Party was divided over the Iraq war and my predecessor as a Lords Health Minister had resigned over it. I had some unease about joining the government but felt that Blair had been let down by Chirac at the last moment over a second UN resolution on Iraq which would have provided a stronger legal basis for the war. At the time I thought it reasonable to believe that Saddam Hussein still had chemical weapons that he was willing to use. As the Chilcot Inquiry is showing, hindsight is a wonderful thing but few of us then could have known how inept the US would be at securing the peace.

The reality was that I was a Blairite appointment whether I liked it or not and that I would be doing this job when Tony Blair's political share price was falling rather than rising. The full extent to which he was going to be continually sniped at internally by his own ambitious and disloyal Chancellor – or 'friends of Gordon' as they were often described - was only to become fully apparent when I was in office. Back in 2003 I did not realise that Brown's commitment to public service reform was as intermittent as it turned out to be or appreciate the dysfunctionality of the Blair/Brown relationship.

On a personal level I liked Tony Blair from my work with him before the 1997 election and my later experience as the Home Secretary's Senior

Policy Adviser. Fresh from reforming the youth justice system I totally supported his public service reform agenda. I thought then, as now, that the NHS was an over-bureaucratic public monopoly that needed a healthy dose of reform and modernisation if it was to develop and to justify the huge investment of taxpayers' money being made in it. I had no problem about keeping my foot on the reform accelerator but then I had no trade union links or sponsorship to worry about. Unlike most of my elected colleagues I had managed big organisations at a time of change. These included a large Social Security Region (Wales and the South West of England) in the 1980's during the Thatcher efficiency programme; after that a large Social Services Department, Kent, spearheading community care reform; and from 1998 to 2003 I had reformed the youth justice system from the Home office and chaired the new Youth Justice Board for England and Wales to drive the reforms. I was well aware of the ways that government departments and public sector organisations can thwart reform and avoid change.

As a former senior civil servant I was well-versed in mandarin behaviour. I have never considered that the British civil service was quite the Rolls-Royce machine that many in it liked to claim. Nor was I as paranoid about civil service manipulation as some former Ministers I have encountered. As a former Cabinet Secretary, Lord Butler, said in a recent interview, "the job of a civil servant is being a mercenary."[1] So they can be directed. My perspective provided me with a healthy scepticism about much of the advice I was given and the confidence both to look for alternative sources of ideas and help and to reject some official advice. This experience and perspective undoubtedly made it easier to be a reforming Minister in government. But however much I could claim to be a politically-savvy technocrat rather than an ideological politician I could not escape the fetters and distractions of Ministerial life. These impose considerable constraints on reforming Ministers whatever political party they belong to. They need to be better understood.

Life as a Minister

There is a large amount of routine in the life of a Minister which has little to do with changing the world: correspondence, Parliamentary business, speeches, duty Minister rosters, voting, Cabinet committees, EU business and dealing with the media. Elected Ministers have to nurture their constituencies and manage their small Parliamentary constituency offices. As an unelected Lords Minister I had some of these distractions but also different ones – namely the business and preoccupations of an unmodernised House of Lords.

Most people, including elected Ministers, do not understand the role and workings of the House of Lords as a scrutiny and revising second Chamber. They have little sympathy with the fact that as a Minister you cannot rely on a whipped majority, as in the House of Commons, to get the Government's business through because in the Lords no government usually has a majority. With the Foundation Trust legislation in 2003 John Reid – who liked to refer to the House of Lords as the 'Eastern Front' – had to accept negotiating with the opposition parties to secure the legislation. From the Prime Minister downwards Commons Ministers underestimate the time that Lords Ministers have to spend on House of Lords business.

As the Lords Health Minister I had to cover all aspects of the Department of Health (and Food Standards Agency) work in the Lords as well as handling my own portfolio of responsibilities. This meant appearing regularly to answer oral questions, signing off all written health answers in the Lords, dealing with frequent debates and taking all DH legislation through the Lords. These duties did not exempt me from my share of the normal Ministerial slog of signing hundreds of Ministerial replies to MPs a month; being a duty Minister over weekends and in Parliamentary Recesses; and covering for Ministerial colleagues when they were away on overseas visits. My own portfolio produced the usual share of Cabinet Committees, media appearances, overseas visits and speeches to conferences.

Looking back over my time as a Minister I find I gave about 60 speeches at various conferences and events; averaged one or two media appearances a week; probably signed the best part of 10,000 letters; undertook EU Ministerial meetings and about five or six other overseas representational visits; and acted as Duty Minister for about 40 weekends and some 15-20 weeks of Parliamentary recesses. As the only Minister who both lived in London and had no constituency I was particularly vulnerable to the Duty Minister roster! All this took considerable time away from policy work, thinking and the difficult task of implementing change.

Admittedly these diversions (such as a visit to China to sign health agreements with that absorbing country) could be both interesting and even dramatic. As a Duty Minister in November 2006 I suddenly found myself embroiled in COBR meetings in the Cabinet Office concerned with the poisoning of Alexander Litvinenko with Polonium 210. This had everything one needed for a TV drama – foreign agents allegedly poisoning a person on UK soil in a public place with a radioactive substance; FCO diplomacy with a powerful foreign country in a state of denial; a police investigation fraught with intelligence implications and new scientific challenges; and concerns about public and NHS staff exposure to radioactive dosages. A bemused public and hyperactive media also needed to be kept informed on what was going on in a fast-changing drama. This is when one learns what Government is all about – "events, dear boy, events" as Harold Macmillan said. As a Minister you end up taking decisions with imperfect amounts of reliable information and trying to keep people informed without raising anxieties unnecessarily or jeopardising a possible criminal prosecution. Events like this were not much to do with my day job but it was what you turned your hand to as a Minister, reforming or otherwise.

Whatever else one does as a Minister, keeping your political boss informed and happy is critical. I found John Reid and Patricia Hewitt easy to work with. Both were accepting of the fact that I lacked their Labour Party contacts and that some Labour backbenchers found me too managerialist for their taste. Patricia defended me staunchly at a Parliamentary Labour Party meeting when some Labour MPs went on a rant about unelected Ministers taking contentious decisions.

Keeping the Prime Minister on side is even more important. This was never a problem with Tony Blair providing he was convinced that you were driving the reform vehicle as fast as possible. He was accessible on a regular basis, unlike his next-door neighbour cocooned in the Treasury. Blair was skilled at keeping himself sufficiently informed through his staff without becoming submerged in detailed documents. So keeping the No. 10 apparatchiks informed and on side is key for any adventurous Minister trying to achieve change. This is one of the best time investments any reforming Minister can make.

The biggest distraction from my main Ministerial portfolio was the House of Lords itself. Apart from my role as a Health Minister I was part of the Government's payroll vote for all its legislation in a Second Chamber in which it had no majority. If the Liberal Democrats and Conservatives joined forces – as they regularly did - they could defeat the Government on its legislation unless the Crossbenchers sided with the Government, which they rarely did. This meant that for parts of the year either I based myself in the House of Lords during afternoons and evenings or I rushed from meetings in the Department, jumped in a Ministerial car and sprinted up the Lords' stairs to get into the division lobby in the 8 minutes allowed to me.

One of the greatest problems was oral questions. Unlike the Commons the House of Lords does not have set days for particular Departments and oral questions. It starts each day (i.e. Monday – Thursday) with four oral questions (which can be on anything) lasting 8 minutes each. This means, as happened to me on occasion, you could end up having three or even four questions on totally different topics on the same day on matters outside your main portfolio – and sometimes with little notice. You spend the evening or morning before the questions becoming an instant expert on anything from avian 'flu or contaminated blood to obscure cancers or mixed-sex hospital wards. Fragments of the voluminous civil service material mugged up for these Lords appearances served me well when appearing in the media as a Duty Minister. I found that odd factual pieces of information could at least slow down Jeremy Paxman or John Humphreys even if they did not totally distract them from their pursuit of you.

By the time I became a Minister in 2003 the House of Lords had become more politically confrontational following the removal of most hereditary peers and the realisation by many campaigners that the main place to sandbag the Government was in the Lords where the Government did not have a majority. Sometimes civil service accuracy failed. On 25 October 2006 I was asked an oral question about the costs and justification for tattoo removals under the NHS, following an answer in the Commons suggesting that the NHS removed 187,000 tattoos a year. I did not believe these figures and asked the DH statisticians to check them. Silence reigned until just before I went into the Chamber to answer the question when I was told that the correct figure was not 187,000 but about half a dozen! I had to acknowledge the figures were wrong; use jokes about a surgeon on the Conservative benches having to use his skill to remove 'I love William', 'I love Iain' and 'I love Michael' tattoos from Conservative MPs because of their frequent change of Leader; and be rude to Lord Tebbit which always went down well on the Labour benches.

Debates and legislation in the Lords took up a lot of time. Apart from secondary legislation I piloted through five major Health Bills: the Health and Social Care Act 2003 (which set up Foundation Trusts and new inspectorates/regulators); the Human Tissue Act 2004 (which reformed the law on the removal, storage and use of human organs and other tissues following scandals over the widespread misuse of children's organs at Alder Hey Children's Hospital); the Health Protection Agency Act 2003 (which provided a proper statutory basis for the body); the NHS Redress Act 2006 (which reformed the Clinical Negligence Scheme); and the Health Act 2006 (which amongst other things banned smoking in work and public places). Three of these were very controversial and occupied a lot of time on the floor of the House, sometimes until late into the night or even early morning.

Your quality of life as a Minister depends a great deal on your Private office. I chose the Principal Private Secretaries I wanted, not always what I was offered. Ministers have only themselves to blame if they put up with Private Office personnel who are unsuitable. If you cannot trust your Private Secretaries – and I have been one – you are in trouble. The frenetic lifestyle makes a sense of humour important. Your Private Office have to be able to cope with you applying to official submissions a stamp which reads "I haven't got time to read this CRAP"; and accept that your gym and theatre engagements are high priority diary commitments.

Because health was a 'hot' issue in my time as a Minister there were many debates which could require you to sit on the front bench for hours at a time. The temptation to let your attention wander was enormous. During one interminable speech by an opponent of a smoking ban in public places I was in a private reverie and was accused of not paying proper attention to the speaker. Rather ill-advisedly I told him his endless repetition must have caused me to doze off: but after a bit of uproar business speeded up. My personal record was $8^1/_2$ hours on the front bench for the Second Reading of Lord Joffé's Assisted Dying Private Members Bill in 2006 when I had to pretend to be neutral (the Government's position usually on private members bills) even though people knew I supported the Bill.

This brief sketch of Ministerial life in the Lords is not intended to excuse my mistakes – which I acknowledge freely – but to demonstrate how much time can be diverted away from a Minister's main job and priorities. The time spent by Ministers on Parliamentary matters is often little understood either by the public or the commentariat. In terms of Ministerial accountability this time may well be important but we should not pretend that it does not come at a price in terms of tiredness, rushed decision-making and distraction from implementing change. The more we tie up Ministerial time in Parliamentary and media activity – important though they are – the less time Ministers have to think through the policy, legislation and implementation implications of changes they are trying to make.

The NHS culture and reform

The NHS is a great achievement and publicly popular. It tends to produce good intentions in politicians but also frustration that it is not as good as it could be. The 'public monopoly' culture of the NHS is something that any reforming Health Minister has to be prepared to deal with. Monopolies have their own ways of doing things and can be slow to innovate and respond to the changing needs of services users. Yet healthcare is an area where science and technology keep producing new treatments and care regimes that make older treatments and approaches to care obsolete with increasing rapidity.

As a monopoly the NHS has struggled to respond to medical advances and adapt to changing public expectations. As a public monopoly the NHS has behaved much like private monopolies but the public hostility has been less and there has been no market or regulator to force change. The scale of this monopoly is huge, spending over £100billion a year and employing over 1.3 million people. There are 300 million GP and community consultations a year; 20 million A and E attendances; and 300,000 people receiving mental health services. Denting its complacency is difficult.

This monopolistic power shows in the attitude of many NHS staff and their resistance to external providers and reform. While I was a Minister, the health team regularly had meetings with groups of NHS staff, with everyone from porters to consultants, but with no senior managers present. When asked what they would most like me as a Minister to do, they invariably asked me to stop change. There was a touching belief that I could insulate the NHS from changes in society and the public's rising expectations of the NHS, particularly when it was consuming more of their taxes. At these meetings few people saw themselves as having much by way of an obligation to the taxpayers – as distinct from patients – who were funding their jobs. Some simply wanted to be left alone, unchallenged, because they were professionals.

As a Health Minister you are required to pay tribute to the hard-working commitment of NHS staff; and I genuinely believed that was true for many staff. However I often came away from many 'staff engagement' meetings depressed by the unwillingness of so many people to accept the inevitability of change in the way they did their jobs or to embrace ideas of innovation and new ways of working. George Bernard Shaw's line in 'The Doctors Dilemma' that "all professions are conspiracies against the laity" came too often to mind for comfort.

Monopoly service providers and powerful vested professional and union interests – combined in the British Medical Association – cause particular problems for a tax-funded healthcare system with free patient access on a basis of clinical need. This model of healthcare funding is excellent in terms of controlling overall costs and providing universal coverage at a reasonable price. It is not so good in terms of guaranteeing choice and responsiveness and avoiding long waits. Yet like all healthcare systems the NHS has to reconcile heavier demand for services from an ageing and longer-lived population, more rapid medical advances and rising public expectations. Reconciling these systemic features with the monopolistic and change-averse culture of the NHS is the challenge faced by reforming Health Ministers of all political hues.

I recognised that the NHS monopolistic culture and powerful vested interests needed to be engaged with and challenged. Many of those interests were bound to oppose challenge mechanisms that involved making the NHS a more open market, with greater diversity of providers competing for contracts. More patient choice and empowerment would make that greater competition more responsive to patient preferences. A marketised NHS required an effective purchaser/provider split with powerful commissioners driving change in patterns of service delivery. Providers with high overheads like acute hospitals needed only to be used when really necessary and in the most economical configurations. Economies of scale needed to be looked for, together with higher productivity in what is a high-cost labour-intensive industry. Robust inspectorates and regulators were required to provide reliable performance information, guarantee quality and deal with the inevitable failures when weaker providers needed to be replaced.

This was the reform agenda of the second and third Labour governments, with much of it set out in Labour's 2005 election manifesto – appropriately a little red book, entitled "Britain forward not back". It was the agenda I signed up for as health reform Minister. I was confident that it was what Tony Blair had in mind but he hadn't left himself much time to deliver it, with his anointed successor breathing down his neck. It was the brooding presence in 11 Downing Street that was the uncertain factor.

This book provides my account of the pursuit of NHS reform and Labour's stewardship of the NHS. The NHS is a Labour icon that has survived 60 years as a popular, civilising influence in our liberal democracy. It cannot be preserved in aspic if it is to survive another 60 years. It has to demonstrate adaptability and continuing value for money and not atrophy into a monopoly requiring more and more of the national wealth to prop it up. Markets are not popular at present but then nor are monopolies. Some greater measure of challenge and change is required if the NHS is to meet the demands it will face. This will require political leadership and courage to take the NHS where is needs to go. Will the Coalition Government be able to provide the necessary Star Trek crew and Captain Kirk?

1

The NHS reform inheritance

For the first 25 years of its life there was little change to the NHS organisational structure and its approach to service delivery. From the 1970s onwards successive governments and Ministers tried to reorganise it or reform it. Richard Crossman, Keith Joseph and Ken Clarke all had a go before Alan Milburn returned to the subject in 2000. The reason that reform or reorganisation continues to be attempted is I suspect because when you get up close to the NHS you quickly realise that it could and should perform better, especially at times of increasing investment of public money. You come to believe that better performance would come if only you could find the right structures and processes.

More recently those interested in public service reform have become more attracted to ideas like increasing competition and patient choice as ways of shaking up complacent public monopoly. One of the attractions of these ideas is that they offer an alternative vision of self-balancing local systems with more decisions in the hands of service users rather than the traditional method of politicians trying to drive change from the centre. In the past two decades a raft of new instruments and approaches have been tried: purchaser/provider splits, targets or guarantees, more inspection and regulation, increased managerialism, more diversity of providers, tariffs, increased patient voice and choice, markets and competition. All have their supporters and opponents with a debate that ebbs and flows between more or less centralism and localism.

The Conservative inheritance

When I took over the NHS reform baton from John Hutton in 2005 I was well aware of Labour's mixed history on NHS reform and the hostility in many parts of the Labour party to the Conservative reforms of Ken Clarke. Personally I was much more sympathetic to those reforms than I ever dared admit to my colleagues. Until the 1970s the NHS had made do with a simple structure which had Regional Hospital Boards supervising local hospital boards, with medical directors, matrons and hospital secretaries running individual hospitals. Executive Councils ran all the primary care services (GPs, dentists, pharmacists and opticians); with local authorities running health centres and community nursing and health visitor services. Prior to Alan Milburn, Dick Crossman was probably the only Labour Health Secretary who considered major organisational change with his attempt at greater NHS integration in a White Paper published in 1970. It had been the Conservatives who had made all the running on NHS reform and reorganisation until Alan Milburn arrived.

Keith Joseph made the first serious attempt at a reorganisation driven by managerialism in 1974. This created Area Health Authorities with wider responsibilities; he removed local authorities from involvement in healthcare; but retained a regional tier and separate Family Practitioner Committees to run primary care – mainly because GPs wanted an administrative system they had more control over. This reorganisation had as underpinning a management 'grey book' largely produced by a team at Brunel University led by Professor Elliott Jacques. As a young civil servant I had worked on the grey book and implementing this reorganisation. It was nearly aborted by Labour when it came to power in 1974 two months before the Joseph reorganisation was due to go live on the 1 April 1974. Barbara Castle, Labour's new Secretary of State, only went ahead with it reluctantly because she feared that Labour would be blamed for the chaos and wasted money that would ensue from a last minute cancellation when thousands of NHS staff were already in place with new employers.

After the Conservatives returned to office in 1979 they used Sir Roy Griffiths of Sainsbury's to help them introduce the concept of general management into the NHS to improve efficiency and secure better value for money. This was part of a wider and in my view praiseworthy attempt by the Thatcher Government to improve management efficiency across the public services. The final sentence of Sir Roy's October 1983 report to the then Health Secretary, Norman (now Lord) Fowler summed up the introspective nature of the NHS and its resistance to change: "……….the Health Service can ill afford to indulge in any lengthy self- imposed Hamlet-like soliloquy as a precursor or alternative to the required action."[1] Roy Griffiths and Derek Rayner of Marks & Spencer's were Margaret Thatcher's two management gurus of choice, with retail as her business model for the public services. The NHS remained reluctant to accept the idea of customers who could take their business elsewhere and preferred to continue in its self-preoccupied way of spending taxpayer's money without too much scrutiny or local accountability.

Part of Thatcher's wider agenda was to make Ministers take more responsibility for managing their Departments. From my own civil service experience this was met with mixed enthusiasm by most of her cabinet colleagues, with the exception of Michael Heseltine and Ken Clarke. Labour throughout the Thatcher and Major years misguidedly took little interest in the management or efficiency agenda for improving public services. It ended up in 1997 promising to cut 'the men in grey suits' in an already under-managed NHS. This anti-managerialism still infects parts of the Labour Party, including some former Cabinet Ministers; and has now seems to have spread to the Conservatives. In my more gloomy moments I sometimes think that parts of the Labour Party believe that the NHS could run itself perfectly well as a kind of workers' cooperative, while the Conservatives looked to have moved on to a touching faith in self-improving professionals listening to the voices of patients.

Throughout their time in government between 1979 and 1997 the Conservatives struggled to convince the public that they cared about the NHS and supported its basic tenet of healthcare available to all on the basis of clinical need and free at the point of use. They seemed, for the most part, more interested in encouraging people to opt out of the NHS with tax incentives for private health insurance to buy care from the private sector. They also played with the idea of extending co-payments beyond prescription charges to hotel charges in hospitals and fees for GP's visits to reduce use/abuse – depending upon your political point of view. A Treasury-initiated CPRS Report in 1982 when Leon (now Lord) Brittain was Chief Secretary had proposed options of this kind. It was the leaking of this Report – allegedly by one of the Cabinet "wets" – that led to Margaret Thatcher telling the Conservative Party Conference in October 1982: "Let me make one thing absolutely clear. The National Health Service is safe with us".[2] This is a view that David Cameron has been keen to emphasise as the Conservatives tried to woo disenchanted NHS staff before the 2010 Election.

For the rest of their time in government the Conservatives continued with their public mantra that the NHS was "safe in their hands". However while Thatcher remained Prime Minister she continued to hanker after higher patient charges (which to be fair had fallen as a proportion of NHS finance so some increase could have been justified); and for tax incentives to encourage more people to take out private health insurance and so reduce demand on the NHS.

It was not until the ebullient Ken Clarke arrived as Health Secretary in the summer of 1987 that plans for financing the NHS other than through general taxation were effectively killed off politically. The proportion of the population with private medical insurance continued to grow – up from 5% in 1979 to about 11% in 1990 – but the services covered shrank as treatment costs rose. Public funding for independent hospitals and nursing homes increased considerably under the Conservatives chiefly through payments from a loophole in social security regulations. These payments were for long-stay care rather than acute care. On the whole – apart from occasional crises, usually in winter, investment in NHS buildings and equipment stagnated through the 1980's and 1990's, despite rapid changes in medical technology and rising public expectations. For some in the middle classes private health insurance was the safety valve that reduced pressure on the NHS.

Nevertheless some Conservatives were genuinely interested in making the NHS more efficient. Clarke was to be a creative Health

Secretary not afraid to stand up to Mrs Thatcher and the BMA. On his summer holiday in 1987 he came up with the idea of GP budget-holding. Family doctors would be given budgets to purchase a range of operations and outpatient treatments from hospitals and to pay for the drugs they prescribed. GP's would be expected to make savings that they could spend on their own practices or other services. This was fed into a secretive review that Thatcher has been chairing (involving Nigel Lawson and John Major from the Treasury and John Moore and Tony Newton from Health). That Review was pursuing the idea of money following patients (as was being pursued in education) with an internal market in which health authorities and now GPs would commission services from hospital trusts that were to become self-governing. This last idea was to restore the old Boards of Governors of teaching hospitals like Guys and St Thomas's.

At the end of January 1989 Ken Clarke had himself transported by riverboat from the Commons to Limehouse to launch the Review's findings in a White Paper "Working for Patients". According to one commentator, Nick Timmins, "a million pounds was spent on a staff video and a laser-lit closed-circuit telecast from Limehouse to 2,500 managers, doctors, chairmen and nurses who had been assembled in television studios and hotels in six cities."[3] If only such an event was as cheap today!

This White Paper had three big ideas that were to shape much of the NHS reform agenda for the next twenty years whether Labour opponents liked it or not. As a Minister I was not ashamed to draw upon them. These ideas were an internal NHS market with a purchaser-provider split, with health authorities doing the purchasing (or commissioning as it was later to be called) and a range of public and private hospitals providing the services; secondly those hospital trusts who wished could become self-governing (later to re-emerge as Foundation Trusts); and third those GPs who volunteered could become budget-holders later to be re-named fund-holders and by me as practice-based commissioners. These ideas remain at the centre of NHS reform thinking today.

The BMA had not been consulted on these changes and there was a major conflict with them, with Labour joining in this opposition. Opponents fought the government vigorously complaining – as they did when I was a Minister – that changes of this kind were the first steps to privatising the NHS. Thatcher – then nearing the end of her time – pressured Clarke to postpone the changes but Ken Clarke kept his nerve as Tony Blair was to do later. This legislation was passed despite Labour opposition and in April 1991 the new NHS trusts (now including community and ambulance services as well as hospitals) started to come into being along with the first GP fund-holders.

By the time of the 1997 election about half the country's population was covered by GP fund-holders. By easing the eligibility conditions – a mistake which Labour did not repeat with Foundation Trusts – the Conservatives had all service providers (except GPs) in NHS Trusts. The reforms were seen as more managerial than clinical; and the BMA and NHS came to accept them – however reluctantly – for the most part. But with little extra money being made available to the NHS, these reforms never received the backing they deserved. To many they looked more like moving the organisational furniture around than the potentially significant changes that they represented.

Labour's first term

In the 1990s Labour got themselves totally on the wrong side of the argument over the Clarke reforms. The late Robin Cook, then Shadow Health Secretary, made blood-curdling remarks – "by God the government is going to get it in the neck" – and lined up Labour with a BMA hostile to Clarke's reforms.[4] Successive Labour spokesmen (and women) were to waste their time attacking the Conservative reforms and NHS managers ("men in grey suits") rather than devising credible policies of their own. Labour opposed the internal market and GP fundholding, both ideas that were finally adopted in modified form in the Labour 2005 manifesto and that I was more than delighted to implement.

Strangely enough the 1997 manifesto with which Labour won a landslide victory had little to say on the NHS. Conservative unpopularity allowed Labour to travel policy-lite - as David Cameron did in a period of Labour unpopularity. Labour's ideas were confined to cutting waiting lists and bureaucracy (again, "men in grey suits"); rejecting the internal market; and replacing GP fundholding with "GP commissioning to give all GP's a voice in shaping local health services".[5] This last promise was never really delivered until I pushed on with practice-based commissioning in 2005.

This unpromising background for NHS reform under Labour was made worse by two years of inaction after the 1997 election. As the Millennium approached the political priority for the NHS was an investment plan. Alan Milburn, the new Health Secretary delivered this in 2000 in The NHS Plan which set out ideas for a huge expansion of NHS capacity but it also resurrected the idea of reform. For the first time it linked the two ideas of investment and reform and brutally pointed out that "The NHS is a1940's system operating in a 21st Century world".[6]

For the first time since Dick Crossman at the end of the 1960s, the NHS Plan started to map out a distinctive Labour view on what NHS reform involved. "The principles of the NHS are sound but its practices need to change". The proposed reforms included "a big expansion of quality-based contracts for GP's" and consultants would "be expected to increase their productivity while working for the NHS." Patients were to have more say and "their views on local health services will help decide how much cash they get." The previously thought "Great Satan" - otherwise known as the private sector - was to be involved. "For the first time there will be a concordat with private providers of health care to enable the NHS to make better use of facilities in private hospitals......"[7]

Looking back however it is far from clear that the idea of reform was really taken seriously by that many people in the NHS. It was still an acute sector, provider-driven health care system that could now salivate over the prospect of unexpected riches. The implications of this reform agenda only really sunk in much later for many people in the NHS when a reform-minded Prime Minister was running out of time and patience and Simon Stevens had shifted to his elbow from that of Alan Milburn. Only then did the words in the NHS Plan start to move from political rhetoric to reality.

Labour went into its 2001 election campaign mentioning reform but in a low key way and with its distinctive political narrative being primarily about NHS investment and increased capacity and performance. There was a commitment in its Manifesto to creating new elective surgery centres, some of which could be managed by the private sector. For the first time there was mention of failing hospitals being taken over by successful NHS ones. These cautious steps towards a health care market in which private providers might play a part were also accompanied by some low key promises on patient choice over hospital bookings and maternity services.[8] The big messages however were more money for the NHS, more staff and some national targets on improving health. Even the NHS reorganisation that Milburn had started work on before the 2001 election was reassuringly but misleadingly described as devolving more autonomy and cutting bureaucracy. Unfortunately it was to be a reorganisation that did not help NHS reform and was to come back to haunt Labour and make delivery of the reform agenda much more difficult.

The 2002 NHS reorganisation

After the success of the NHS Plan, securing more money for the NHS and opening up the prospect of a more diverse provider market, Alan Milburn rather spoilt things with the 2002 NHS reorganisation. I struggled to find any coherent explanation for it when I took over NHS reform in 2005. I had, for some time, thought that we had created a totally unsustainable structure - in terms of cost and management capability - for running the NHS. Essentially what Alan did – no doubt with advice and good intentions – was to scrap the remaining 4 regional bodies - he had already abolished most of them - and the 90 health authorities. He replaced them with 28 Strategic Health Authorities (SHAs) and 304 new Primary Care Trusts (PCTs). The PCTs were to commission services from the untouched acute and mental health trusts, let contracts for primary care and provide and manage community services.

Without much acknowledgement the reorganisation effectively reintroduced the Conservatives' internal market with a purchaser-provider split at least as far as the hospitals were concerned. In principle this was the right thing to do but unfortunately this was not the best way to do it. The reorganisation took away a strong regional tier that could have helped PCTs performance-manage the hospital provider side and deliver the NHS Plan while commissioning skills were developed. The change repeated the Conservatives mistake of not investing enough in the development of high quality commissioning skills in the new PCTs. It exacerbated that problem by hopelessly overestimating the capacity of the NHS to find 304 senior management teams capable of doing the commissioning job and also running community services well. The purchaser-provider split was left incomplete because the provision of community services was left with the PCT commissioners, with all the conflicts of interest that involved, and still involves. As I was to discover not only were these new PCTs not very good commissioners they were not great at managing community services either.

While the rest of Whitehall was concentrating its regional presence on 9 standard government regions the NHS was going in another direction under the 2002 reorganisation. The 28 new SHAs had no co-terminosity with any other regional services that were important to the government's public health agenda. Public health itself was strategically cast adrift from the NHS by being left in the 9 government regional offices. The London changes were totally misguided, with five SHAs replacing a single strategic body for the capital, 31 PCTs and a huge growth in staff that was in inverse proportions to strategic effectiveness. Sadly the 2002 reorganisation was a major mistake that was a significant waste of management effort, money and manpower which had to be corrected three years later at a considerable cost in money, effort and political capital. Labour's first real venture into NHS reorganisation since the inception of the NHS was a disaster.

The emerging reform agenda

Two other, much more successful, policy changes in 2002 had created divisions within the NHS, the Government and the Labour backbenches – Foundation Hospital Trusts (FTs) and the 2001 election commitment to use the private sector. The reform-minded parts of the NHS wanted more autonomy and wanted to take the Government at its word and press on with change. It wanted to do this outside the Whitehall-controlled performance management system which too often led to good performers handing over financial surpluses to bail out other poorly-performing hospitals. Alan Milburn was keen on local autonomy and pressed for the new FT hospitals to have far more autonomy from Whitehall so that they could innovate and plan ahead for future changes. FTs were to have a governance structure based on the Coop mutual model, with a lot of local accountability. The then Chancellor, Gordon Brown, and the Treasury, feared losing control, particularly if the new FTs could borrow in the private financial markets as Milburn and Tony Blair wanted.

There was a heated debate between the Chancellor in one camp and the Prime Minister and the Health Secretary in another. Labour back benchers became very excited that FTs would become agents for more private practice, privatisation and semi-detachment from the NHS. The row broke out into the media and became part of the Brown/ Blair factions' regular arm-wrestling. Although a fragile peace between the two sides eventually broke out the dispute led to the legislation introducing FTs becoming extremely controversial, as is described in Chapter 3.

Alongside this controversy and partly fuelling it was the central letting of contracts for Independent Sector Treatment Centres (ISTCs). This was both to increase capacity to cut waiting times and, as became increasingly obvious, to introduce competition with local NHS monopoly providers of day surgery and diagnostics. How this developed is also described in Chapter 3 but the blue touch paper was lit by the establishment of a Commercial Directorate in the Department of Health, led by a Texan, Ken Anderson; and the publication in December 2002 of "Growing Capacity: Independent Sector Diagnosis and Treatment Centres" which invited expressions of interest from the independent sector to run a number of ISTCs.

Paranoia in the NHS trades unions and parts of the Labour back benches rose, even though this merely implemented the 2001 Manifesto promise. (Some Labour MPs have come to be very selective about which parts of manifestos on which they are elected they regard as suitable for implementation). The NHS, allegedly, was going to be privatised in a way never previously foreseen and the driving force for this was none other than the Prime Minister. Tony Blair made little secret of his impatience at what he regarded as the slow pace of change in the NHS in response to rising public expectations. He met overtly with private sector players to encourage their participation in the NHS.

By 2003 there was a growing reform agenda developing alongside investment and delivery targets. This was not only about FT hospitals and ISTCs and the associated concerns about privatisation, competition and markets. As access and performance improved as a result of the extra money and staff, issues of quality and efficiency began to be part of the public and political debate. The public turned out to want not only faster and better clinical services they wanted the 'hotel' services and the clunky administrative systems to improve.

Although new buildings and equipment were coming on stream, the greater intensity of bed use was making it more difficult to stem the rising tide of health care-acquired infections, especially MRSA (see Chapter 11). Although average length of stay was dropping, with more procedures done on a day basis, the quality of people's hospital stay was attracting more public concern. People expected better, healthier food and more choice. They noticed when the wards and toilets weren't cleaned properly. As more people came by car the paucity of hospital visitor car-parking was exposed. Why couldn't NHS hospitals have access to TV, telephones and even the internet as patients had in private hospitals? If NHS patients could now be treated in private hospitals, why could not NHS hospitals provide the same quality of 'hotel' experience? Choosing when you had your operation or could see your GP rose up the public wish list, especially amongst the working population who were paying for all these improvements through their taxes.

The growing interest in the quality of the healthcare experience brought an increasing focus on the issues of standards, regulation and choice which are discussed in later chapters. The further NHS reorganisation and growth of managers and arms-length bodies was raising concern that too much of the extra money was going on a growing NHS bureaucracy. Alan Milburn was coming under pressure on these issues as well as from the discontent within the Labour Party over FTs and the greater use of the private sector. NHS reforms started to distract attention from the political benefits of the extra investment in the NHS.

Suddenly in mid-June 2003 in the middle of the passage of the FT legislation and with the Department of Health sitting on a pile of expressions of interest from the private sector in building ISTCs the Prime Minister decided to reshuffle his cabinet. The architect of the growing programme of NHS reform left DH for personal reasons and was replaced by Dr John ("oh Fuck, not health") Reid. John was given the contradictory remit of calming things down without taking his foot off the NHS reform accelerator. Strong rumours had circulated that influential figures in the NHS had complained to No.10 about Alan Milburn's energetic style. To help maintain reform momentum in an acceptable style the more emollient John Hutton stayed on with the reform brief as John Reid's deputy but otherwise there was a new team of ministers of which I was one.

During the summer of 2003 there was a period of calm apart from the controversy over the FT legislation in the Commons. The new financial year – 2003/4 – was the first of the five years of 7% a year real terms growth for the NHS. At the local level NHS trusts were busily engaged in spending more money and delivering their targets. John Reid settled the dispute with the BMA over the new consultants' contract but without imposing centrally the productivity requirement that Alan Milburn had been pursuing. These improvements were left to local negotiation which suited the consultants fine but not necessarily the NHS finances – see later chapters.

The new star-rating system for hospitals showed a respectable picture. Mr Fixit, as John Reid became known, had a calm and personable manner with the public and the NHS. His competent deputy, John Hutton, was respected in the NHS. Ministers were able to go off on their summer holidays in a climate in which, however reluctantly, the NHS seemed to be moving to some kind of acceptance that change was the price to be paid for the extra investment and staff. Doctors might think managers were getting above themselves but there was a growing number of NHS people behind a modernisation agenda. There was continuing anxiety about the role of the private sector and the new tariff system being drawn up for paying hospitals but it was hitting their targets that remained the big issue of the day for most people in the NHS.

2

Investing in the NHS: money and targets

The story of the NHS between 1997 and 2003 is essentially one of a massive injection of money, people and equipment and the creation of a raft of targets as the basis for demonstrating the results of the huge increase in expenditure. By the end of this period the mantra had changed however to "Investment and Reform". Yet with the exception of FTs, most of the NHS reform had not started and was to come later, with the proposals in the 2005 Election Manifesto. It is easy now to criticise this period of increasing expenditure and targets but some of the criticism is unfair and simplistic, given the circumstances Labour faced. There was - and remains - a good case for some central targets. At the end of the 1990s the case for extra NHS investment was overwhelming but there were few ways of showing improvements for patients in return for the extra expenditure.

The NHS funding inheritance

Whatever the mistakes the New Labour Government made, the NHS it inherited was under-funded and neglected. What Labour found in May 1997 was an NHS in very poor shape after a lengthy period of underinvestment stretching back in some ways to its earliest days. The NHS had a revenue deficit for 1996-1997 that was 1.5% of the annual turnover. This was far worse proportionately than the 2004/5 financial deficit that Patricia Hewitt and I dealt with and which caused so much political furore, as described in Chapter 9.

The legacy of underinvestment had to be tackled and could not be resolved simply by reform and better management, although both were needed. The investment would have to show improvement otherwise public support for continuing with it would evaporate. Targets were an important part of demonstrating that improvement was taking place, however much professionals, political opponents and commentators may choose now to criticise them. The extra money may not always have been well spent and there may have been too many targets or ill-defined ones. But without both the investment and some key targets to provide focus we would not have seen the NHS improvement that even critics acknowledge has taken place over the last decade.

Money and the NHS have always been intertwined. The birth of the NHS itself took place only after a bitter struggle with the medical profession and after Nye Bevan – as he put it – had stuffed the doctors' mouths with gold. (The Blair Government may have done too much of that as well.) Right from the outset the funding and financial underpinning of the NHS has been a problem and a political issue. The plant and equipment that the new NHS inherited in a bankrupt, post-war Britain was poor but the public expectations of the new service were very high and were to remain so. This mismatch has turned out to be a continuing political problem for successive governments and remains an issue today as we face a difficult public expenditure climate. A good quality health and healthcare system does not come cheap and requires sustained investment and modernisation.

As early as 1949 Bevan was telling the Cabinet that hospitals had underestimated the number of beds they needed, thereby ruining his budget. (So there is a history of health Ministers having to take decisions about the NHS on the basis of dodgy figures!) Prescription charges had to be introduced in 1951 to bolster the shaky NHS finances, leading to the resignation of three Labour Ministers, including the future Prime Minister, Harold Wilson. It was to be the 1960s before the first NHS hospital building programme even started as a result of a Conservative Health Minister, Enoch Powell. Successive Governments have struggled to balance the NHS books, maintain an adequate workforce and invest in new buildings and equipment. The march of scientific discoveries and new medical technologies posed major problems for the NHS budget through the 1970s, 1980s and 1990s and continues to do so.

The Conservatives had for the most part declined to engage with the NHS investment issue during their 18 years in office. They tried managerialism and system reform (both worthwhile in themselves) together with playing around with the idea of incentivising private health insurance. What they did not do was develop any credible investment programme for the NHS. Buildings were dilapidated with many from the pre-NHS era and too often from the 19th Century. In many acute hospitals modern diagnostic equipment was not available and there were no plans to install it, even though imaging technology was changing rapidly. In some areas and specialties doctors and nurses were in short supply and there was a heavy reliance on overseas clinical staff. There were no plans to cope with reductions in the working week of doctors being driven by the European Commission. Administrative systems were cumbersome; and waiting lists and waiting times were long and growing for all but truly emergency care. Even there, in some Accident and Emergency Departments, it was not unusual to find elderly patients waiting 12 hours on trolleys for treatment. Use of IT was extremely limited outside general practice and none of it was networked.

In 1997 compared with other major EU countries the UK's expenditure on health care was a much lower proportion of its

GDP – about 6% compared with an EU average of 8%-9%. Compared with other similar countries mortality and morbidity rates were not declining as they should have been for killer diseases like cancer. For many people with these conditions accessing diagnosis let alone treatment was a major issue. Yet Labour was curiously cautious in its 1997 Manifesto as to what it promised to do about this parlous state of affairs. A promise to cut waiting lists by 100,000 was made but this was to be funded by reducing bureaucracy. More ominously the Manifesto also said: "In Government, Ministers will be asked to save before they spend."[1] To demonstrate Labour's responsible attitude to taxation and spending – historically thought to be a Labour political weakness – the new Iron Chancellor, Gordon Brown, promised to live within Conservative spending plans for 2 years. Even the outgoing Conservative Chancellor, Ken Clarke, was willing to admit breezily after the Election that he would not have done so. After nearly two decades of penny-pinching it was difficult to see where the NHS was to make the savings to generate new investment. And the men (and women) in grey suits had hardly been wooed by Robin Cook and Margaret Becket as Shadow Health Ministers to come up with any bright ideas.

To make matters worse the then young and inexperienced new Prime Minister had promised his Shadow Ministers one go on the Ministerial merry-go-round. This may have produced collective harmony in the run up to an election but it left Frank Dobson in charge of the Department of Health, with little appetite for NHS reform. By 1999 the inexperience of the Government and the absence of any health plans prepared in opposition were showing. The worst aspects of waiting lists and waiting times were being tackled but little had been done to improve investment in the creaking NHS services. An election was little more than 2 years away and people were beginning to notice the absence of significant improvement. Something had to give and it was the Health Secretary. Frank Dobson was moved aside and left to run disastrously against Ken Livingstone for the new mayoralty of London. His No.2 the more dynamic Alan Milburn was promoted to Health Secretary and with his expert special adviser Simon Stevens and the ear of the Prime Minister was let off the leash to galvanise health policy.

The NHS Plan – extra money and increased ambition

With the prospect of a 2001 election the Government's level of ambition to improve the NHS went up several notches under Milburn. Using a process of wide-ranging consultation with a diverse group of interests – clinicians, patients' groups, the unions, voluntary organisations, managers, local government and others – Alan Milburn secured buy-in to a major change programme for the NHS for the next 10 years. Much more to the point the Prime Minister and Alan Milburn secured a loosening of the purse strings for the NHS. In the March 2000 Budget the Chancellor announced that the NHS budget would grow over the next 5 years by 50% in cash terms and a third in real terms. More immediately in the financial year starting in April 2000 the NHS received its first substantial budget increase for a very long time with the prospect of more to come in future years.

In July 2000 Blair and Milburn were able to launch the first major development plan for the NHS since Enoch Powell's Hospital Plan of the early 1960s. The NHS Plan promised a mouth-watering level and range of development and investment for an NHS that had waited nearly 60 years for this amount of growth:[2]

- 7000 extra hospital and intermediate care beds
- 3000 GP premises modernised and 250 new scanners
- Over 100 new hospitals by 2010 and 500 new one-stop primary care centres
- Cleaner wards overseen by modern matrons and with better food
- A modern IT system in every hospital and GP surgery
- 7500 more consultants and 2000 more GPs
- 20000 extra nurses and 6500 extra therapists
- 1000 more medical school places
- By the end of 2005 the maximum waiting time for an outpatient appointment would be 3 months and for inpatients 6 months
- Shorter waits for heart operations
- Rapid-access chest pain clinics across the country by 2003
- A big expansion of cancer screening programmes
- An end to the postcode lottery on prescribing cancer drugs
- Breast screening for all women 65-70 years
- By 2004 new intermediate care packages costing nearly £1billion to allow older people to live more independent lives

After decades of neglect the NHS needed this scale of investment and development. It is difficult to do other than admire both the way the Plan was put together and its ambition and coherence. What is now clear is that the planning and financial management systems were not in place to execute it successfully within budget; and nor was there the management capability in the DH or NHS to handle effectively such a large-scale programme. Nevertheless with the 2000 NHS Plan the era of targets was born.

Implementation problems and concerns were to become matters for later. As the 2001 Election approached the NHS Plan's ambitious proposals and the extra money and staff promised had turned things round for the Government. Labour was able to say in its 2001 Manifesto that compared with 1997:

> "Today waiting lists are down by over 100,000 in numbers and waiting times are falling. There are 17000 more nurses, over 6500 more doctors and over 9000 more therapists, scientists and technicians working for patients. The biggest-ever hospital building programme is under way. NHS Direct, the 24-hour helpline is available across the country."

In the NHS offer that the Government was making to the country the narrative was still mainly about investment and cutting bureaucracy, rather than reform. From today's standpoint the offer looks fairly modest:[4]

- "Decentralise power to give local Primary Care Trusts control of 75% NHS funding and cut by two-thirds the number of health authorities.
- Reform the appointments system so that by 2005 every hospital appointment is booked for the convenience of the patient.
- Cut maximum waiting times by end of 2005 for outpatient appointments from six months to three months and inpatients from 18 to six months.
- Work with the private sector to use spare capacity, where it makes sense, for NHS patients.
- Create a new type of hospital – specially built surgical units, managed by the NHS or the private sector – to guarantee shorter waiting time.
- Allow successful NHS hospitals to take over failing ones."

For the first time Labour, rather like a prim Victorian lady, was showing a little ankle in relation to the private sector. But overwhelmingly back in 2001 the story was about the NHS itself delivering improvement through increased investment, reducing bureaucracy and more devolution. Apart from the modest nod towards more private sector involvement there was nothing in the 2001 Manifesto to signal the scale of the reform agenda that was to come later and cause such a furore with unions, NHS staff and Labour backbenchers. FT hospitals, payment by results, commissioning and practice-based commissioning, patient choice and a national programme for IT were not mentioned. The public narrative was still that the NHS needed more investment to secure improvement; and Labour would deliver both with a bit of reorganisation and performance management using targets.

Changing the crew

The 2000 NHS Plan represented a massive expansion of inputs – money, staff, buildings and equipment - with an expectation that there would be some measurable improvements in waiting times for operations and particular services such as cancer, together with shorter waits in Accident and Emergency Departments and speedier access to GPs. It required organisational stability, improved and coordinated project and financial management systems and a tougher accountability regime for delivery than is usually associated with the public sector. What the NHS got instead was a major managerial upheaval. This had been promised before the 2001 Election and was delivered in 2002. This 2002 reorganisation is discussed in more detail in Chapter 5 but in essence it was the wrong reorganisation at the wrong time. It placed in charge of the extra money 304 new, inexperienced and often too small commissioning bodies, Primary Care Trusts (PCTs) and a new intermediate tier of 28 Strategic Health Authorities (SHAs).

This change distracted the NHS management cadre from implementing the ambitious NHS Plan as they sought jobs in a reorganised NHS. This left the NHS ill-equipped to hold in check 200 or so powerful acute hospital trusts. These trusts were ready to absorb all the extra money the Government sent their way in support of the NHS Plan's aspirations. Unaffected by the reorganisation, they were free to expand staff as rapidly as they liked while a disrupted and shaky intermediate tier tried to pursue the DH performance targets at almost any price. As a result the NHS experienced an expensive and inflationary burst of supplier-induced demand as it dashed for service growth after decades of investment famine. Much of the acute hospital sector behaved like lottery winners splurging money to increase outputs irrespective of input costs and productivity.

To complicate matters Alan Milburn had grown impatient with the joint command at the top of the Department of Health. He decided to combine the posts of Permanent Secretary and NHS Chief Executive and go after a powerful private sector person to drive change in the NHS. Alan Langlands, the NHS Chief Executive, was the biggest loss. An able and popular figure in the NHS Langlands had been the Chief Executive since 1994 and was not a person whom Milburn could easily afford to lose. He became Vice-Chancellor of Dundee University and is now Chief Executive of the Higher Education Funding Council; while Chris Kelly, the Permanent Secretary (now Sir Christopher Kelly reviewing MPs' expenses as Chairman of the Committee on Standards of Public Life) departed as well. Things then fell apart when the proposed replacement pulled out at the last moment. Alan Milburn still decided to merge the two posts but with a shortlist of one. He brought in as his new supremo the London NHS Regional Director, Nigel (now Lord) Crisp who unexpectedly found himself not only the NHS Chief Executive but the Permanent Secretary as well.

The Health Department now lacked a traditional Permanent Secretary to protect its interests across a Whitehall increasingly jealous of the huge riches coming its way. The NHS lost a leader it respected and liked in Langlands. Instead it got someone who owed his position entirely to a powerful Minister who expected him to deliver his agenda. Much traditional civil service analytical capability and political nous was lost as faststream civil servants moved away to be replaced by NHS managers. This was the context in which the Government took forward the new targets-driven approach to improving the NHS.

Delivering improvement through targets

Labour has been much criticised by clinicians and others in the NHS over targets. The Conservatives – spotting a bandwagon of internal NHS dissent – jumped on it. Academics and commentators have weighed in. Examples of gaming targets delivery by some senior managers were highlighted in the media. When things have gone wrong clinically as in the Mid-Staffordshire Trust targets have been blamed in preference to facing up to straightforward clinical and managerial failure and incompetence. So was the Government wrong to use targets and did they work?

20-20 hindsight is a wonderful thing. It is easy now to forget that at the time of the 2000 NHS Plan, with an election beckoning, there were not that many tools in the Ministerial delivery tool box. What Alan Milburn had on his hands was a tax-funded, monopoly NHS that was used to a 'make do and mend' approach under Conservative governments that had kept it desperately short of money for two decades. The NHS had little experience of managing growth. Large parts of it – including many clinicians – accepted long waiting lists as a fact of life and a reasonable way of rationing a tax-funded healthcare system. There was little patient choice. The doctors were doing the rationing with some doing very nicely thank you from private practice that benefited from an under-funded NHS with long waiting times. Most of the NHS did not see itself as publicly accountable. The NHS had a poor track record in accepting innovation and was often reluctant to change its clinical and administrative practices. It lacked a modern, data-rich financial management system of the kind needed for the scale of the investment being made.

In these circumstances it made a good deal of sense to use centrally-driven targets as a basis for implementing the NHS Plan. There was a chain of command – albeit disrupted by the 2002 reorganisation – through which centrally-devised and driven targets could be enforced. For a government pouring money into the NHS and wanting to see results quickly the targets approach was more likely to show improvements speedily than waiting for other reforms to mature. And nobody, including the Opposition, had any other suggestions for ensuring rapid delivery of change.

Targets also fitted Treasury requirements to see what happened to the extra money; a Prime Minister anxious for evidence of results; and a DH senior management keen to show the Minister it could deliver. In these circumstances probably any government ploughing in this level of extra money to the NHS would have done the same. This does of course beg the question of whether it was wise to pour as much money as went into the NHS between 2000 and 2004 with such weak delivery and accountability mechanisms.

Selection of targets

What was true however was that Alan Milburn had correctly identified for targets areas of real public concern. The public were rightly fed up with long waits. Leaving elderly patients on trolleys for 12 hours in A and E Departments was a national disgrace. People did not see why they should wait a week or two to see their GP. The long waits for elective surgery may have done much for hospital consultants private practice income but they were a continuing source of complaints by patients who, on occasion, were waiting up to 3 years for an operation. The UK had some of the worst cancer survival rates in Europe because of the length of time it took to see a specialist, achieve a diagnosis and secure treatment.

Measurable improvement in all these areas and others were needed if people were to see the benefits they were to receive from the extra taxpayers' money being injected into the NHS. Whether one called them "targets" rather than "standards", "entitlements" or "guarantees" – as now seems fashionable – seems to me a semantic rather than a substantive matter. Anyone who has managed a large organisation – which excludes most elected politicians – knows that whatever gets measured gets done. Some way of measuring and demonstrating improvement was required if public support for a tax-funded NHS was to be retained, with such large amounts of extra money being invested.

Many staff in the NHS thought the targets were too demanding. However owever there is some evidence that the Government let the NHS off lightly and the public themselves would have been more demanding. A 2006 Report by the IPPR, "Public Expectations in the NHS"[5] shows the public's expectations running ahead of the

Government's in relation to waiting times and access. The Government's target was to see a GP within 48 hours but the public's average "reasonable" wait was less. For A & E Departments the public's average "reasonable" wait was $2^1/_2$ hours, not the Government's maximum wait of 4 hours – with two thirds of people thinking they should be seen in A & E in two hours or less. The public's view of a reasonable wait for a non-serious outpatient appointment was up to five weeks on average, not the thirteen weeks of the Government target, with nearly half the public thinking two weeks was long enough. So those in the NHS who think the Government was too tough on them and those politicians who wish to abolish targets for waiting times and access would do well to check with the public before getting too carried away.

In my view Labour Ministers made a reasonable judgment to drive improved NHS performance through central targets in exchange for the extra investment. If anything they calibrated the NHS waiting-time and access targets on the generous side compared with what much of the public considered appropriate. The NHS was also given a reasonable period of time to achieve the targets. It could well be argued that many in the NHS were slow to develop the systems and processes that made it more likely that these targets would be achieved, given the large amount of public money they were given to tackle the problems of long waits and poor access. An objective view of the key targets would say that they delivered considerable change but rather expensively and with some adverse consequences for management cultures. The real problems arose when targets became seen by the Treasury and others as the way of delivering change across a wider range of public services, irrespective of their appropriateness and adverse impact on organisational cultures.

What targets delivered

When I became the Minister responsible for NHS Delivery, targets had helped produce good progress in key areas like heart disease. By the end of 2001 about 108 people out of 100,000 died of heart disease and strokes compared with 140 in 1997 and the figures continued dropping further. There was a 30% increase in NHS heart operations between 1999/2000 and 2002/2003. The maximum waiting time for heart operations had fallen from 18 months to 6 months in four years and was well on the way to 3 months in March 2005. Over 80% of patients who had just had a heart attack now received clot-busting drugs within a half hour of arrival at hospital compared with only 38% in 2000. Approaching 2 million people were receiving cholesterol-lowering drugs to reduce their risk of a heart attack. A major killer disease was being tackled and death rates from coronary heart disease were dropping, even allowing for the increased use of statins.

On accessing services the patient experience was improving significantly. At their peak NHS inpatient waiting lists had contained nearly 1.3million people and were private health care's best recruiting sergeant. In March 2004 waiting lists were down to 906,000 and would drop by another 100,000 or so by the time of the 2005 Election. The maximum waiting time had reduced from 18 months to 9 months for inpatient treatment and this was accelerating further towards a maximum of 6 months in March 2005. The number of people waiting more than 3 months for an outpatient appointment had fallen by about 200,000 since 2000 and the maximum wait was now 17 weeks compared with 21 weeks in 2003. The NHS Plan had set a target that the maximum waiting time in A & E from arrival to admission or discharge should be 4 hours. By March 2004 services had improved to the point that nearly 94% of patients were treated within 4 hours. By March 2005 this was to reach 98% - the effective target accepted by John Reid on medical advice given that 100% could never be achieved for clinical reasons relating to emergencies.

The ability of patients to access their GP or practices quickly had been – and continues to be – a long running source of complaint from the public, despite all protestations to the contrary by the BMA. Targets had been set for people to be able to see their GP within 2 days and a primary healthcare professional within 1 day. By March 2004 the percentage of patients able to see their GP within 2 days was just over 97% compared with about 75% two years previously. It was the same for accessing a primary health care professional within a day compared with 72% two years previously.

When the NHS Improvement Plan was published in June 2004[6] with a foreword by Tony Blair and a preface by John Reid they could demonstrate, using the targets information, major NHS improvements. They could show significant improvements in relation to the killer diseases – particularly cancer - because often for the first time, activity and change were being measured consistently and in a timely way. Death rates from cancer were falling steadily by about 3% a year. An additional 200,000 women had been invited to breast screening in the 3 years since 2001. Virtually every patient with suspected cancer was being seen by a specialist within 2 weeks of referral by their GP, compared with 63% in 1997. There were 1000 more cancer consultants than in 1997 and over 1000 more MRI and CT scanners, linear accelerators and pieces of breast screening equipment. Many more new cancer drugs were available on the NHS. As Labour approached the 2005 Election it was clear that targets were doing the job they had been asked to do – show that the NHS was improving access and healthcare performance for patients, using the extra money invested.

The preoccupation with targets

Although targets helped produce major service improvements for patients alongside the increased investment, they created their own problems. Some unforeseen consequences flowed from the targets culture. As the only show in town for delivering improvements in the aftermath of the 2001 Election was centrally-driven targets these became the major preoccupation of Ministers, DH and the NHS between 2001 and 2004. As the extra money was poured in so the machinery for ensuring delivery was cranked up, both in DH and in No.10. A Prime Minister's Delivery Unit had been established under the leadership of Michael Barber, fresh from making David Blunkett look good from his time as Education Secretary. The DH and SHAs and the Clinical Czars (as the National Clinical Directors became known) all became deeply absorbed in targets and in improvement measurement. "Delivery" became a new term in the political, civil service and NHS lexicons. This political and managerial preoccupation and the management culture that grew up in DH after Nigel Crisp's appointment had some far reaching consequences. The top management of DH and the NHS became obsessed with delivery through targets almost irrespective of the cost and other important policy agendas.

As NHS Chief Executive Nigel Crisp had the authority for approving the accountable officers of each NHS trust. The local NHS chief executives knew who they were really accountable to and who called the shots on their career advancement – the NHS Chief Executive and his Deputy John Bacon, not their local Boards. What had been created – intentionally or otherwise – was a rather closed management system which was preoccupied with targets but was also over-supportive of chief executives when things went wrong. Another managerial slot was usually found for them and over the next 5 years one sensed that quite a few NHS chief executives became like Flying Dutchmen wandering the high seas of the NHS – or if they were really lucky paid off and then returning as consultants on generous daily rates. Yet despite all this delivery management effort the financial and information systems were still extremely creaky for the sums of money being poured in and were poor at relating activity levels to expenditure and workforce effort.

Crisp slimmed down the DH Management Board to four (excluding the Workforce Director among others) with John Bacon becoming increasingly the intermediary between this small Board and the NHS. Although the Chief Medical Officer, Liam Donaldson, was on this Board he appeared detached from running the NHS. To some extent this was offset by the appointment of some extremely talented National Clinical Directors who helped drive improvements in their particular specialty areas – especially the killer diseases – but they were not always well connected to DH top management. Over the years following the 2001 Election when money was being poured into the NHS, clinical buy-in to the service delivery targets reduced. Delivery through targets was too often seen as a chief executive's agenda in which managers ruled the roost locally and ran things through a parallel management universe that often seemed to exclude clinicians and Board non-executives. After 2001 the NHS was increasingly managed down the chief executive line through 28 SHA chief executives down to local trust chief executives. Gradually many local trusts started to look upwards rather than outwards to their communities. Apart from those trusts with a thirst for autonomy who moved to become Foundation Trusts, the chairs and non-executives were often sidelined and disengaged from trust management by executive management teams taking their orders from the centre. Quite a few trusts chairs and non-executives were to talk to me about this disempowerment both when I was a Minister and when later I became the Chairman of the NHS London Provider Agency.

I do not think that any of these side effects of targets were inevitable or deliberately planned but they happened. Targets could have been managed more through clinicians and local boards if there had been a different approach by the DH top management who often seemed to me disconnected from NHS criticism and day-to-day reality checks. The way targets were implemented led to a considerable loss of goodwill across the NHS which only became fully revealed in 2005 and 2006 when Patricia Hewitt and I were confronted with the financial crisis described in Chapter 9.

Sustaining improvement

Despite these problems it is important not to sell targets short on what they achieved in sustaining improvement. They improved NHS data collection and use and became embedded in the annual performance regime and the NHS regulatory framework. The Healthcare Commission (and its successor the Care Quality Commission) have used target data to assess the NHS performance locally and nationally. Monitor, the Independent Regulator for Foundation Trusts, has target-achievement as part of its licence enforcement. The measurement of progress in key areas where targets have been used has been impressive and in my judgement justifies their use. In 2007/8, 99.5% of people with suspected cancer were seen by a specialist within 2 weeks; and 99.6% diagnosed with cancer began treatment within 1 month. These are still not good enough; and

Britain has a problem with early diagnosis compared with France, but without the target data comparisons would be difficult. The UK figures are a huge improvement on the situation a decade ago, as the death rates for cancers and other killer diseases show.

The rate of premature death (before age 75) from all cancers was 116 per 100,000 people in 2006, a drop of over 18% compared with 1996. Without Labour's targeted approach to cancer, many more people would have died. The picture on survival is even more dramatic with coronary heart disease. There were 91 deaths per 100,000 people in 1996 but this had dropped to 45 per 100,000 in 2006. Early deaths due to stroke have also fallen markedly to 15 per 100,000 people – a fall of 44% in 10 years.[7] Not all these improvements can be attributed to targets, but better access to GPs and shorter waiting times for specialist appointments have played a major part.

Targets have produced major improvements in emergency care. In 2007/8, 98% of people were seen within the 4 hour target, compared with 91% in 2003/4. Admittedly there were still about 15% of acute hospitals not hitting the target but the NHS overall was. Ambulances have played their part in improving access to emergency care through the target regime. Again in 2007/8, 77% of top priority 999 calls to ambulance trusts were responded to within 8 minutes. Moreover both ambulance trusts and acute hospital trusts were ensuring 80% or more of people with heart attacks were receiving thrombolysis within an hour of a call for help.[8]

The A and E target has forced acute hospitals to look at how they use beds and avoid delayed discharges. They have been forced to increase their efficiency as a result. When I was a Minister a group of A & E clinicians came to see me to ask me not to drop the four hour A & E target, despite the calls to do so from many medical leaders. They said that the target had forced the NHS to take A & E work more seriously, improve the status of emergency staff and improve services to patients, including saving lives. These improvements in the way hospitals were run and the closer working of ambulance and acute hospital trusts also made a contribution to one of the regular features of the NHS a decade ago – winter crises. Now the NHS copes better with the winter surge of patients.

Probably the jewel in the crown for targets has been the commitment John Reid made in 2004 that for the NHS in England by December 2008 there would be a maximum waiting time of 18 weeks from GP referral to hospital treatment. This had to take in the first outpatient appointment, diagnostic services and admission to hospital. When I arrived as the responsible Minister in June 2005, many DH officials thought this could not be achieved. I did not agree with them but I accepted that we might not be able to do this for areas where there was no data base like psychological therapies, physical therapies and audiology. This would mean some criticism of "hidden waits" but it also meant attention had to be given to improving access to these neglected services – and it was.

I monitored progress on the 18 week target monthly at regular meetings. We set milestones for various stages along the journey. We were always lagging behind but by sending in teams to help trusts improve their performance and getting poor performers learning from high performers we started to get closer to the milestones. There were problems with specialist hospitals like Great Ormond Street Hospital who often received their referrals for highly specialist treatments very close to the 18 week deadline. Despite all this we made better progress than I expected despite the financial problems of 2005/2006.

The NHS is a bit like journalists with deadlines – it meets them but only just. About two-thirds of acute trusts had achieved the 18-week target by March 2008, 9 months from the deadline. When the Care Quality Commission (CQC) came to look at performance on 18 weeks at the end of 2008/9 it found that 89% of acute and specialist trusts had consistently achieved its indicator in the 3 months January to March 2009, with 6% underachieving it and 5% failing it. However in crude terms the December 2008 deadline for 18-week waits had been achieved for the 840,000 admitted patients and 2.3 million non-admitted patients in that 3 month period. Perhaps more to the point the average time for patients on the journey from GP to hospital admission was down to around 7 weeks and "hidden waits" in services like audiology had virtually disappeared.[9] This was a level of improvement in service access for patients through use of targets that could not have been contemplated by the NHS in 1997.

Targets have come with downsides and a hefty price tag but linked with investment they have achieved major improvements for patients. They have been used with some success in areas other than those I have mentioned like smoking during pregnancy, incidence of healthcare-acquired infections (discussed more fully in Chapter 11) and with mental health trusts. They have not worked well with teenage pregnancy and Chlamydia screening where individual behavioural change is required rather than NHS performance improvement. Our knowledge on how to secure behavioural change by individuals and groups is still far from complete.

It is striking that during this era of targets staff satisfaction ratings have remained consistently over 80% in all types of trust. Patient satisfaction ratings are high; and the latest one from the CQC for acute and specialist trusts - 2008/9 - was at 88%. Despite the noise from the BMA and Conservative politicians about targets, they seem more popular with patients than their critics recognise because people then know what to expect from the NHS. Targets may also not be as unpopular with staff as some have suggested.

A recent study by the Nuffield Trust discussed more in Chapter 15 suggests that targets combined with naming and shaming have improved

NHS performance in England. Coalition Ministers should think carefully about a bonfire of targets before they have other convincing measurement tools for explaining NHS performance to the public. Outcomes are fine if they can be defined and measured but in the health field they are usually long-term measures and some shorter-term measures may well be needed in the politically-charged world of healthcare.

Adding reform to investment

Targets have helped justify the extra investment in the NHS. In the 2001 Election Labour had shown that it had refurbished this faded national icon, the NHS, and had secured a mandate to spend even more money on it. After that Election, a Prime Minister in his pomp outflanked his Chancellor by announcing on television that by 2008 the UK would be spending at the EU average on healthcare. This meant an increase in the proportion of GDP spent on healthcare in the decade to 2007/8 of nearly 50%. This required a massive increase in NHS expenditure in the last five years of the decade. The NHS budget was to rise from about £36billion in 1997 to over £100billion in 2007/8 – a threefold increase in cash terms.

There would be an 8 year period of sustained growth across the NHS, unprecedented in its history and unique in length across advanced healthcare systems. The final 5 years of the period meant growth of some 9% annually in cash terms and 7% annually in real terms. Although there were a few public sector accountancy wrinkles that made these figures lower in terms of cash that actually reached local level, this was treasure on a never to be repeated scale for the NHS. The politicians were doing what NHS staff had asked for by delivering more investment, with most of it going on more staff.

The increase in the NHS workforce under Labour has been dramatic as Chapter 6 details, with an annual rate of growth of about 3%. However as I and other Ministers were to discover this largesse was to produce little gratitude from many working in the NHS. In large part this was because it increasingly dawned on them that the extra investment was to be accompanied by wider reforms and these would bring more challenge to the business processes, models and culture that had prevailed in the NHS since its inception. These new approaches would transfer more power to patients and challenge monopoly NHS service providers and were first expressed in the 2004 'NHS Improvement Plan'. In that document John Reid set out a list of what would be required from the NHS "in return for this investment", including a wider range of providers, more Foundation Trusts, more services in primary care and great focus by the NHS on health rather than sickness. So the mantra became "investment and reform", as the next few chapters explain.

3

Creating an NHS market – foundation trusts, competition and tariffs

Competition, the Labour Party and the NHS

The 2005 Election manifesto buried Labour's opposition to competition in the NHS and to the idea of a healthcare market. The groundwork for creating a more diverse group of providers had been laid with Foundation Trusts and the opening up of NHS elective surgery and diagnostics to private providers. These initiatives had been done piecemeal and without a clear narrative but they had been opposed from the start by NHS trades unions, who put a different label –"privatisation" - on these reforms. The BMA joined in the fun later, epitomised by a 2006 Sunday Times article by their chairman, Jim Johnson, entitled "Privatisation by Stealth is Bad for Your Health".[1] More sophisticated critics preached the virtues of cooperation between service providers and between providers and commissioners, reluctant to recognise the inherent contradiction in the latter idea and what collusion had done to patients over many years. The critics did not accept the views of the Prime Minister and reformers that competition and choice could change an NHS that was too lethargic and too reluctant to make changes quickly enough to match rising public expectations and scientific advances.

Most of the Labour Party and union hostility to markets was a doctrinal opposition to the private sector and to profit being involved in healthcare. This was despite the fact that NHS buildings, equipment and drugs were provided by the private sector and GPs were small businessmen operating profit and loss accounts. This political hostility was encouraged by the NHS's own innate resistance to competition from outsiders. For 60 years the NHS had effectively been able to operate on a basis of monopoly with a gateway system to specialist care that heavily constrained patient choice as well as rationing demand. The GP gatekeepers had tightly controlled access to general practice by new entrants and had prevented the over-supply that might generate more competition. The default-setting of the NHS was – and continues to be – local monopoly and central control. The latter is the favoured position of many civil servants (especially in the Treasury), NHS managers and elected Ministers - with some honourable exceptions – even though this is rarely acknowledged publicly.

Most NHS staff prefer this approach - provided enough money is made available - because it reinforces professional control and keeps patients in a state of dependency. This attitude was brought home to me time and time again on my Ministerial visits but never more graphically than at a packed audience of doctors at the Royal College of Surgeons in the 2005 Election campaign. After listening to me advancing the virtues of choice, competition and other works of the devil, an angry orthopaedic surgeon burst out "Lord Warner, my patients don't need choice, they know I am the best".

The person who was spoiling the NHS party was none other than the Prime Minister who had provided the extra funding. He had tried centrally-driven targets but they had not produced enough change at sufficient speed. Now Tony Blair was on an impatient mission of public service reform focussed on health and education with choice and competition as the main drivers but without abandoning national targets. He drove change through a small cadre of Ministers and advisers in No.10 and the main Departments, with some key civil servants in both places. In DH it had been Alan Milburn, John Reid and John Hutton with Simon Stevens, Paul Corrigan and Julian Le Grand as the advisers. The starting point for reform had been Foundation Trust (FT) hospitals which were inflaming the Labour Party when I first became a Minister in 2003.

Foundation Trusts (FTs)

My summer of 2003 was spent mastering my first portfolio as a Minister. Most of this was concerned with matters other than NHS reform: mainly the pharmaceutical industry, NHS research and development and healthcare acquired infections. All of which I discuss in later chapters. However it was clear that in the autumn I would have to pilot through the House of Lords the legislation establishing FTs. This was included in a portmanteau bill: the Health and Social Care (Community Health and Standards) Bill. This Bill had limped out of the House of Commons after much noise and some amendments to the FT provisions, with the attack led by Tony Blair's first Health Secretary, Frank Dobson. Frank was still sore from being ditched from the Cabinet and losing out to Ken Livingstone as Labour's candidate for London Mayor.

The Bill that arrived in the House of Lords still retained the provisions giving financial freedoms to FTs and placing them outside Ministerial and DH direction. FTs were clearly an integral part of the NHS but they had the capacity to make their own decisions on adapting services more speedily to local needs. So what was all the fuss about?

The diehard statists in the Labour Party did not like the idea of independent hospital trusts outside Ministerial control. This was despite the fact that the proposed governance of FTs as not-for-profit public benefit corporations was based on Cooperative movement principles of mutualism, with a lot of local involvement and accountability. The critics were unconvinced that these hospitals would remain part of the NHS. Dobson had orchestrated an amendment to insert a restrictive cap on the private patient income that FTs could generate. In order to appease Labour critics the Government accepted this amendment – unwisely as it turned out. This not only infuriated the Conservatives in the House of Lords but was something of an own-goal. It reduced the private income that FTs could generate from overseas and UK patients to increase NHS services; and because of the arbitrary nature by which the cap was calculated it made it more difficult for some high profile trusts to become FTs.

The issue of the private income cap continued as a problem long after 2003 legislation was passed, with Unison challenging the legal basis of the Regulator's computation of the cap for individual FTs and finally winning a High Court judgement in their favour. Some of us tried to remove the cap in the 2009 Health Bill and the Labour Government had to concede a review and allow mental health trusts to raise private income in a limited way. The private income cap remains an unnecessary restriction on FTs with a Labour government unable to face down the unions and its backbenchers to achieve a sensible solution that benefits the NHS financially. The Coalition Government rightly now intends to remove it.

During the passage of the 2003 legislation Labour critics, egged on by trade unions, worked themselves up into a lather over NHS privatisation, which they were convinced was Tony Blair's secret agenda. They lumped FTs into that agenda on the grounds that once these hospitals were outside Ministerial control it would be easier, it was claimed, to hand over their management to the private sector. Being able to raise their own capital for development would put non-FT NHS Trusts at a disadvantage and would lead to a two-tier NHS. At one point there had even been the suggestion that the assets and liabilities of FTs should be removed from the public sector balance sheet but after a robust debate Gordon Brown and the Treasury had prevented that.

In the eyes of critics of FTs it was even worse that the Government seemed willing to contemplate a mismanaged FT hospital going broke and being handed over to someone else to run. (I made that point very clear during the passage of the Bill in the House of Lords which I fear won me few Labour friends.) FTs were another step along the road to the very internal market that Labour had opposed in its 1997 Manifesto. There was some truth in the argument that non-FTs would be disadvantaged but that was the whole purpose of the scheme which was to incentivise higher performance by hospital trusts by giving them more local freedoms. Too many in the Labour Party prefer soggy mediocrity in the NHS to the best performers providing more of the services.

The Conservatives supported the idea of FTs but wanted to exploit Labour divisions by teasing the Government that it didn't have the courage of its convictions because it wanted to restrict the autonomy of FTs more than was originally intended. Gordon Brown had opposed the original more independent form of FT with no limits on borrowing. He was known to be concerned about their level of autonomy, particularly if their borrowing made public sector borrowing difficult to control. Despite the fact that FTs are required to operate within a prudential borrowing code, the issue of borrowing has remained an unresolved issue in the sense that if all FTs chose to make large borrowings and were able to do so at the same time this could, theoretically, cause some problems for the public sector borrowing requirement. The evidence so far, however, is that FTs have been very prudent borrowers and spread their borrowing requirements over time.

Against this background I celebrated my 63rd birthday on the 8 September 2003 moving the Lords Second Reading of the Bill. The Conservatives and Liberal Democrats worked together to embarrass the Government and moved a large number of amendments, many of which I had to concede in some form. The Committee stage lasted 6 days between 7 and 23 October and many of these days were very long ones ending late into the night. There were three days of Report stage covering many, many hours between 6 and 11 November and a day on Third Reading on the 18 November. During this period of two months or so I moved over 200 amendments to try to placate a joint Opposition that could always outvote us. The point of these concessions was to minimise the risk of losing the Bill in a Parliamentary session that was to end by the 30 November. Eventually things came down to an Opposition amendment that would have delayed the start of the process for approving the queue of applicants that now existed for the first two waves of would-be FTs.

When the Commons rejected the Lords' amendments on 19 November a furious game of 'ping pong' between the two Houses took place through the night of 20 November. I found myself shuffling between the Lords and the Commons to try to agree with John Reid cosmetic concessions that I could make in the Lords without doing too much damage to the Bill. John's patience with the House of Lords diminished considerably during that night but finally he agreed a concession. After Monitor – the new FT regulator – had considered and approved successful applications from the first two waves of applicants, there would be no more applications until there had been a review of the impact on the NHS of the two waves by the new Healthcare Commission. I ended up on my feet at 5am on the 21 November furiously arguing with the Opposition.

But with everybody exhausted, I finally secured agreement to the legislation, with the amendment on a review included. Shifting gear between emollient Minister and attack dog during that night did much for my street-cred with John Reid and my elected Ministerial colleagues.

Once the Parliamentary tempest had blown itself out the move of trusts to FT status went ahead relatively smoothly. The first tranche of 10 were authorised in April 2004 and were for the most part highly committed high performing hospitals. Like their successors they were very keen to escape Ministerial direction and Whitehall's control and performance management through Strategic Health Authorities. They favoured the ability to access capital on the basis of affordability instead of the old system of centrally controlled allocations and lengthy capital approval processes. If they made revenue surpluses they could invest these in developing new services locally rather than having them removed to prop up failing hospitals elsewhere. Although the concessions made during the Parliamentary process made the governance of FTs more cumbersome than it need have been, FTs still ended up as membership organisations of local people and staff. Their boards of governors were made up of patients, staff and local people elected by members as well as local stakeholders. In some cases the turnout for these elections was higher than in local government elections. However one looked at it, the level of local involvement with FTs was far greater than in ordinary NHS trusts.

The peace process of the Healthcare Commission review took place in 2004. When the Commission's report was published it found that contrary to the view of critics of FTs the rest of the NHS had not been noticeably affected, although it was recognised that it was probably too soon to make a final judgement. The Commission's report was sufficient to clear the way for further FT applicants to come forward.

I took over responsibility for FTs in May 2005 as part of the competition brief. Having created a social care market in the late 1980s under the Conservatives I had no problems of principle with building up a market of diverse healthcare providers. If providers met NHS standards and operated within sustainable prices my approach was that any willing provider – public, private or voluntary – should be able to compete on a level playing field to provide services under NHS contracts. There was not - and is still not – much evidence that the public cares which sector the provider comes from providing the care is safe and competent and free at the point of use. Indeed the patients I spoke to as a Minister visiting ISTCs thought their experience much better than their previous experiences of NHS hospital care. Back in 2005, however, the problem I faced was that we had no pipeline of FT applicants now that 32 FTs had been approved from the first wave of applicants.

With the officials who had done the policy work on FTs I developed a process for producing a more steady flow of applicants to Monitor – the regulator - who rightly wanted to have a smoother flow of applicants than the initial burst followed by no applications at all.. The first five waves were to be given free assistance to get themselves in a good state to become FTs. All applicants first of all needed to satisfy the responsible Minister – me after mid-2005 – that they could go forward to Monitor for a rigorous assessment of their business plan. Some would fail to satisfy Ministers; others would fall at the Monitor hurdle. Experience has shown that only 60%-70% of applicants get through at the first application. It became apparent very early on that those who failed in their application were likely to do so for financial over-optimism, poor risk assessment in their business plans and overall doubts about the robustness of their governance and financial management capability.

The enthusiasts for FTs had somewhat discounted the limitations of many acute and mental health trusts and their inability to make successful applications. The new Regulator, Bill Moyes, did not want to seem a soft touch or to repeat the Conservative mistake of the early 1990s of letting through inadequate hospital trusts to a higher status. He was certainly not going to indulge the tendency in some parts of the NHS to regard all geese as swans in order to avoid confrontation. Nor was I. It was also clear to me that letting candidates go forward to Monitor on the basis of three-star ratings based on historical performance would not do. Although this past performance indicator was useful in part it was no guarantee that a trust had thought about and planned for a very different future trading environment or had the governance capability to support much more independence.

Using the data that we had it seemed to me that by the end of 2008 – 3 years hence – we might with hard work achieve about 100 FT approvals. However that would still leave the majority of hospital trusts outside the FT magic circle. I had to make it clear to the Prime Minister and Patricia Hewitt that it was going to take a lot longer than they thought to get the whole of the NHS to go on the FT journey; and that we could not get them all into FT status by the end of 2008 in time for a 2009 or even a 2010 election. A bit reluctantly, Tony Blair accepted this but also to his credit agreed that we should not lower the bar and let applicants through inappropriately.

In 2005 the main reasons why such a large proportion of NHS hospitals could not become FTs were fourfold: high reference costs (i.e. they were too expensive and inefficient); poor financial management; their performance ratings from the Healthcare Commission were inadequate; and they lacked the business planning and other skills to get them through the Monitor authorisation process. This was a considerable indictment of the state of an NHS's governance and management into which we were pouring huge sums of extra public money. These problems were at the heart of the 2006 NHS financial storm described in Chapter 9. However it was the FT applications process that forced the DH top management to start confronting some deep underlying problems of poor financial management and control and inadequate governance across the NHS that had been glossed over by them for far too long. Endless wittering about the virtues of the "NHS family" in the top echelons of DH was no substitute for an effective financial and performance management regime.

I ensured that DH agreed with Monitor a process that was likely to produce a higher success rate. We commissioned a diagnostic tool that allowed SHAs to assess each acute trust's state of readiness to apply, together with an action plan process in two pilot SHA regions for getting people up to speed to apply. This approach was then rolled out across the country as a whole. We invested money in it and also gave financial help to those trusts who would go forward to Monitor in the first five waves. I asked for candidates for the next wave to come forward by December 2005 to go to Monitor for approval from April 2006 and for a further wave from July 2006.

This injected some momentum into a process that had stagnated as the NHS awaited the evaluation of the early successful applicants by the Healthcare Commission. Frank Dobson and his fellow critics had introduced sufficient uncertainty into the minds of the NHS, that together with an election, much of the momentum of 2003 had been lost. However by the time I left office at the end of December 2006 there were 54 fully operational FTs – 59 by the end of March 2007. In the financial year 2006/7 these 59 FTs generated a surplus for reinvestment of about £130million. They had generated efficiency savings of 3% of operational costs - equivalent to about £270million - compared with the 2.5% assumed in the 2006/7 tariff. These FTs had consolidated cash balances of nearly £1billion and only four of them had poor financial risk ratings on which action was being taken by Monitor.[2] In 2006/7 only 48 hospital trusts across the NHS were rated 'excellent' in their use of resources by the Healthcare Commission and all of these were FTs.[3] On any basis FTs were better financially managed than the rest of the NHS, thereby providing security of services to patients and the scope, in most cases, for investment in service development and improvement.

The pipeline I had established continued to produce a steady flow of candidates after my departure. By July 2007 the FT Network reported that there were 70 FTs with 200,000 staff, 600,000 members and over 1000 governors.[4] I was satisfied when I left office that we had a development programme that provided the prospect that by the end of 2008 Monitor would be able to approve about 100 FTs, many of whom would be mental health trusts as well as acute hospitals. This would mean however that more than half of the acute hospital trusts in England were still not good enough to achieve FT status.

In the event Monitor reported that in September 2008 there were 105 NHS FTs, 31 of them mental health trusts. They were generating revenues at an annual rate of about £20billion. Their financial risk ratings were still very sound with only one FT below par. Just over 10% were struggling a little with their performance on health care acquired infections (MRSA and C.Diff) but overall their service performance was well above that of the non-FT sector of the NHS. What was clear however was that geographical enthusiasm for becoming an FT was varied. London, West and East Midlands and the South East Coast SHAs had only a third or less of potential FTs approved when five other SHAs had over 50% with one of them reaching 80% of Trusts being approved as FTs.[5]

After a difficult birth FTs have proved successful. They are producing the local hospital autonomy that the Conservatives had promised in the early 1990s but they have done so after a much more rigorous assessment process. It is not easy to become an FT as many trusts have discovered. Monitor's processes were rigorous and some trusts fail or withdraw. I was prepared to reject weak applicants before they got to Monitor and the civil servants took their cue from me. There was considerable pressure from No. 10 to get more trusts into FT status faster but I was determined not to repeat the Conservatives' mistake of dropping standards so that more trusts achieved the higher status unjustifiably and then failed their patients.

Regrettably too many NHS Boards, clinicians and managers have not been prepared to put the effort into becoming an FT and have preferred watching and waiting. Too many non-FTs still have weak governance structures, inadequate clinical performance and poor financial management. They are not fit to become FTs. These situations have not been gripped by most SHAs and DH Ministers. The 2008/9 Care Quality Commission ratings demonstrate this. Those trusts who have gone through the Monitor process often found it tough and then that the new environment was demanding. One FT Chief Executive, Nancy Hallett of the Homerton Hospital, put it well: "It's a tougher environment, very different but better. I certainly would not want to go back".[6]

Not every FT has been a total success, Bradford (financial) and Mid-Staffordshire and Basildon and Thurrock (clinical) have shown that achieving FT status is not an absolute guarantee of quality. However problem FTs have been a small percentage of the total – certainly compared with non-FTs. Overall the Monitor processes have proved robust both in approval terms, in continuing to hold FTs to account and in acting quickly when things start to go wrong. Unfortunately Monitor's regulatory system is not used to tackle failing acute hospitals who are not FTs. That is for SHAs who seem to prefer looking nervously over their shoulder at equally nervous Ministers who are unwilling to face down local opposition to hospital changes that are inevitable eventually.

In his Next Stage Review, Lord Darzi said: "It is our clear ambition that in future hospital care will be provided by NHS foundation trusts."[7] At the end of 2008/9 Monitor had approved 114 Trusts who had recruited over 1.2million members; employed approaching 400,000 staff; and had a combined turnover of over £22billion a year.[8] As businesses FTs are in rude financial health compared with non-FT hospitals. The gap between FTs total income and their operating costs in 2007/8 was about 8%, way beyond what the rest of the NHS was achieving. And their cost improvement plans in the same year at 3% were above the 2.5% sought in the payment by results tariff set by DH Ministers. They are improving their efficiency and profitability much faster than the rest of the NHS at a time of reduced public expenditure. This bodes ill for those hospitals that have sat on their hands and failed to engage with the FT approval process. It is now for the new Coalition Ministers to tackle these failing and under-performing hospitals.

FT financial solidity is key to improving the quality of services as the 2009 Health Act requires. The Healthcare Commission's annual health check results have shown that organisations that are not financially strong are frequently not able to focus on clinical quality. In 2008 the Commission's final report showed that of the NHS trusts rated "excellent" for use of resources, 91% were rated "good or excellent" for quality of services – as were 86% of trusts who were rated "good" for use of resources. Compared with these figures the Commission's data shows that of those rated "weak" in the way they manage their finances, only 45% were said to have "good or excellent" services.[9]

In five of the ten SHAs the majority of acute and mental health trusts have simply not applied for FT status. These included more than half the 25 hospital trusts with the largest annual turnovers in the NHS (over £400million a year).[10] If trusts with turnovers of over £400million a year cannot achieve the preferred model for NHS hospitals of all political parties it is an indictment of their competence and commitment. Not surprisingly the NHS Chief Executive, David Nicholson, asked SHAs to identify those Trusts who will not be FTs by the end of 2010. The question that remains unanswered is what the Coalition Government will do about those trusts who are not FTs by 2012/13.

At the end of 2008/9 the Care Quality Commission's annual report showed that only about half the 230 hospital trusts had become FTs. The pipeline of applications to Monitor has almost dried up. Nearly 90 acute trusts, including major hospitals like the Oxford Radcliffe, Great Ormond Street and Barts and the Royal London are still not FTs.[11] A good number of these non-FT trusts are simply not robust enough financially, whatever their clinical performance, to be standalone FTs. What has been lacking is the political will to tackle the issue of failing and financially unsustainable hospitals and to require the mergers and realignment of hospital services that are needed. FTs have been successful and proved their worth and are providing a superior service to many if not most of the non-FT hospitals. A significant proportion of NHS patients are now expected to put up with NHS providers who are operating within an inferior model for financial management and, as a consequence, often have lower clinical quality. An important question for the Coalition Government is how they will bring the advantages of the FT model to all parts of the country without reducing the standards for becoming an FT.

The Independent Sector Treatment Centre (ISTC) programme

Alongside FTs the key battleground for establishing an NHS market of providers was the creation of new ISTCs managed by private sector companies that NHS patients could use as an alternative to lengthy NHS waits for operations. The ISTC programme drew on some aspects of the Private Finance Initiative but was very much a centrally-driven programme aimed at breaking NHS monopoly and providing alternative providers for NHS patients. It was intended to provide choice and was a clear statement of Tony Blair's intention of forcing public sector reform through greater competition. Periodically private sector providers were brought into No.10 and given encouragement and support in front of DH Ministers and officials. Whether they all wanted to be Tony's shock troops remained less certain. As time progressed these private sector providers became increasingly anxious in conversations with me about whether Gordon Brown would continue with Tony Blair's policies on use of the private sector. I did my best to be honest without depressing them too much but I knew they had good reason to be nervous.

Enthusiasm for the ISTC programme within DH was stronger in the political cadre than the senior bureaucracy with its over-representation of former NHS managers. I was hampered by the fact that despite No.10's strong support, there was little Labour enthusiasm for talking too openly about 'markets' or 'competition' with 'contestability', more the phrase of choice. One thing was clear – if we were to create a true NHS market we had to succeed with ISTCs.

The ISTC story began with a change of clinical practice that started in the 1990s when some NHS doctors began advocating the separation of elective surgery from emergency surgery. Mixed emergency and elective lists had led to many patients with less serious conditions being "bumped" for operations by emergencies. Repeat cancellations were a significant issue and the loss of productivity for hospitals was a problem. In 1999 the first treatment centre in England dedicated to elective surgery – the Ambulatory Care and Diagnostic Centre – was opened at the Central Middlesex Hospital in West London. Left to their own devices the NHS would probably have moved eventually to separate elective and emergency procedures but in their own leisurely and piecemeal way.

However the even tempo of NHS life was disturbed by two events in 2002. First the DH under Alan Milburn's leadership announced in April 2002 that it was creating a programme of NHS Treatment Centres in order to have a more systematic approach to the separation of electives and emergencies. But it was the second initiative at the end of 2002 that was to prove much more controversial. This was the announcement that DH would be commissioning a number of Independent Sector Treatment Centres "ISTCs" to treat NHS patients who required relatively straightforward elective or diagnostic procedures. The justification for this engagement of the private sector was provided by a planning exercise the DH had conducted in October 2002 with SHAs and PCTs in which they were asked to identify any anticipated gaps in their capacity needed to meet the new waiting time targets.

The results of the planning exercise revealed capacity gaps across the country, particularly in specialties such as cataract removal and orthopaedic procedures – the latter being a very healthy source of private practice income for consultants as a result of long NHS waiting lists. In December 2002 the DH invited expressions of interest from private providers in running a series of treatment centres to speed up access to surgery for NHS patients.[12] In advance of the actual procurement of new centres a joint venture between the NHS and BUPA – the Redwood Diagnostic Treatment Centre – opened in Redhill in January 2003. So the private sector now had a foot in the NHS door in addition to the spot-purchase care in its own facilities that it had long provided to the NHS – at high unit prices – when the NHS suddenly needed extra capacity.

When I became a Minister in June 2003 the procurement exercise was still in progress under the direction of Ken Anderson's new DH Commercial Directorate. Ken, who had considerable US health care experience, was technically a civil servant but with a salary, style and access to Ministers (including the Prime Minister) very different from most Whitehall mandarins – which irritated many civil servants. In an early meeting of the new 2003 Ministerial team John Reid wanted to settle what we were going to call these new beasts which at that time were called Diagnostic Treatment Centres – DTCs. We settled on Independent Sector Treatment Centres and thus the term ISTCs was born.

In September 2003 DH announced the preferred bidders for the majority of ISTCs. Contracts were subsequently awarded on the basis that bidders met the core clinical standards required by the NHS, provided high standards of patient care, offered additional staffing capacity (i.e. they would not simply recruit NHS clinical staff) and provided good value for money. The first contracts were signed in September 2003 - some involving new builds and some the adaptation of NHS premises. The first ISTC opened in Daventry in October 2003. This first wave of ISTCs involved renewable five-year contracts and was worth some £1.7billion in total. I became responsible for this programme in mid-2005; and by mid 2006 there were 19 fully operational ISTCs; 6 partially operational and 4 still under negotiation. The specialties covered included ophthalmology, orthopaedics, urology, general surgery, gynaecology, plastic surgery, gastroenterology, oral surgery, rheumatology, and many diagnostic procedures such as endoscopies.

Alongside the Wave 1 ISTC programme the Commercial Directorate negotiated another system of private sector NHS elective care. This was the General Supplementary Contracts (GSsupp). Under this contract Nuffield and Capio provided extra activity on a call down basis in ENT, general surgery, urology and orthopaedics in areas with long waiting lists. A further GSsupp 6 month contract later in 2005 concentrated on orthopaedics. These contracts reduced the unit price of procedures to the NHS. By the end of 2005 about 250,000 NHS patients had been treated by the private sector as a result of these various contracts, over 50,000 of them in new ISTCs.

The reaction within the NHS and the BMA to the Wave 1 ISTC programme was for the most part hostile. The ISTCs were said to be cherry-picking easy patients, they didn't do any training, they diverted money from the NHS, they didn't contribute much to reducing waiting times and their standards of patient care were lower. This latter point was driven mainly by the British Orthopaedic Association (BOA) who seemed ill-disposed to the foreign-trained doctors brought into the ISTCs even though their qualifications had been recognised by the General Medical Council. The Health Select Committee's report of 2006 on ISTCs chastised the BOA for "the strident and alarmist criticisms of clinical standards" when the data for comparing NHS and independent sector performance on elective surgery was not available.[13] About the only thing on which everybody was agreed was the wisdom of the 'additionality' rule which stopped the new ISTCs poaching NHS clinical staff.

Perhaps the most significant and persistent criticism was that the local NHS had been forced to accept these ISTCs against their wishes because the Government was determined to force private sector competition on the NHS. That issue was to dominate much of my time as a Minister when

I had to launch and handle Wave 2 of the ISTC programme. Although the criticism had some substance it is less than convincing when applied to Wave 1. Ministers had a number of goals when they decided to bring in the private sector. Alongside increasing capacity they wanted to bring down the price of spot purchasing by the NHS of private sector services, inject some innovation and stimulate NHS reform and efficiency through outside competition. Later patient choice was to join the list.

The critics of ISTCs too often overlooked the need to increase capacity, improve throughput and reduce waiting lists in 2002/2003; and that the plans for extra capacity were drawn up locally. The point was well made by Ken Anderson in his evidence to the Health Select Committee in 2006;

> "The capacity planning was done at the local economy level. It was not for us [the Commercial Directorate] to try to determine at our level. We would not have had the capability because we don't have the granularity of data to go out and make those decisions for a local health economy."[14]

If the numbers were wrong that was more the fault of the local PCTs and SHAs than the paranoid views ascribed to Ministers and DH.

Of course Ministers were interested in bringing in the private sector to galvanize a reluctant NHS; and DH and SHAs may well have indulged in a bit of gentle arm twisting of uncooperative PCTs who claimed they needed no extra capacity. But it is totally fanciful to believe that the Commercial Directorate could have achieved 147 expressions of interest from the private sector and over 25 contracted ISTCs after a lengthy, arduous and costly contracting process if there had not been a genuine capacity gap to be filled. If the local figures were wrong that is more to do with NHS ineptitude than anything else. What is possible – but less easy to prove – is that as the reality of what Ministers were doing dawned on the NHS they speeded up the productivity of their own elective services, aided and abetted by a cumbersome public procurement process that slowed the ability of the new private sector competition to go live as quickly as possible. Whether the NHS would have changed much or quickly without a real threat to them is in my view highly doubtful.

Alongside the Wave I ISTC programme a tendering and contracting process had been initiated for private sector Walk-in Centres – some of which had opened before the 2005 Election – to help particularly commuters who lived in one place where their GP was located but worked elsewhere. Just before the Election a further substantial procurement of elective surgery and diagnostic capacity from the private sector had been launched in March 2005 to more than double the size of the Wave 1 procurement. When the new Health Ministerial team arrived in May 2005 the scene was set for the next stage of the battle over competition within and with the NHS – the Wave 2 ISTC programme. Wave 1 had been justified primarily on the ground of increasing much-needed capacity to reduce waiting lists and this made it more difficult for Labour and NHS critics to argue against it. Wave 2 clearly had a wider purpose – more competition with NHS providers and extending patient choice.

Wave 2 of the ISTC programme

Wave 2 covered two areas - elective procedures and diagnostics. The latter had been added to the programme because diagnostics had become a major blockage to progress for the Government's commitment to reduce to 18 weeks the period from a GP referral to receiving hospital specialist treatment. Too many patients were experiencing long waits for hospital diagnostic procedures before the specialist could decide what action to take. Extra capacity was still a driver of the Wave 2 ISTC programme. The plan I inherited was ambitious. It involved delivering up to 250,000 new procedures a year and creating an Extended Choice Network (ECN) of independent sector providers who would deliver up to an additional 150,000 procedures a year on a call-down basis. The additional capacity would be provided through a variety of facilities such as existing ISTCs, new build centres, refurbishments and existing NHS facilities. At the time this part of the programme represented an investment of £3billion over five years. Alongside it was a diagnostics element of over £1billion over the five years. However the timescales involved in procuring this volume of service were considerable and the processes complex. The diagnostics element was moving the fastest.

When I arrived in May 2005 all the invitations to negotiate had been sent out to those who had qualified from the expressions of interest. The hope was that some contracts would be signed in the summer of 2005 and the first service delivery would commence in 2006. The diagnostics were less contentious than ISTCs because there was a clear lack of NHS capacity and these additional diagnostic procedures were less threatening to an NHS hospital's tariff income than the ISTCs. It was to be ISTCs and elective surgery that attracted most of the criticism. What became clear to me was that DH top management commitment to this programme – outside the Commercial Directorate – was less than whole-hearted. Lurking in the background was the Treasury keen to use value-for-money arguments to scale back the programme. Gordon Brown had never bought into the arguments on extra private sector capacity to facilitate choice and competition.

The elective surgery projects in Wave 2 were a mixed bag in terms of their quality, judged by need, NHS commitment and clear business plans. To justify Wave 2 progress I was using three key arguments – the extra capacity needed, greater choice for patients and the scope for the NHS to learn from more innovative processes in the ISTCs – in terms of layout, patient experience and speed of response. I was able to show that if the NHS was buying about 100,000 operations a year from private providers – as it was – then these new contracts were much cheaper than spot purchasing a 100,000 operations at premium rates 40% to 100% more than necessary. So a value-for-money argument was another string to my bow.

The critics in Parliament, the unions and the media continued their attacks. The doctors didn't have UK qualifications; patient safety was inferior; and ISTCs didn't do any training of the next generation of clinical staff. Driving most of the arguments were xenophobia and resistance to competition. Once ISTCs were established we required them to take on training responsibilities which for the most part their doctors were keen to do. ISTCs did make mistakes but there was no evidence that they made any more than their NHS counterparts, as the Health Select Committee said in its July 2006 report.[15] The ISTCs provided more up-to-date information on their clinical performance than the NHS centres did although the data were not strictly aligned for comparison purposes. The "British-trained doctors are best" arguments rumbled on with little convincing evidence that the overseas-trained doctors used by ISTCs were inferior, except occasionally in terms of their mastery of English. Effectively there was a stand-off on the clinical arguments but patients continued to give high satisfaction ratings for their ISTC experiences and these were higher than their general responses for NHS care.

I pressed on with opening new centres. In July 2005 I travelled to the Trent region to open the new Barlborough Centre which would provide 22,000 orthopaedic operations over the next five years. This £9million purpose-built centre had 36 beds and another 4 critical care beds for any complications and an impressive physiotherapy gym. The patients loved the experience and it was proving very popular: it was to do 5,000 operations in its first year. Its South African owners were delighted to be working for the NHS but some of the local NHS were suspicious. Another ISTC I opened later in Kent, close to the Medway towns, was to prove less popular because the owner/operator had failed to persuade the local GPs to refer patients because they preferred not to upset their local NHS hospital consultant colleagues. Restrictive clinical practices were alive and well in the Kent NHS and this ISTC struggled in occupancy terms rarely above 50% a year after opening.

Over several months I had regular meetings on Wave 2 projects and reported progress to the Prime Minister. In total the schemes amounted to about £550million of ISTC business a year for five years when fully operational, with another £200million plus a year of diagnostics work for the same period. A lot of market analysis had been done to try to identify how much business the government needed to commit to overall in order to convince the private sector that there would be a continuing NHS market of sufficient scale for the sector to remain committed managerially and in investment terms to competing in this market.

There was a view in the Commercial Directorate based on their analysis that with Waves 1 and 2 you needed a market of nearly £1billion a year of business for a reasonable period of time for the private sector to remain convinced that there was sufficient business to compete for. The more I probed these numbers the less resilient they looked, although it was clear that if Wave 2 was too small the greater was the risk that the private sector would lose investment and managerial interest. They needed a reasonably stable market with a guaranteed investment return to convince their investors to stump up money. The cumbersome and costly public sector procurement processes were winning few private sector friends. What I lacked was a clear and reliable set of figures on the scale of the private sector provision I had to generate to guarantee continuing competition with NHS providers. It was that competition the Prime Minister rightly wanted to see.

I found myself caught between No.10, the Commercial Directorate and the private sector wanting a minimum total programme of about £1billion a year and a sceptical Departmental/NHS viewpoint, with the Treasury behind them, insisting on no target figure and signing off each project one by one in terms of value-for-money. The Office of Government Commerce (OGC) was brought in to do a Gateway Review of the programme and I worked hard on them. Its October 2006 internal report showed the Wave 2 programme was well matched to the requirements of the NHS and represented good value-for-money. But I was still faced with a Wave 2 programme whose individual projects were variable in quality and local commitment.

The processes of the Commercial Directorate depended on local assessments of service needs and the underpinning data which were decidedly shaky in some places. So I decided to break Wave 2 into three groups of projects with the weaker ones to be dealt with last and some further work done to bolster them. Our public position remained that we were determined to deliver a Wave 2 worth £550million a year. This minimised agitation from the Prime Minister and an industry with access to him. Patricia Hewitt supported the approach and the DH top management and Treasury were unwilling to seriously challenge it given Tony Blair's commitment.

In the first half of 2006 we had over £200million worth of projects moving through the contracting process. I dropped a few smaller projects in South Yorkshire and elsewhere as sops to NHS critics but without too much agitation from No.10. I was able to say I was preventing the private sector making poor investments in these cases – which had the advantage of being true. We got through a review by the Health Select Committee whose report was published in July 2006. This was hardly flattering about the ISTC programme but accepted that the "threat of competition from the ISTCs may have had a significant effect on the NHS".[16] We headed off trouble from the professional medical bodies about quality of comparable international clinical standards by announcing a review of ISTC care by the Chief Medical Officer, Liam Donaldson. The Select Committee pressed us for an assessment of the impact of the ISTC programme on NHS facilities but we were unresponsive.

MPs were starting to put pressure on Wave 2 projects in particular areas where ISTCs would have a significant impact on the income of their local hospitals and the viability of some hospital departments. Some of this pressure came from Patricia Hewitt's own Cabinet colleagues lobbied by local hospital consultants – in Blackburn for example. I had a few adjustments made to projects by using some of them more for clinical assessments of hospital referrals rather than elective surgery and cancelled a few projects that were clearly not viable such as one in South London.

The financial problems in the NHS in 2005/6 which carried over into 2006/7, made trimming and adapting the programme inevitable to reduce the pressure for abandoning the programme altogether. The diagnostics part of Wave 2 was holding up well because the NHS so obviously needed the extra capacity to achieve the 18 weeks manifesto commitment. Many hospitals and doctors also liked the idea of access to some modern diagnostic kit. But Wave 2 elective surgery projects remained under considerable pressure from a reluctant NHS and consultant cadre. By the time I left office at the end of 2006 the Wave 2 programme in its entirety was still heading towards a total value of over £400million a year – compared with the £550million we had originally envisaged. The private sector became restive as their champions left government: the Prime Minister in mid-2007 and Ken Anderson and I had gone at the end of 2006. After Ken and I left the contracts in the system drifted and were eroded by the opponents of ISTCs. A new Commercial Director was not appointed for six months and when he was, he lacked the commitment and political backing of his predecessor.

A new Prime Minister and Health Secretary in the summer of 2007 had little enthusiasm for the ISTC programme. Alan Johnson's speech to the Labour Party Conference in September 2007 made no mention of markets, competition or choice and Unison expressed public delight at their absence. The FT headline was "Johnson signals end of NHS Reforms."[17] In the same month the Commercial Advisory Board – a group of business people that had supported the Commercial Directorate in bringing in the private sector – resigned with a blast at Ministers in their resignation letter about scrapping the Wave 2 ISTC programme.[18] The Commercial Directorate was reduced in scale and authority and much of it transferred to SHAs, most of whom were unsure about generating competition. This did not go unnoticed in the NHS and the private sector, whose anxiety about Gordon Brown's commitment to competition turned out to be all too prescient. In December 2007 the FT obtained a DH report on ISTCs that had been withheld from publication. This made clear that the ISTC programme had forced the NHS to become more productive and had helped to contain cost increases in elective surgery. It argued that even if the whole Wave 2 programme had gone ahead there would have been only "localised pressure" on NHS providers; and that without a sufficiently large private sector "there will be no competitive tension" to drive down cost, raise quality and improve accessibility.[19]

For most of the first year of the Brown premiership there was pretty much silence on the subject of the private sector and the NHS. The messages seeping out from Richmond House were that Alan Johnson had been appointed to calm down the NHS. Quite how this squared with the appointment of Lord Darzi to conduct the Next Stage review was never fully explained. Nevertheless the private health care sector conversations I had suggested that the sector had taken away the clear message that Brown and Johnson did not want their help. There was a mixture of silence and endless tinkering with what was left of the Wave 2 ISTC programme – most of which increased private sector costs with no income in return.

When I left as a Minister I had approved 9 fairly large new projects and ruled out five, mainly small ones, as unviable both in NHS terms and commercially. Most of the remainder were, in my judgement, likely to be viable with commitment from Ministers and the Commercial Directorate. After an enormous period of silence Alan Johnson announced on 15 November 2007 that 6 further schemes were cancelled and 7 more were under review. Only 3 new independent sector schemes, worth about £200million, were announced to deliver nearly 20,000 PET-CT diagnostic scans and over a 120,000 kidney dialysis sessions a year.[20] Negotiations on the outstanding 7 ISTC schemes were still limping on in mid-2009 so Wave 2 of the ISTC programme ended more with a whimper than a bang. In February 2008 the Financial Times claimed that the DH had suppressed evidence from independent review teams looking at local plans for Wave 2 ISTCs that these "should be well-matched to the [NHS's] requirements " and were "very good value for money."[21]

In his November 2007 announcement Alan Johnson did pay tribute to the role the private sector had played in improving NHS services by "helping speed up treatments and galvanise the NHS to raise its game". By then Wave 1 projects, worth £1.4billion, had provided 800,000 elective procedures diagnostic assessments and episodes of primary care through 23 ISTCs, a mobile ophthalmology service, a mobile MRI scanning service, a chlamydia screening service and six Walk-in Centres.[22] The private sector had a base camp in the NHS but had not advanced as far as it should and would have done under the previous Ministerial regime.

Alan Johnson did not totally dispatch the private sector to outer darkness: a new forum for independent providers was established to advise DH on local procurement practice; the NHS Clinical Negligence Scheme was extended to non-NHS providers of NHS services; and new guidance to the NHS was promised on how it should work with the private and voluntary sectors. But the agenda was changed from elective surgery to diagnostics, screening and primary care – for the most part cheaper services and less threatening to acute hospital income. It was clear that the pioneering days of trying to create an NHS market with robust competition ended in early 2007 as the Blair premiership came to a close. Before that happened, a private sector NHS presence had been established as a basis for greater competition when political enthusiasm for this returned. In establishing this competition in the acute hospital sector the role of price had to be determined.

Constructing an NHS tariff

Unlike in local government the private sector would not, for the most part, be competing in the NHS on price. For most of the services the NHS provided there were benchmark NHS prices and increasingly an acute hospital tariff. Competition initially was more about quality, patient convenience and making available new capacity more quickly – although over time competition could drive down price. Alongside ISTCs there was a growing internal NHS market with an increasing number of FTs competing with each other and non-FTs for patients who were increasingly able to exercise choice. In this more marketised NHS the decision in principle had been made to make payment for the bulk of acute hospital work on the basis of a new tariff system called Payment by Results (PbR). This was to enable payment to follow the patient and to break out of the block grant system of funding acute hospitals that had been in existence since the beginning of the NHS.

When I took over Ministerial responsibility for PbR in May 2005 the new tariff system had been under development for about three years and was in its second year of limited trialling. There was considerable NHS anxiety about PbR and the threat to viability it might pose for some hospitals. When I looked at the international experience on tariffs I thought the evidence was encouraging but potentially challenging to poor performers. The international experience with activity-related funding of hospitals goes back to 1983 when the US Medicare system introduced Diagnosis-Related Groups (DRGs) as a basis for paying for inpatient services for elderly people. In the 1990s, Sweden, Italy, Germany, Norway and Victoria State in Australia had all introduced a version of DRG payments for hospital care, with Finland and The Netherlands following in 2000 and 2003 respectively.

The international evidence supported the view that activity-related funding promoted greater cost-efficiency in acute hospital services. Studies in Sweden and Australia suggested that the costs per case were about 10% lower in places that operated funding based on a case-mixed averaging DRG system. An OECD study in a number of countries suggested that activity-based funding raised health service activity levels, which was an important consideration for reducing NHS waiting times. The US evidence suggested that when you introduced case-mixed funding hospitals improved their management information systems, especially their medical coding. This was important in the NHS where the Audit Commission had shown that 14% of hospitals did not even bother to code some of their activity – which under PbR would have meant no payment for the work done.[23]

Introducing PbR across the NHS was not risk-free. Hospitals might "cream-skim" by trying to avoid treating the sicker, more expensive patients; they might try to reduce costs by discharging patients too early; they could openly 'game' by trying to code people within higher tariff DRG groups; and they could engage in a higher level of activity that would bust local NHS budgets. But there were ways of reducing these risks through protocols to regulate admissions and quality of care; independent audit of coding data; and risk-sharing agreements between purchase and providers that set a limit on levels of hospital activity attracting higher prices.

I needed to do a deep dive on these issues with officials. From mid-May 2005 I had a series of meetings to clarify my own thinking on PbR. It was clear from these that, using US experience, in the first year there would be extra costs to cover coding and transition costs. There would also be problems for specialist children and orthopaedic hospitals where patients had more complex and more expensive treatments, not adequately covered by the case-mix averaging of the DRG system. Other services were also trying to exclude themselves from PbR for fear of income loss. Whenever we introduced PbR across the NHS there would be problems. My view quickly crystallized to one that despite all the reservations we had to introduce PbR and then refine it over time. No country had started with a perfect system or with perfect data and coding. In most countries governments had imposed the system to improve efficiency and then amended it over time. The NHS would be no different. However

I thought it best to see a comprehensive DRG system in operation so I decided to visit Germany to look at the system they had been working on since 1996 and which had gone live in all hospitals in 2004 and 2005.

I made the German visit with the official who had been working on PbR, Bill McCarthy; and in the British Ambassador's residence in Berlin I recruited him to run the new DH Policy and Strategy Unit that Patricia Hewitt and I had decided to set up. The Germans had approached PbR with scary Teutonic efficiency, including establishing an independent central agency for setting the tariff. (However at dinner with the Agency's head and Health Department counterpart it emerged that there was a level of consultation and information exchange that made me a little more sceptical about some of the independence claims.) 10% of hospitals were sampled each year, on a paid basis, to update cost data. The Germans were operating a system with nearly 1,100 DRGs (and growing) whereas we would be using one with about 650 DRGs. This meant they had a far more ambitious and precise reimbursement scheme than we were envisaging. Even more impressively they cancelled all leave in the tariff-setting agency for the 3 months before the start of each financial year in order to assimilate all the new cost data and calculate the new tariff. Despite this more elaborate machinery the Germans still found it difficult to absorb into the system highly specialist hospitals without making supplementary payments. Nevertheless the German experience encouraged me to go for full implementation across the NHS.

I agreed with officials that we should buy-in some help from Australia and we hired a person who had worked on the Victoria State system. They had a better DRG system than the UK but I could see another half a decade passing if we waited for what was to become known in the trade as "HRG4". The DH boffins who had been working on PbR would have preferred to wait for the more refined HRG4 case-mix system which was a better currency for healthcare than the HRG3.5 system we were using in 2005. However it took DH until 2009/10 to introduce HRG4 into NHS use - and then not completely – so I feel vindicated by my 2005 decision not to delay implementation.

In the summer of 2005 we were part way through a 4-year transition phase for introducing PbR by 2007/8. The NHS was extremely twitchy after the first year's experience and there were strong DH and NHS voices suggesting that we should abandon the whole idea. After seeing the German experience my view was that we should accelerate implementation and in 2006/7 extend PbR to all NHS elective and non-elective inpatient care, outpatients, and A & E and critical care. I could see little point in trying to bring in mental health – about 10% of NHS spend – very quickly because these services had a poor track record of case-mix classification. They had variability of treatment patterns; care pathways that spanned numerous settings; and they lacked data collection and clinician buy-in to the DRG system. New Zealand and Australia had managed to introduce a classification system for mental health but we were a long way from being able to do so.

Holding up acute services PbR for the slowest ship in the NHS convoy seemed pointless.

Patricia Hewitt agreed that we should accelerate expansion of PbR in 2006/7 and that we should settle the tariff no later than January 2006 so that it was issued in good time for the new financial year. This provided us with just enough time to do some "road-testing" of the new extended tariff before we settled on firm figures for 2006/7. This "road-testing" was done with a number of cooperative trusts and we commissioned work on lessons to be learned from the PbR experience so far. We enlisted more help from the Audit Commission for a PbR assurance framework to support good behaviour by NHS Trusts, following the work that the Commission had already done on PbR. We needed an authoritative independent body like the Commission to be involved because regular monitoring of payments and behaviour would be crucial to ensuring that PbR operated as intended. The Commission have continued to play a key role in validating the operation of PbR in the NHS and their auditors have been an important force in checking 'gaming'.

The most difficult part came when Patricia Hewitt and I sat down for two hours with massive spreadsheets and the PbR experts to settle the acute hospital tariffs for 2006/7. We could see who would be losers and winners and the impact of various options for securing efficiency gains and approving inflation factors. For the time being I had rejected the German idea of an independent body to settle tariffs although we had an Advisory Committee on Resource Allocations that could have been adapted to take on setting the PbR tariff. However given the state of the NHS finances in 2005 and 2006 and the political reality of Ministerial accountability for the NHS budget, I considered that it was unrealistic to hand over PbR tariff-setting at this stage to a separate body.

Although it was hard work fine-tuning the 2006/7 tariff it was very clear that the PbR system had huge potential for driving efficiency and quality in the NHS if we concentrated on improving and expanding it and did not become too obsessed with its early-stage limitations. When we issued the 2006/7 tariff we made it clear that down the track the system would be modified to cover more areas, to embrace a quality dimension and to incentivise non-hospital provision of care by unbundling the tariff. We encouraged local experimentation in these areas, although not a lot took place. When Lord Darzi's NHS Next Stage Review, "High Quality Care for All" was published in 2008 it made several clear commitments to building on PbR and improving it. It wanted to reflect quality more in the

PbR tariff and to cover other services. By the time Darzi's report was published the average hospital (in 2008/9) received over 60% of its income through PbR.[24]

By the time I left office the PbR tariff was part of the NHS furniture, with a new tariff for 2007/8 signed off as part of the NHS Operating Framework for that year. People had learnt that Ministers could use it to set efficiency gain requirements and to some extent control healthcare's inflationary tendencies. It was flexible enough to make special payments to a limited number of highly specialist hospitals to avoid bankrupting them, provided you controlled the homogenising tendencies of the PbR purists. Work had begun on preparing for HRG4 changeover which would make the tariff more sophisticated. We had completed implementation of PbR in the projected timescale of 2007/8. All talk of the NHS abandoning PbR had disappeared. The issue now was how rapidly it could be expanded to a wider range of activities, made more sophisticated and handed over to an independent body for tariff-setting.

In February 2008 the Audit Commission published a report on PbR which found that "PbR has undoubtedly improved the fairness and transparency of the payment system. It has, perhaps, had a positive effect on activity and efficiency in elective care. Day cases have increased and the length of stay for elective inpatients has fallen". The Commission recognised however that other factors, like targets, had played a part in these improvements. It considered that "PbR has now been largely mainstreamed by the NHS"; that "overall, interest in information and improving data quality within the NHS has increased as a result of PbR"; and that "in general there is no evidence to date that trusts are 'gaming' the system to gain unwarranted payments".[25]

When I read the Audit Commission and the Darzi Reports I felt totally vindicated in pressing on with PbR implementation when critics said Ministers should give the NHS more time and that we had too much reform going on simultaneously. PbR did not get the media attention of other parts of the NHS reform agenda – mainly I suspect because it was too technical for journalists to write a snappy story about – but it was a key part of NHS reform and creating a healthcare market. As it develops with the new HRG4 currency and the expanded scope set out for it in the 2009/10 Operating Framework, PbR is becoming a key part of driving efficiency and improving quality in the NHS. The tariff is being used to reward desired practice but also restrain costs with a 1.7% increase uplift only in 2009/10; and it was planning expansion into mental health in 2010/11. As the NHS moves from feast to famine future Ministers will appreciate the additional levers PbR provides for cutting costs and driving efficiency, providing they carry on refining the tariff within an independent governance structure..

Conclusion

Between 2003 and 2007 three key reforms were effectively established in the NHS: more autonomous hospitals, Foundation Trusts; some semblance of an NHS market with competition between providers, some of whom came from outside the NHS; and a tariff system for paying hospital providers on an activity basis rather than a block grant. Patients could get their NHS treatment outside an NHS hospital; and the payment for that treatment would be made on the same tariff whether provided in an NHS or a private hospital. The NHS was now part of a public sector which had a third of its services delivered by the private and voluntary sectors according to the DeAnne Julius Review commissioned by John Hutton when Business Secretary in December 2007.

None of these changes were perfect instruments of competition. All needed further refinement, extension and support but they would be difficult to withdraw from the NHS despite continuing criticism from a variety of quarters. They all provided some challenge to the NHS legacy of complacency and monopoly. Public sector unions might not like it but the elements of competition among providers were established, although at nothing like the 15% level for ISTCs that many of us wanted in order to produce a tougher challenge to NHS providers.

Under Tony Blair the messages had been clear from 2003 onwards. The private sector was encouraged to compete for business within an NHS market that was part of a wider reform process. Under Gordon Brown the messages were unclear and mixed. Too often he seemed preoccupied with not upsetting Labour's paymasters in the public sector unions. Then he would make a speech saying how important the private sector was to public sector reform, particularly when John Hutton was Business Secretary. Not surprisingly the private sector has been confused about where they stand with the NHS, particularly when the costs of bidding were so high and the outcomes so uncertain. The messages from Brown's Health Ministers were rarely encouraging, particularly when Andy Burnham made a speech to the King's Fund in September 2009 about the NHS being the preferred provider of services.

The NHS now has some degree of marketisation and scope for more competition but lacks a strong economic regulator to enforce competition, as discussed later. However it is now easier to apply a good dose of competition to the NHS if the Coalition Government and their successors have the appetite for it.

4

Choice and commissioning a patient-led NHS

The political and public debate about the NHS over the years has been full of well-meaning utterances about services being patient-focussed and patient-led and giving patients more say and choice over services and the way they are delivered. Professional bodies have continued to exhort doctors and nurses to listen to patients and respond more to what they say. Patients continue to complain about their voices not being heard and having too little say over services. The new Coalition Government assures people that patients are to be given more power and say at the local level. Their intentions are good, like those of their predecessors, but at the heart of the matter is whether service commissioning responds to patient needs and whether the NHS systems and behaviour facilitate patient choice.

Producing a patient-led NHS involves difficult practical issues around information, choice and commissioning that no political party has yet resolved but Labour was the latest to try. Important in their efforts was the start-stop attempt to create an NHS market of diverse providers described in the last chapter. Without greater provider variety and adequate capacity it is difficult to make choice meaningful to patients. That absence of variety, capacity and choice was very much a feature of the NHS before the recent Labour government and was one of the reasons why people were willing to pay to secure private treatment. Convenience and speedy relief of pain and discomfort have been too often matters to which the NHS does not respond effectively.

To make the NHS patient-led those who commission services – whether they are GPs, local commissioning bodies or more remote specialist commissioners – need more clearly to be seen as responding to patient views and needs across the whole country, not just parts of it. Creating high quality commissioning skills and ensuring their even geographical spread is a long way from achievement across the NHS but some progress was made by Labour and there are lessons to be learned from their attempts to improve choice and commissioning.

Choice and the road to the 2005 election

The NHS Plan of 2000 had a strong patient focus and talked of giving people 'a real say in the NHS'. But the aspiration in that plan was more about seeking patient views, having advocates, patients getting copies of doctor's letters and patient surveys. The only real service choice patients were offered related to cancelled operations.[1] In mid-2003 the choice agenda began to change significantly with the arrival of John Reid as Health Secretary. While John was no longer the Clydeside firebrand of his youth, patient choice appealed to his egalitarian instincts. He took some delight in the idea that choice had as much, if not more, appeal to working-class Labour voters who historically had had little choice in public services, as it did to the middle classes that New Labour had been wooing. Shortly after John's arrival a major public consultation was launched, led by Harry Cayton, the DH Director for Patients and the Public.

There were three main strands to this consultation: a national consultation led by Expert Task Groups across eight themes; a Choice Consultation Survey so that public, staff, patients, users and carers could contribute their ideas; and SHA-led local consultations. Over 100,000 people were involved, as were many hundreds of bodies and organisations. Several recurring themes came from the consultation. All classes of people wanted to share in decisions about health and healthcare and to make choices about that care; 90% of people said they needed more information to make their choices over treatment or care, and people said clearly that their health needs were personal and they didn't like being expected to fit into a system. I was to find these messages repeated with even greater emphasis in the public consultation Patricia Hewitt and I set up in 2005 for our White Paper 'Our Health, Our Care, Our Say' (see Chapter 12).

There were big messages for the NHS that involved major cultural change. People wanted extra NHS capacity to be provided, especially for long-term conditions, and they supported continuing reform. More power should be devolved locally but system changes had to deliver more choice. The NHS had to do a better job of listening to patients and the public. For me – and I think for other Ministers – there was however a considerable gulf between what the public wanted and where the local NHS – staff and systems – were in their thinking. As I went round the NHS on Ministerial visits and held local staff engagement meetings it was clear that most NHS staff were not on the same page as the public and DH Ministers in terms of more patient choice and voice. Hoping that local staff would have a change of heart without more intervention was wishful thinking.

John Reid's response to this consultation was the publication in December 2003 of a White Paper that identified six main changes:

- Giving people a bigger say in how they were treated with the provision of their own Health Space linked to the electronic health record which would enable people to make their preferences known to the clinical team.
- Increased choice of access to a wider range of services in primary care
- Increased choice of where, when and how to get medicines

- Enabling people to book appointments at a time that suited them from a wider choice of hospitals, with a promise that by the end of 2005 patients requiring surgery would have a choice of four or five hospitals.
- Widening choice of treatment and care, starting with maternity services and end of life care (relating to where they wished to die and how they wanted to be treated)
- Ensuring people had the right information at the right time.[2]

These changes would take time but the December 2003 document laid down a credible choice agenda that one could press the NHS to engage with. Political 'bite' was provided in a personal foreword by John Reid that related the 2003 document to the 1944 White Paper on the creation of the NHS: "Choice has to be real rather than just theoretical. It has to be available to the many not just the few. And it has to be the route to equity as well as excellence." The Foreword made it clear that "without an increase in capacity in the NHS, we cannot deliver the degree of choice that we want for patients" and that the ability to offer patients "real choices goes hand in hand with the better use of capacity"[3]. The Ministerial message on the link between choice and capacity was clear in 2003 but as I found over the next 3 years many in both the Labour ranks and the NHS were not keen on hearing this message.

John Reid kept his foot firmly on the choice accelerator and egged on by No.10 he followed up the December 2003 document with another blast in June 2004 when the "NHS Improvement Plan" was published. The Prime Minister was now in full flow on public service reform, with patient choice as another weapon in his armoury. A Foreword by Tony Blair made it clear that there would be no slowing down on NHS reform and no apology for driving reforms from the centre. The NHS Improvement Plan contained some new and radical proposals that were not fully grasped by the NHS at the time of publication:

- "Patients will be admitted for treatment within a maximum of 18 weeks from referral to their GP and those with urgent conditions will be treated much faster."
- "Patients will be able to choose between a range of providers, including NHS Foundation Trusts and treatment centres."
- "They will be able to be treated at any facility that meets NHS standards, within the national maximum price that the NHS pays for the treatment they need."
- "We anticipate that by 2008, the independent sector will carry out up to 15% of procedures per annum for NHS patients, paid for by the NHS."

- "By 2008 all NHS acute trusts in England will be in a position to apply to become NHS Foundation Trusts, working as independent public benefit corporations, modelled on cooperative and mutual traditions."
- "The Healthcare Commission will inspect all providers of care and provide assurance of quality of care wherever it is delivered."[4]

Improving delivery through central targets was extended with a new demanding target of a maximum of 18 weeks from GP referral to specialist operation. There was more emphasis on personalisation and devolution to counter the criticism of an over-centralised 'command and control' NHS. More personalised care was promised and more care was to be delivered closer to home, with a better deal for people with complex long-term conditions. Local communities would have greater influence and say over how their services were run. All hospitals were to be taken out of Whitehall control by becoming FTs by the end of 2008. This was a hopelessly optimistic claim, as described in Chapter 3.

NHS patients would be "able to choose from a growing range of independent providers" who by 2008, would "provide up to 15% of procedures on behalf of the NHS." The expansion of private sector capacity was linked to choice unequivocally for the first time. Two future choice benchmarks were laid down. "From the end of 2005 patients will have the right to choose from at least four to five healthcare providers." "In 2008 patients will have the right to choose from any provider," subject to meeting NHS standards and keeping within NHS tariff price. The 15% figure was immediately attacked by the unions, outraged that someone with John Reid's Labour pedigree could agree this. He ducked and weaved and said it was an estimate not a target but the private sector was delighted. Tony Blair continued to regard 15% as a target.

The commitments in the December 2003 and the June 2004 documents were carried through into the 2005 Election Manifesto which promised to expand capacity and choice in primary care, not just hospitals. By 2009 all women would "have choice over where and how they have their baby and what pain relief to use". More patients with cancer would have a choice to be treated at home. In social care there would be "personalised budgets" so, "people can decide for themselves what they need and how it should be provided."[5] However when I arrived in my new job after the 2005 Election my induction pack made no mention of choice or indeed of competition, apart from a single slide on the independent sector. Senior civil service enthusiasm for the choice agenda was muted and little work had been done on delivering our choice of 4 or 5 hospitals by the end of 2005.

As I read myself into the literature on patient choice I found there was a compelling case and it could not just be dismissed as a fad of Ministers.

There was good survey data showing that over 60% of patients thought choice of hospitals was very or fairly important. This compared with over 75% in relation to schools where there had been more public debate on parental choice. Choice was more important to women than men, so there were some gender politics involved as well. The 2005 British Social Attitudes Survey revealed that support for choice of hospitals was spread throughout the socio-economic groups. If anything support for choice was stronger in the poorer groups who often received a worse deal from the NHS than the sharp-elbowed middle classes. Armed with this information and the arrival of a few, more enthusiastic, civil servants I was able to go on the stump around the NHS about choice being a key issue. We set up a raft of seminars with PCTs to push the agenda and found some PCT champions – largely women - who were enthusiastic about choice.

Back in the DH there was the critical matter of giving people the information they needed to exercise choice. A duff pilot effort and booklet for each area had to be aborted, at some cost. There was endless debate about what measures for each hospital should be included and tortuous discussions about the reliability of the local data. I wanted to use published data and agree the material with local trusts. I was able to persuade the Healthcare Commission to help us with data provision. We settled on a traffic-light system for each of seven hospital measures (including waiting times and infection scores) so that it was easier for the public to understand. We had to pressurise some areas to include private sector providers so that people had a wider choice. There was a printing screw up which added to the costs and my woes. After some months' work we distributed booklets around the country at the end of 2005 so that, at least in theory, people could exercise choice of hospital as we had promised. I authorised a publicity campaign in early 2006 and we set up later an NHS Choices website when we brought in Dr. Foster to do this. (I had entered into a joint venture with Dr. Foster to improve dissemination of the mountain of data the DH had on performance.)

Although we had enabled people to exercise choice of hospital, many clinicians (including GPs) and managers were less enthusiastic and found choice very threatening. Some NHS staff tried to scare local people about going to a hospital outside their area on the grounds that loss of income would threaten the future of local hospitals. Some acute hospitals and their consultants refused to put available appointments on the Choose and Book computer system so that patients couldn't exercise choice. Some GPs said the data on quality was unreliable. The tensions and conflicts over choice within the NHS were reflected in the views expressed in professional journals and by the media, with many journalists siding with professional self-interest. Although the civil servants working directly to me on choice were very supportive, the top echelons of the NHS and SHAs were much less keen on projecting the case for more patient choice.

Despite having public opinion on our side, the government received little credit for pushing on with choice. Many in the media presented choice as something Ministers were inflicting on a hard-pressed NHS and that the public didn't really want. There was virtually no coverage of the view that parts of the NHS were simply engaging in restrictive practices to suit provider convenience. The mantra "people just want good local hospitals" appeared repeatedly. We surveyed the public later in 2006 to see how many people had a sense of increased choice.

This survey showed considerable local variation. In the new SHA areas that came into operation in July 2006, 6 out of the 10 had between a third and a half of people reporting a choice of hospital with the remainder reporting under a third. About a quarter of the new PCTs reported over half their population saying they had a choice and about a dozen reported over two-thirds. We were able to compare this data with unoccupied and available beds. With the exception of East Anglia, Devon and Cornwall, Cumbria and parts of Northumberland and a few other rural areas, most parts of the country had reasonable bed availability within an hour's travel time of people's homes. So when I resigned as a Minister at the end of 2006 we had delivered some reality of choice of hospital to at least a third of the country and in some places over a half of the population.

Despite some scepticism the evidence is that parts of the public have an appetite for choosing the hospital they go into and are prepared to travel to receive treatment quicker. But King's Fund research published in 2010 shows that many patients do not get a choice of hospital. Many GPs were resisting patients' entitlement to choice and rarely pointed patients towards performance data to help them choose. Although information was available to help people choose they did not always know about it or find it easy to use. The public were relying for help with choosing on NHS personnel who were often far from helpful.[6]

There is still a long way to go before patients can exercise choice easily so that poorly performing hospitals will feel unsettled enough to change. There are still information, professional and technological obstacles to be overcome before choice is as universally and easily available as it should be. Some in the NHS who resist more patient choice argue that patients do not want to go to a non-NHS hospital but the survey information available to me when I was a Minister did not support this viewpoint, as I repeatedly told NHS audiences. In April 2005 a Mori Survey indicated that 71% of the public were happy to use the independent sector to provide NHS treatment: 16% had no preference and only 11% were unhappy with the idea.[7] Patient satisfaction levels on ISTCs were consistently higher than those with NHS hospitals overall;

and every ISTC patient I spoke to was delighted with their care and treatment but often surprised that they could get this level of service on the NHS. They liked the customer-focus of the private providers and compared their previous NHS experience unfavourably with the ISTC.

Labour Ministers planted the seed of patient choice in the NHS. As access to meaningful information improves more people should feel more confident about exercising choice and challenging health professionals who are resistant. Although the notion of choice is an intrinsically appealing idea it was never likely to be powerful enough on it is own to drive the NHS reform agenda. However it remains an important part of the armoury of challenge mechanisms that shift the NHS towards patient preference and greater efficiency. Barriers to choice and its companion, competition, continue to need removing. That will be easier to do by strengthening the work on commissioning begun under Labour.

The challenges of NHS commissioning

At the heart of many NHS problems is the 20-year muddle over commissioning – what it is and how best to do it. We have created a system whereby most of the money spent on the NHS is sent by the DH direct to a large number of Primary Care Trust (PCT) commissioners. The allocations to PCTs are on a weighted population basis that attempts to reflect local health needs by for example providing more money to areas with high numbers of elderly people, who, generally, consume more health care than other groups. Over the years there have been endless debates about the fairness of the allocation system and these continue. Some of the criticisms are justified; others are special pleading. If the basis of a fair allocation system is health need then the system is likely to favour poorer areas (i.e. Labour) rather than wealthier ones (i.e. Conservative). This is because poverty and lower income have a stronger correlation with ill health than almost anything else. Inevitably the basis of the allocation system becomes political as well as statistical. More recently the Conservatives have suggested this allocation formula needs a further review, as indeed it may.

When I was a Minister I concluded that spending a lot of time devising "the perfect" allocation system was less useful than creating more competent groupings and organisations to do the job of commissioning itself. If we could improve the functionality of the bodies handing out most of the NHS budgets, patients were more likely to get better services and the tax-payer better value for money. Easy to say but not easy to do from where we were in mid-2005.

Commissioning health services is undoubtedly complex. It requires striking a balance between the varied and sometimes conflicting needs of particular populations. If you spend too much on acute hospital care – the biggest spender – you may have insufficient resources to meet for example a community's needs for mental health, care of chronic conditions or health promotion and disease prevention. Overdosing on preparations for swine or pandemic 'flu leaves less money for everyday healthcare. Commissioning some services is likely to require operating over larger territories and populations than fit neatly into organisational boundaries. Some commissioning is very local and some ought to operate over the health/social care divide.

Commissioning embraces a range of functions: identifying a variety of needs; specifying requirements to meet those needs; identifying service providers to respond to those needs at an acceptable price; contracting with those providers; monitoring their performance; dealing with performance failure and being able to bring in new providers; forecasting future needs and providers; paying providers; and dealing with disputes. Commissioning is much more than contracting and far more complicated than drawing up a shopping list and popping down to the supermarket. Yet some PCTs seem to operate as though it is not much more and once they have found a convenient supplier why bother to change them.

Commissioners have to live within their allocated budgets; cooperate with each other for commissioning specialist services with high unit costs; and manage service demands so that their budgets remain in balance over time. For responding to the everyday needs of individual patients it makes more sense for PCT commissioners to hand over a proportion of their budgets to GPs to purchase some services for their patients (i.e. micro-level commissioning). High class commissioning requires a set of specialist skills and the nerve to stand up to powerful big spenders like acute hospitals and to seek better value from them. Commissioners need the courage to switch providers when they do not perform but many PCTs seem unable to do so particularly when the provider is powerful. They are almost totally unwilling to change the provider of particular services, such as maternity, within an acute hospital.

There has been a long standing debate about whether those who commission services can also be service providers themselves because of the inherent conflict of interest that this can pose. How can you get the best services for your population if you decide to provide them yourself without any competition? The idea of a purchaser/provider split in the NHS has been around for nearly 3 decades now. I had pioneered such a purchaser split in social care in the late 1980s as Director of Social Services in Kent. This had been supported by the then Conservative Government in developing community care nationally. Ken Clarke, as Health Secretary, had favoured a purchaser-provider split for the NHS but had used GP fundholders and health authorities as commissioners, with the latter still running community services as well.

Labour had opposed GP fund-holding and the whole idea of a healthcare market, as described already. In 2002 Alan Milburn established 302 PCTs as commissioners of services including GPs and other primary care contractors but also left them as providers of community health services. Both Conservative and Labour attempts to establish health commissioners have had considerable shortcomings, with commissioners continuing to provide services and being deflected from their commissioning role. More significantly commissioners were never properly trained for commissioning. To add complexity a version of practice-based commissioning (PBC) by GPs had been initiated by Labour just before the 2005 Election but on a voluntary basis, so that GPs could decide whether they wished to commission and PCTs could decline to cooperate. This was the situation on commissioning that I inherited in May 2005.

Most of the 302 PCTs were far too small. Other countries commissioned on a bigger scale. In California, Kaiser Permanente commissioned services on a state-wide basis. In Australia hospital services were commissioned and paid for on a state-wide basis. In New Zealand the 21 District Health Boards came together in four shared service organisations covering over 1 million population each to commission specialist services. PCTs remained conflicted by being providers of community services with many feeling threatened by the prospect of GP commissioning. Many of the PCTs did not know how to do their jobs effectively and were reluctant to control excessive demands for cash from big acute hospitals or change underperforming providers. A fundamental problem in 2005 was the absence of an agreed and clear definition of what commissioning involved. This problem continues today.

I tried to get across within DH the three essential elements of PCT commissioning. First a local needs analysis which involved understanding and measuring an assessment of the health needs of the local population served. Second identifying and defining the services required to meet those needs in some order of priority. And third, within the resources available, contracting for the services needed from the most appropriate providers (whether in the NHS or not), monitoring performance against those contracts and changing providers when they did not perform. The great majority of PCTs in 2005 did not know how to make a market so that they could attract good new providers and most had little interest in doing so. Most still do not know how to do this and have been given little political encouragement since 2007 to learn. Indeed the former Health Secretary, Andy Burnham, in September 2009 told the world that for him the NHS was the preferred provider, a blatantly anti-competitive move that made it more difficult for PCTs to commission from the private or voluntary sector.

In 2005 most PCTs had some form of contract system in place but whether it was always based on a prioritised local needs analysis was highly doubtful. In most areas PCTs were still attached to cosy contracts with their local acute hospitals and let these hospitals shape present and future spending patterns. Most PCTs lacked the bottle or skill to change providers, whether it was underperforming GPs or hospital services. As a government we were pouring increasing amounts of money into a failing commissioning system with targets as the only weapon in our armoury. Unfortunately most of these targets strengthened the position of powerful acute hospitals to seek more money to implement them. The more hospitals who became FTs the worse the situation would become with surging provider-induced demand and weak commissioners unable to control demand or commission alternative, more appropriate services and providers.

A report from the Health Foundation in October 2004 had found that: "There is little evidence to show that any primary care-led (or other) commissioning had made a significant impact on the way hospital care is delivered, except in relation to waiting times for treatment." It also concluded that: "Primary care-led commissioning has been shown to be effective in the area of primary and intermediate care and in encouraging greater responsiveness in elective hospital services."[8] In other words PCTs had not made much of an impact on the big battalions of the acute hospitals but GPs might be more promising.

I used the 2005 Manifesto commitment to streamline the NHS to tackle two aspects of commissioning weaknesses: the excessive number of PCTs and their continuing responsibility for provider functions. This exercise led to a document entitled "Commissioning a Patient-led NHS", published in July 2005. My aim had been to reduce the 302 PCTs to 60 or so. Unfortunately, as described in the next chapter, my proposals unravelled and we ended up only halving their number. There remain far too many small organisations without the capability to be effective commissioners. The result is that too many local NHS plans continue to be dominated by how much money the local hospital claims it needs, often using national targets to justify their financial demands. Among most PCTs there has been little appetite for shifting service delivery outside hospitals. Powerful figures in the NHS and at the top of DH have built their careers in managing acute hospitals so many had little real interest in commissioning - either in theory or practice – until Mark Britnell came along after I left DH.

The PCTs have remained conflicted because they are still both commissioners and service providers. It is much easier to concentrate on managing community services than mastering the more difficult task of learning to commission and making enemies among local acute hospitals and other service providers. The idea of reappraising and shifting resources from acute hospitals and making them more efficient has not come naturally to most PCTs. It required an expertise and resolve that was usually absent, and it might well not prove popular with MPs, SHAs and the DH. People tended to view commissioning as a word to use when trotting out the mantra on NHS reform rather than as something you took seriously. After the 2005 setbacks on reducing the number of PCTs and hiving off their provider arms I decided to get practice-based commissioning better established as a way of shaking up PCTs.

Practice-based commissioning (PBC)

The Conservatives had been through their own mixed-experience with NHS commissioning. Ken Clarke had tried to progress commissioning with his innovative idea of fund-holding under which GPs would hold budgets and commission some hospital services; but he had been unable to cover more than about 50% of the population with fundholders. Foolishly Labour had been opposed to fundholding and had let it die after 1997. Then a variant of it – practice-based commissioning (PBC) – had been encouraged on a voluntary basis by John Hutton just before the 2005 election. Some technical guidance on PBC was issued to the NHS in February 2005. I found in June that the DH had little by way of a plan to ensure that PCTs cooperated with or helped GPs who wanted to do PBC. Many PCTs seemed to see both PBC and me as a threat to the way they operated, both of which were true because I thought PBC needed to be pursued with more vigour.

I decided that we should move from a voluntary approach – which was going nowhere fast – to incentivising GPs to the point where we achieved virtually 100% of practices undertaking PBC. I set myself the target of achieving this by the end of 2006. It was clear from the outset that DH officials and PCTs were going to be reluctant participants in my PBC drive so I looked for friends outside DH. Two of my allies were Dr James Kingsland of the National Association of Primary Care (NAPC) and Dr Michael Dixon of the NHS Alliance. The BMA's general practitioner committee were cautious and operating in trade union mode to see how this would benefit GPs financially. Their mood was sweetened by my agreeing with the negotiators a Directed Enhanced Scheme to reimburse practices for the cost of engaging with PBC at a rate of 95p per registered patient. The Royal College of General Practitioners were also cooperative. Sir John Oldham, a reforming Peak District GP, was a tower of strength and agreed to set up and run a network system for training GPs in PBC through the National Primary Care Development Team that he managed. He did this despite some bureaucratic resistance in DH.

The DH culture was reluctant to empower GPs in this way. They could always flourish the smaller practices that struggled with commissioning under fund-holding and would do so again with PBC unless they joined with other practices. There was resistance to my ideas of setting a deadline for requiring all GPs to participate in PBC and giving them cash incentives for doing so. No. 10 were supportive, although I was to learn at one meeting with Tony Blair that his support was based on a sketchy grasp of what was involved when I had to conduct an impromptu tutorial on PBC. In the end Ministerial will and internal and external GP support trumped bureaucratic inertia, at least temporarily. I launched in January 2006, with a personal foreword, a document setting out what needed to be done to achieve full GP coverage of PBC by December 2006. It instructed PCTs in some detail on what to do to provide GPs with the standards and information they would need to make PBC a reality and how to set indicative budgets for PBC. The issues of accountability, governance and arbitration between GPs and PCTs were laid out.[9]

The most contentious issue was my decision to follow the Nye Bevan route of giving doctors money to do what you wanted done. I incentivised GPs to take up PBC by allowing them to redirect the lion's share of any resources freed up by PBC. The sentence I insisted on and that was resisted by the civil servants, prompted by PCT interests (and probably the Treasury) read: "we recommend that for 2006/7 individual practices should be entitled to access and redirect at least 70% of any freed up resources; the remaining 30% to be used by the PCT to meet a wider need across the whole PCT area".[10] I was backing the strand of financially shrewd entrepreneurialism in general practice against the bureaucratic caution of most PCTs.

Although I was to have my differences with the BMA negotiators over GP remuneration I have never been in any doubt that if we want more NHS resources diverted to services outside hospitals, chronic conditions and preventative health services we have to put GPs more in the commissioning driving seat. If we are to tackle health inequalities and make services more personalised, it is critical that service commissioning becomes more localised with a stronger dose of GP involvement. GPs understand money and its power. Many politicians and most of the public do not realise that GP practices are small businesses with a profit and loss account and they have been so since the beginning of the NHS. GPs respond to financial incentives and, for the most part, also to the clinical needs of patients. They have a potential to drive efficiency in the NHS which has never been fully harnessed and exploited. Conservative Ministers have understood this on the whole, much better than Labour politicians who tend to prefer public organisations that provide public sector jobs rather than small businesses that cut corners and are more individualistic in their responses. Corner-cutting, entrepreneurial GPs make rule-bound civil servants and public sector managers nervous, sometimes with good reason; but it remains my view that it is better to risk overpaying GPs to do more commissioning than it is to sink larger and larger sums of public money into inadequate PCTs and through them into the black hole of acute hospitals. Although PBC can give some encouragement to GPs to feather their own nests, personally I would prefer to risk that if it can prevent so much money going unnecessarily into inefficient and inappropriate acute hospital services who, in their own way, are also feathering their own nests at the taxpayers' expense. For these reasons I was in this alliance with GP professional leaders on PBC against the forces of resistance in the DH bureaucracy and vested PCT interests. It is not a position without political and accountability risks as the Coalition Government will find as they pursue GP commissioning, but the potential public benefits are likely to justify the risks.

I got my way with the January 2006 guidance and a subsequent clinically-focussed document which I asked professional leaders to produce. These leaders were immensely supportive and their guidance showed where clinical gains for patients could be produced quickest through PBC. The forces of opposition to PBC continued for the rest of my time as a Minister to fight a delaying action with a variety of excuses. PCTs couldn't provide the data; GPs could not be trusted when they were both providers and commissioners; PBC would wreck demand management; and so on. Most of the resistance amounted simply to an unwillingness by PCTs and their supporters to share commissioning power with GPs. I ensured that the battle of principle was over when we published in July 2006 a fuller document on commissioning for PCTs and SHAs. This made it clear that "PBC will play a central role in the future health systems as the integrator of services for patients". It went on to say that: "To achieve this, practices will have indicative budgets for most services."[11]

The annex to this document stated unequivocally that "PBC will be critical in enabling PCTs to achieve the best value for patients". It continued: "Through PBC practices will have indicative budgets and the freedoms and incentives to exercise devolved responsibility for aspects of the commissioning and redesign of services."[12] An Appendix tried to lay to rest the arguments over governance and an accountability framework for PBC that had rumbled on since my January document. The proposals in effect achieved a workable balance between public accountability for taxpayer's money with freedom for clinicians to innovate and deliver improvements for patients.

PCT resistance to PBC continued. The battle with the DH bureaucracy was to some extent over but the acute hospital and targets-preoccupied DH top management never enthused over commissioning – PBC or otherwise. It was the alliance of committed Ministers and professional leaders that had ensured that PBC was to continue to be an integral part of future annual operational frameworks for the NHS. PCTs were pressured to share commissioning power with GPs, some of whom were to form sizeable consortia to do the job more effectively and to keep overheads low. But the know-how and will to make PBC work well was a long way from being established in many PCTs, as Coalition Ministers will find as they attempt to transfer greater commissioning responsibility to GPs.

The Audit Commission published in November 2007 a report on PBC in 16 PCTs which "found that the engagement of practices was variable". However they also found that "The combination of an incentive payment to practices, together with the requirement on PCTs to provide a supporting infrastructure has helped to introduce and implement PBC."[13] I felt vindicated over my robust approach to incentives but PCT infrastructure support was still unreliable. Some GPs were not participating significantly, leaving the effort to enthusiasts who were often the old GP fundholders. Working with public health professionals on preventative strategies was poor.

I had established PBC universally but there was a long way to go before it could play its full part in a commissioning-led NHS. Although DH attitudes towards PBC have improved there continue to be problems with PCT attitudes. Bodies like the NHS Alliance have continued to champion PBC but the experience of too many GPs is captured by the remarks in July 2008 by a Birmingham GP, Dr Fay Wilson: "In the majority of areas in England, PCTs don't want PBC to happen. GPs are interested but they turn up to a PBC meeting and realise it is a talking shop. There was a lot of energy but GPs are disillusioned."[14] PCTs have continued to give inadequate support and information for PBC and to reject the majority of GP plans for new services under PBC. Many PCTs have failed to hand over real budgets to GPs. A £100million of incentive payments to GPs has produced insufficient innovation in the services commissioned according to a King's Fund study. Nevertheless despite shortcomings in PBC this two-year study argued in 2008 that the Darzi Review was right to commit the Government to persevering with PBC.[15]

In December 2008 a national framework to provide practical support to PBC groups and PCTs was established but progress has not been speedy. In July 2009 I asked a Parliamentary Question about the proportion of GP practices engaged in PBC and the proportion of PCT commissioning budgets spent on PBC. The answer I received on 8 July

2009 was that the proportion of money spent on PBC was not collected nationally but the DH was carrying out quarterly surveys of 2000 GP practices (nearly a quarter of all practices). The March 2009 survey showed that 92% of practices were part of a PBC group.[16] Although PBC has been established as part of the NHS operational landscape it has not been pushed strongly since 2007, probably because handing more power and budget to GP commissioning undermined any residual rationale for so many small PCTs. Labour Ministers would have been forced to merge PCTs, a course they have been reluctant to pursue.

Taking forward the commissioning agenda

Despite the 2005 setbacks on implementing a full purchaser-provider split it was clear that we had to enhance the commissioning skills of the reduced number of PCTs and to integrate commissioning properly into the NHS operational annual cycle. In 2006/7 about 30% of the NHS spend would follow patient flows with choice and the PbR tariff, so the era of controlling NHS demand through block grants was coming to an end. PCT commissioners would have to manage demand in order to balance the NHS budget overall. Through the autumn of 2005 Ministers worked with officials to produce a document showing how the various strands of NHS reform fitted together. It set out a timetable for specific reforms that looked ahead to 2008/9 and was a reform route map for the NHS, something that had been lacking previously as one change was piled upon another, usually to the bafflement of most of the NHS.[17]

An appendix to this document explained to PCTs what the purpose of commissioning was and that PBC would be a key part of their future, along with joint commissioning with local authorities. In the summer of 2006 the new PCTs would be in place and they would be expected to run their affairs with a view to achieving a small surplus. To help the new bodies do this the NHS was provided in January 2006 with a set of operating rules on how commissioning, contracts, PBC, payment by result and performance management would work during the financial year 2006/7.

For the first time the NHS was issued before the start of a new financial year (2006/7) with an operational framework that showed it how reform would start to work and would influence their day to day activity. These documents were far from perfect but they were a genuine attempt to move NHS reform from Ministerial rhetoric and exhortation to some nitty-gritty operational reality. This flurry of operational activity was aimed at keeping the NHS show on the road during reorganisation whilst pointing firmly in the direction of reform. We received some credit for this operational work from within the NHS but it was clear that PCTs had, for the most part, a low knowledge-base on commissioning. Many were struggling to contain the expenditure of their major acute hospitals that were busy spending the higher NHS budgets pursuing government targets – in many cases almost irrespective of cost. Many PCTs claimed to be uncertain about what the Government expected them to do about budget overruns or how to manage demand when they were being bullied by powerful, overspending acute hospital trusts.

A review of PCT resource allocations in 2003/4 had revealed that quite a few PCTs were still some distance away from their target budget allocations based on assessments of health needs. For some PCTs this was a perfect excuse for not balancing their books. There was nothing for it but to settle down and produce comprehensive guidance on how commissioning would work in practice and to relate this to the annual operational framework for the NHS. Following the holding document in January 2006, Patricia Hewitt and I worked closely with the new Strategy Policy Directorate and the special advisers to construct what was to become the July 2006 commissioning framework document already mentioned - 80 pages in length. In the first half of 2006 I was meeting the new Directorate's head and his staff weekly on a range of NHS reform issues but particularly on commissioning and PBC. These meetings teased out the detailed operational consequences of the Government's reform intent alongside the financial issues emerging in the NHS. Using commissioning to manage demand was an integral part of this work but new for most managers and clinicians in the NHS. Much of the work was tested out informally with a raft of NHS contacts to assess understanding, acceptance and workability. I had access to a small cadre of reform-minded people who could help operationalise NHS reform, an essential component of any politically-led reform in the public services, as the Coalition Government will discover. Too often 'public service reform' remains a Ministerial mantra rather than a set of operational systems that show public bodies how to change.

This work in 2005 and 2006 brought home to me how little the NHS understood what commissioning was all about and how few powerful champions there really were for it. This remains the case I suspect. The collective memory at the top of DH seemed to have forgotten what had been done on purchaser/provider splits and GP fund-holding in the Conservative years – or else they weren't telling! Nevertheless we ended up in July 2006 with a workmanlike document that explained what commissioning was all about and how it would help PCTs to achieve the best value within the resources available if they chose to use it. It attempted to terminate the endless arguments about resource allocation with a firm statement; "Some PCTs continue to argue for a greater share of resources. We will keep the funding formula under review but allocations made for 2006/7 and 2007/8 would not be changed. It is the responsibility of PCT Boards to operate within the cash limit".[18]

This robust approach was essential because as I and other Ministers went round the NHS we continued to encounter people saying they couldn't use commissioning to change service delivery because they didn't have enough money. Some PCTs fed stories to the Conservative MPs in areas of lower health needs complaining about the lower budget increases they received compared with areas of much more serious health needs. When money is at stake local public services completely forget about political neutrality. I suspect much of this experience will be repeated with Coalition Government Ministers as they grapple with NHS spending and reform.

To link commissioning better with demand management in the minds of the NHS commissioners we devoted a part of the July 2006 commissioning document to resource utilisation techniques. These included ideas like prior approval (under which hospital doctors confirm the appropriateness of a proposed course of treatment with the referring GP); utilisation management (under which hospital admissions were tested for appropriateness – either in terms of illness severity or appropriateness of procedures); or referral management centres and clinical assessment centres – which were other ways of assessing and challenging hospital referrals and some of which were run by the independent sector. We all knew that hospital referral patterns among GPs were highly variable and some needed challenge: that remains the case and a problem for GP commissioning consortia.

We tried to get commissioners to be more assertive about challenging the status quo on referrals of patients to hospital specialist services. None of this was popular but it is what commissioners should be doing as part of moving the NHS away from its culture of shovelling money into acute hospitals. Some hospital specialists and managers did not like either their clinical judgements or income streams being challenged by the use of these commissioning techniques but they are essential to balancing budgets in a well-run healthcare system without unlimited resources.

I was well aware of the need to build commissioning capacity if we were to use it to drive NHS change. I asked the new NHS Institute for Innovation and Improvement (with which I had replaced the bloated Modernisation Agency) to develop a new Fitness for Purpose Improvement programme for PCT boards and senior managers. We used websites to provide a database of demand management and commissioning initiatives. Much to the annoyance of trade unions we also undertook a national procurement to enable PCTs to call off a range of commissioning skills and services from private sector companies. This produced a lurid Guardian front page story[19] about how we were just working to privatise the NHS. Patricia and I had angry meetings with the trades unions; and I was cross-examined on this by the Health Select Committee. We stuck to our guns and the DH website provided a menu of services and providers that PCTs could draw upon under this procurement, although many declined to use it. This flurry of activity was only a start on improving commissioning know-how. We needed the new SHAs to push their PCTs to improve much more than many of them have done.

One of the most important things for better commissioning was the new national contract for PCTs to use with acute hospital trusts, alongside a more effective disputes resolution system. Many of the acute trusts were adept at incorporating new costs into their contracts and stringing out disputes resolution. The acute hospital bias in DH management made for difficulty in resolving these issues. Some PCTs were foolish enough to enter into very long-term contracts – a 30 year contract came to my attention which had to be reviewed.

Patricia Hewitt and I wanted the default position on disputes to be resolution in favour of commissioners. I wanted firm deadlines so these could be resolved within a financial year for existing contracts or at the beginning of the new year where a new contract was involved. We managed to get to this position, after considerable persistence, in new guidance settling a new draft national contract as part of the operational framework for 2007/8. In practice however many acute trusts have continued to bully and threaten PCTs with loss of local services and too often SHAs have sided with acute trusts, sometimes under pressure from MPs or Ministers. In many parts of the country – especially London – the PCTs are too weak or poorly supported to call the shots with big acute hospital providers and to be effective demand managers or securers of alternative providers. The guidance on disputes resolution we produced in 2006 is too often honoured more in the breach.

Specialist and joint commissioning

Some services that require population sizes larger than that of most PCTs, need consortia of PCTs. These usually work on the basis of a 'lead' PCT so that providers know who to deal with. This is often a cumbersome system which frustrates many specialist providers but it is in part a result of having too many commissioning PCTs. Reducing them substantially would sort out many of the problems of consortia, but having failed in that endeavour I was reluctant to encourage central intervention in particular consortia. However there was growing concern that PCTs, individually and collectively, were paying insufficient attention to commissioning new highly specialised and expensive services and treatments, where relatively small numbers of patients were involved. So alongside the wider work on

NHS commissioning I established in 2005 a review of the arrangements for commissioning specialised services under the chairmanship of Sir David Carter – a former Chief Medical Officer in Scotland. Sir David did a good job in achieving consensus in a disputed area and worked with me to ensure continuing political support for the changes needed. I accepted the recommendations in his May 2006 report.[20]

In the December 2006 operating framework document[20] the 10 new SHAs were required to ensure effective implementation of Carter's new arrangements for specialised commissioning. These involved the establishment of a new National Commissioning Group based in the London SHA and 10 regional Specialised Commissioning Groups (SCGs) composed of PCT representatives that would collectively commission a minimum of 10 specialised services by 2008/9 and continue commissioning most specialised services for their new populations.

After I left DH progress on implementing the new specialised commissioning structure seemed to slow as people argued in classic NHS fashion about financial commitments. In the Operating Framework for 2008/9 the NHS was being told "we expect SCGs to create pooled budgets to commission the majority of specialised services on their patch this year, extending to all specialised services in 2009/10".[22] This is a good illustration of how reform in the NHS slows if the Ministerial foot is not kept on the accelerator. Nevertheless at least I left behind a more coherent NHS structure for commissioning that stretched from micro-level commissioning (PBC) through local commissioning by individual PCTs to 10 regional Specialised Commissioning Groups with PCTs in consortia and a National Specialised Commissioning Group for highly specialised and expensive treatments that could only be commissioned nationally.

The one area where I failed was that of joint commissioning between PCTs and local authorities. This area has long been one of difficulty and contention and continues to be so. This is in large part because of the means-tested nature of social care and the boundary this creates with the 'free at the point of use' NHS. There are powerful incentives on both sides of this boundary to protect budgets, shunt costs across it and leave luckless service users stuck in the middle of bureaucratic struggles over who pays. Dementia with its 750,000 sufferers, and growing, is a good example where the health and social care bureaucracies try to avoid financial responsibility.

In the White Paper published in January 2006, " Our Health, Our Care, Our Say", we had tried to give a push to joint commissioning (see Chapter 12); and in the December 2006 Operating Framework for 2007/8 we said: "a greater focus on joint commissioning between health care and social care and better integration between health care, social care and local government services will bring benefits to patients and service users".[23]

However we failed to find a mechanism that dealt with the cross-boundary problems or incentives that would make the boundary more porous. In most places what Frank Dobson called the Berlin Wall between health and social care remains firmly in place. It was little consolation that our Ministerial predecessors had also failed and our successors continue to do so, despite much rhetoric.

In my time as a Minister I never had any sense that the top brass in DH had their heart in joint commissioning. They preferred protecting NHS budgets even when giving a bit more to adult social care could have helped the NHS a great deal by avoiding unnecessary admission to hospitals and delayed discharges from them. It was striking throughout my time in DH that the top management had little interest in learning from local government or building a stronger relationship with it. Only when the social care capability in DH was strengthened did this improve. I return to the issue of social care funding and integration with health - where demography makes change inevitable - at the end of this book.

Commissioning: a job only part done

When I left the DH at the end of 2006 I had provided the foundations for a commissioning-led NHS but there was much unfinished business. There was a coherent commissioning framework stretching from the GP practice to the National Specialised Commissioning Group. The number of PCTs had been halved but there were still too many commissioners, who were also distracted by being the managers of often indifferent community services. A PCT "Fitness for Purpose Review" was to be completed by March 2007 to develop PCT commissioning capability. And the NHS Operating Framework for 2007/8 that I agreed before I left enshrined commissioning and PBC as part of the operational fabric of the NHS as well as incorporating the reformed arrangements for commissioning specialised services.

I thought things had changed at the top of DH when two months after his arrival the new NHS Chief Executive, David Nicholson, was advising Patricia Hewitt in December 2006 that "a truly patient-centred NHS has to be driven through commissioning and we need to see a qualitative shift in the quality and nature of commissioning in this country". The arrival of Mark Britnell in 2007 as a new and energetic Director of Commissioning enabled PCT commissioning to be driven harder through the "World Class Commissioning" initiative launched in December 2007. This initiative provided a stronger emphasis on commissioning for health outcomes and reducing health inequalities. There was a published set of competencies that a "World Class" commissioner would need; an assurance system for assessing commissioners covering health outcomes, competencies in governance; and more emphasis on building capability, including using expertise from the private sector.

For the first time DH top management was showing the NHS some leadership on the importance of commissioning and a determination to improve PCT competency. PCTs were expected to demonstrate excellence in leadership, knowledge management and strategy development, as well as having outstanding negotiating, contracting, financial and performance management skills. They were required to form closer links with patients, the public, local authorities, clinicians and providers by working on a partnership basis. Looking outwards, strategically developing services and demonstrating competence was what I had been striving for and these messages were now being taken forward in an operational form by the top DH management.

The 2008/9 Operating Framework issued in December 2007 consolidated the work in progress on commissioning that Patricia Hewitt and I had left behind. There was a final version of the national contract for PCTs to use with all acute trusts; PBC was integrated fully into PCT governance frameworks as the best way of generating services for local communities; and the new system of specialised commissioning was embedded. "World Class Commissioning" was to be pushed by SHAs as an important part of NHS development. Britnell did not mince his words, describing PCT commissioning and purchasing skills as "featherweight" compared to the strength of the acute hospital sector. This had been demonstrated in the financial crisis in 2005/6 when 175 PCTs – well over half the PCTs in England – had to be visited by turnaround teams because their finances were in such a mess. In one PCT, two thirds of the ineffective management was made redundant according to the Humana CEO speaking at a conference in October 2007.

PCTs needed to be transformed under the "World Class Commissioning" initiative from bodies that simply handed out cheques to providers of services into bodies that implemented 5-year health and wellbeing targets to improve the health of their local populations. This would enable them, as Britnell said, to "put their money where their ambitions are".[24] However what was revealed was a growing gap between the most and the least competent PCT commissioners and a political reluctance to tackle this by merging PCTs and bringing in more external expertise. Mark Britnell left the DH in 2009 and the drive faltered for transforming commissioning and separating provision from it. Autonomous Provider Organisations have been created by SHAs within PCTs but there has been little political appetite for separating them after a robust process of market-testing.

The case for more radical action on PCTs is clear from the Care Quality Commission's NHS performance ratings for 2008/9. After all the effort to improve PCTs and the huge sums of extra money made available to them, this independent assessment shows an extremely disappointing picture. Although there was some improvement over 2007/8 only 3 out of 152 PCTs were rated "excellent" for service quality, with 71 rated "fair" or "weak" – with all 4 "weak" PCTs in NE London. On financial management no PCT was rated "excellent" and 71 were shown as "fair" or "weak".[25] After 7 years of plenty in which to establish themselves and with the NHS approaching a tougher financial climate, PCT commissioning has not delivered and a more radical reform of commissioning than I was contemplating in 2005/6, now seems inevitable.

This seems to be the view also of the Health Select Committee who looked at the performance of PCTs on several occasions. In a March 2009 report they summed up their frustration. "The Department argued that its World Class Commissioning programme will transform PCTs. While the programme has only been in place since July 2007, there are few signs yet that variations between PCTs in their commissioning capability have been addressed. The NHS purchasing/commissioning function was introduced nearly 20 years ago and its management continues to be largely passive when active evidence-based contracting is required to improve the quality of patient care."[26]

PCTs have had their chance to show their worth and the great majority have not done so. Overall SHAs have been unable to performance manage a sufficient number of them into an adequate piece of NHS machinery or to separate provision from commissioning. Too often PCTs have frustrated the commissioning capability of those GPs who are capable commissioners. The Coalition Government has understandably lost patience as well and is now looking for more radical solutions, with GPs more centre stage. I offer some thoughts on a way forward in Chapter 16. What is now in prospect is a further streamlining of NHS organisations, following my own efforts in 2005/6 described in the next chapter.

5

Cutting bureaucracy
and streamlining the NHS

Reducing bureaucracy

As early as 2003 questions were being asked about whether too much of the extra NHS money was being wasted on 'bureaucracy'. A number of factors contributed to this. The ill-conceived 2002 NHS reorganisation had been dislocating and expensive and had added more managers to the NHS payroll. Targets and stronger performance management increased the demand for data by DH and caused resentment and complaints from the local level. The Conservative Opposition had struggled to find an NHS issue on which to criticise the government but began to land more telling blows on taxpayers' money being wasted on bureaucrats rather than being spent on patients. Labour was the party that had promised to save money on bureaucracy and "men in grey suits" so more attention had to be paid to management costs and overheads. The Government needed to show that it was tackling bureaucracy as part of public service reform; and in the Department of Health John Reid decided to make me the "bureaucracy buster".

There had been no queue of applicants for this job from my elected Ministerial colleagues; and matters were settled quickly when John discovered that I had been a civil service efficiency scrutineer during the Thatcher years. In my new role I took on two tasks that most politicians hate because they require penetrating the opaque world of public sector organisations. The first task was the thankless one of trying to curb the insatiable demands made on the local NHS for information. The second was an NHS version of Thatcher's quango-culling, the Arm's Length Body review. A bonfire of the quangos has now become popular with the arrival of the new Coalition Government but back in 2003 it was a new experience for the NHS and strongly resisted by most of the bodies involved.

As I strapped on my 'bureaucracy-buster's' outfit I realised that DH officials thought that it was pretty quirky for a Minister to involve himself in the number and detail of statistical returns. Yet it was clear from discussions with NHS staff on local visits that two things were a longstanding source of grievance: the rising number of statistical returns and the increasing visits and demands by a growing number of inspectors and regulators. Some earlier attempts to restrain the demands on the local NHS had achieved little but I pressed on with a new programme that I called "Reducing the burdens on the NHS".

With a few civil servants to help me I opened up discussions with the Departmental statisticians tucked away in Leeds. They were devoted to their individual statistical returns and regarded with deep suspicion any politician who wanted to reduce or change them. After a lot of tedious discussions I set in place a system of Ministerial approvals (by me and the responsible Minister) for all new information requests imposed on the NHS. I also had a comprehensive review made of all existing returns with a view to reducing their frequency and scale. I found that the periods for which returns were made often lacked common definitions: for example there were several ways of defining a month! This drove the NHS mad so I started a process of standardising definitions.

Much to the irritation of the civil service I set up a system of 'man years' budgets. Officials had to show how many 'man years' it would cost the NHS to produce a particular return. The Department had to keep within a budget of 'man years' that I established; and this would be reduced over time. Statisticians tend to have somewhat obsessive qualities so I decided to put a statistician in charge of this budget. Gradually the rising volume of returns was curbed and started to decline in 'man year' terms. Most of my Ministerial colleagues entered into the spirit of the exercise. The change was noted in some parts of the NHS although I didn't spot any welcoming banners on the subject on my Ministerial visits. However I subsequently discovered that although a review of NHS data collections in 2005 did indeed show that DH had reduced the number of data requests, there was still on average 600 collections a year.[1] Most of these were at the behest of SHAs who had stepped in to fill the space left by DH statisticians!

Flushed with success I herded DH statisticians into a new Information Centre which had a new governing Board and a brief to make the statistical material more relevant and useful to NHS users. My view was that this expensive statistical resource would benefit from a hefty dose of management and greater focus. The DH and NHS collect a huge volume of data but much of it has simply been used as a data bank for answering questions in Parliament and serving as material for Ministerial briefings, speeches and press notices. Too little was presented in a format that the NHS could use to better manage its affairs. The NHS had been programmed to 'feed the beast' at the centre – which they often did resentfully – rather than using their own material to improve their performance. The NHS could collect data but seemed unable to distil it into usable management information.

A savvy ex-Sunday Times journalist, Tim Kelsey, had spotted a commercial opportunity with all this NHS information lying fallow.

He had set up a company called Dr. Foster that converted NHS data into useful information and sold it back to the NHS. I thought the Information Centre could provide a better service to the NHS and to patients as the reform agenda progressed, if it was in partnership with Dr. Foster. Tim Kelsey saw the advantages in this which naturally made the civil service nervous. I agreed that DH should construct a joint venture company between Dr. Foster and the Information Centre. After a degree of resistance within the bureaucracy Hugh Taylor – later to become the Permanent Secretary – skilfully brought this to fruition; and I launched the new joint venture in 2005. It has had its ups and downs, including appointing the wrong person as its first Chief Executive and some unfair criticism by the Public Accounts Committee. However this change improved the dissemination of information to a wider public and to NHS management. The first 'NHS Choices' website in 2006 - that did so much to help provide the public with useable information about exercising choice - came out of this initiative and was provided by Dr. Foster. Sadly I underestimated the public sector's ability to foul up any enterprising public/private partnership venture once a guardian angel moves on. However the Information Centre has survived as a vehicle for the improving health information for the NHS and the public. The joint venture is coming to an end but there is now a market in health informatics which the joint venture helped to stimulate.

Alongside the statisticians I had the inspectors/regulators in my sights. The Government had set up a Better Regulation Task Force because of the growing demands (and associated costs) of regulators/inspectors on both public and private organisations. The Taskforce's role was to reduce the burden of regulation and was backed by a Cabinet Committee on Regulation of which I was a member. As a result some mergers of DH regulators were inevitable but before this was attempted I decided to bring inspectors/regulators together to discuss how they could coordinate their information demands and visits more effectively. Often almost identical information demands were made by different inspectorates, with little regard for the costs of the demands. Inspectors and regulators organised their visits to hospitals with a total disregard for the cumulative effect of all their visits on the luckless hospital and its staff. This tied up a large amount of senior management and other staff time in dealing with these various demands.

When the inspectors and regulators discussed these issues under my chairmanship there was a predictable prickliness from many of them about their independence; and a deep suspicion of this interfering Minister who was already suggesting fewer organisations and smaller budgets. Was he now going to tell them how to run their affairs? (I must confess that with some of them the temptation was enormous.) It was apparent from these discussions that the prevailing culture was to pay little regard to the cost and burden of demands and visits on those being inspected. 'Independence of judgement' was regarded as justifying almost anything inspectorates/regulators chose to do.

After several meetings, some hard work by officials and leadership from the then Chairman of the Healthcare Commission, Sir Ian Kennedy, we managed to get a 'Concordat' agreed by the inspectorates. This would ensure that they worked more closely together in coordinating their demands on and visits to organisations being inspected. This was a small step on a long march back from a public sector regulatory system that had expanded considerably with little regard to efficiency. The battle to keep public sector regulation cost-effective will be a continuing one but will be assisted by the current dire state of the public finances. Back in the time of financial plenty securing cost-effectiveness was harder work as the review of DH arm's length bodies was to show.

The Arm's Length Bodies (ALB) review

The origins of the ALB Review had an amusing side. As part of its Gershon Efficiency Review, the Government had been pressing on with cutting Departmental overheads and running costs across Whitehall. The DH top management was rather proud of their efforts on this front and had promised to cut the number of Departmental staff by some 38% through organisational change and new ways of working. The Permanent Secretary had sought to impress his new Secretary of State with this high percentage figure when John Reid arrived in the Department in June 2003. I had been made the Minister for DH management issues and I pointed out to John that this was something of a Sir Humphrey manoeuvre. The impressive DH staff reductions looked a little less impressive when one realised that about a half of it was achieved by simply transferring people to Arm's Length Bodies. This produced a predictable Glaswegian response from John, especially when he realised how much these bodies cost and were spending. On 30 October 2003 John Reid announced the ALB Review as a centrepiece of an anti-bureaucracy strategy when he gave evidence to the House of Commons Health Select Committee.

The ALB Review was to take me much longer than I had expected. Over the next year a good number of the bodies affected, their own staff and some DH staff fought a staunch rearguard action to minimise the impact. They were aided in their cause by being able to endlessly recite the fact that Labour had set up many of these bodies since 1997. This tune was sung joyfully by the Tories who in the House of Lords delighted in reminding me that I was smothering Labour's own creations soon after their birth. Fortunately I was not very bothered about being likened to Herod; and being in the Lords I could more easily avoid those Commons Labour colleagues who liked all these public bodies and the employment opportunities they provided. John Reid was immensely supportive of what I was doing, if anything wanting to go further and faster.

The first thing to decide was who to include in the review. We produced a definition that focussed on stand-alone national organisations sponsored by the DH that undertook executive functions. This ruled out a large number of advisory bodies and tribunals with small budgets and few staff. This definition covered 38 bodies, although it included seven who were in various stages of planning for abolition. Some of this seven were to be replaced by four new bodies, two of which were already operational (the Healthcare Commission and the Commission for Social Care Inspection) or about to become so (Dental Special Health Authority and the Human Tissue Authority). This stage of the exercise of deciding the organisations to be reviewed took a little time because there was much ingenuity at looking for definitional escape routes.

Early on it was apparent that there were overlapping and duplicated functions and that some of these functions were questionable in regulatory and policy terms. The ALBs had all decided to set up their own human resources, finance, IT and facilities management departments at considerable cost, so consolidating these back office functions offered the prospect of worthwhile savings. The scope for merging bodies to integrate functions and cut overheads became increasingly apparent. A few could be floated off with interested parties funding them rather than DH.

Volunteers for change and savings were in short supply. I decided we had to bring this first stage of the review to some conclusion by around Easter 2004. At this point we had a review involving about 40 existing or new bodies spending nearly £5billion a year with operating costs approaching £2billion and employing about 22,000 people. There was little doubt that this sector in its then form did not meet current or future health and social care needs relative to the expenditure involved. Left to their own devices ALBs would be employing approaching ten times the number of people in DH if we did not cut back. This seemed to me an untenable position, particularly as their accountability was often obscure or virtually non-existent.

After the 2004 Easter Parliamentary recess I decided to set some tougher parameters around the ALB review in order to make progress. I went to see John Reid with a private secretary and a power point presentation and no officials. I suggested that we conclude the first stage of the review by announcing a 50% reduction in the number of ALBs; an administrative savings target of £0.5billion; and a reduction of 25% in the number of people employed by ALBs. John readily agreed these targets, which were to be achieved by the beginning of 2007/8 financial year. I returned to my room to inform the civil servants of the outcome. They were pleased that we had some levers to pull with the ALBs but rather apprehensive about what John and I had committed us to. There was no point in hanging about with an announcement otherwise it would have leaked, so John Reid made his announcement on the 20 May.[2]

This announcement committed us to consulting individual bodies on a set of proposals for merger, rationalisation or abolition that would be concluded by the end of June 2004. I had agreed with John Reid that the review would unravel if we did not conclude it quickly. In the coming weeks there was intense activity as we completed a narrative for the review. We wanted less bureaucracy and burden on frontline staff, with these bodies intervening less. We defined four functional categories into which all bodies would fit: regulation; standard setting; safety and protection of the public; and central services for the NHS. If new needs arose the aim would be to allocate them to one of the existing bodies in these categories rather than set up a new organisation.

On the 22 July I published the results of our handiwork showing how the 42 bodies involved would be slimmed down to 20 between 2005 and 2008. This would produce savings of at least £0.5billion from a base line of the £1.8billion spent in 2003/4 on operating costs (within a total expenditure of £4.8billion); and reduce by about 25% the number of people working in ALBs.[3] We now faced the challenge of delivering these savings in the following 3 financial years. Bureaucratic infighting resumed with even greater intensity with the ALBs. This focussed on what would be in their 2005/6 budget, together with the detailed timetable for establishing the 20 new bodies - some of which required primary legislation. To help concentrate some minds I offered meetings with John Reid if people preferred dealing with John rather than me: this usually secured reluctant acquiescence.

On 30 November 2004 John Reid published an implementation plan for the review with the supporting political strapline of "redistributing resources to the NHS frontline".[4] This document set the parameters for 20 ALB change projects, saying what would happen to each body and when, with everything to be completed by April 2008. We committed ourselves to setting the 2005/6 budgets for the ALB sector so that they were a £100million less than the baseline year of 2003/4, with a further £200million reduction in each of the following two financial years. Predictably people continued to argue about producing their savings. After the Christmas recess I sat down and simply cut the figures served up by officials so that the 2005/6 budget saved the £100million promised. I also indicated what was expected for the subsequent two years. Without clear Ministerial decisions on budget cuts the review's civil servants could not make the savings targets stick because individual bodies appealed to powerful sponsors inside and outside DH. Arguments continued over the timetables for change and budgets long after I handed over responsibility for this area after the May 2005 election. There was some watering down but most of what I decided stuck.

I checked up on progress with this review with a Parliamentary Question answered on 15 June 2009.[5] Although there had been some delays the number of DH ALBs had been reduced to 20 on 1 April 2009 with the transfer of 3 into the new Care Quality Commission and the merger of the Health Protection Agency and the National Institute of Biological Standards and Control. One new ALB had been transferred from the Home Office to DH – the Alcohol Education and Research Council, so there were now 21. The expenditure of these ALBs in 2008/9 was nearly £900 million (or nearly £800 million at 2003/4 prices) so the cost of running DH ALBs had more than halved since I started the exercise in 2004. With Ministerial resolution quango-culling can be achieved. Civilisation has not ended with the demise of some bodies and running the remainder more cheaply and efficiently.

This exercise was a classic example of how public sector bureaucracies are very effective at resisting change. Once set up in a fit of political enthusiasm a quango is difficult to change significantly, let alone abolish. They develop powerful supporters and sponsors within departments who often lack the appetite for conflict with these bodies by seeking change. Without Ministerial determination, persistence and periodical threats, it would not have been possible to deliver the changes to the DH ALBs within any reasonable timetable and this experience would be repeated across Whitehall. Ministers should think more carefully before setting up these bodies because they develop a life of their own and an appetite for resources that most governments would prefer spending on other priorities. I am less sanguine that this advice will be followed, when public finances improve.

The 2005 Election and reducing bureaucracy

"Bureaucracy-busting" was not simply the work of a DH Lone Ranger. The prospect of a 2005 election was concentrating Ministerial minds on waste and bureaucracy, as Conservatives chose these as political sticks with which to beat the government.ealthHealthHealthHealth Helath The Conservatives had set up a review of their own chaired by the now Lord James of Blackheath as an alternative to the Government's Gershon Review. This had proposed considerable savings from cutting PCTs, DH and ALBs and abolishing SHAs.[6] Tony Blair increasingly wanted to demonstrate that the government was tackling red tape and bureaucracy and spending the extra money on improving public services. To counter the Conservative criticisms the 2005 election manifesto contained a passage reassuring voters that the new investment in the NHS was not being squandered. It reported that the staff in DH were being reduced by a third and that the number of health quangos would be halved, "freeing up £500million for frontline staff". The electorate were promised that "further streamlining measures will allow us to release an additional £250million a year for frontline services by 2007".[7] This new savings target was to preoccupy DH senior management when during the 2005 Election campaign I was left to mind the DH shop.

As soon as Prime Ministers fire the election starting gun most Ministers ditch their red boxes and flee to their constituencies or to whichever marginal seat Party HQ dispatches them. Government still has to govern so unelected Ministers are quite useful in an election campaign because they can deal with unanswered Parliamentary questions and correspondence and urgent operational matters. They can trot off to broadcasting studios to convey some sense that the government is still around and taking decisions. There were the usual electoral spats to deal with, as I had with a Michael Howard round-robin letter to hospital trust chairs telling them effectively how many people their hospital had killed with MRSA. I was able to get out a response showing the evidence that a good proportion of MRSA was brought in from the community and nursing homes and to orchestrate some responses from trust chairs that encouraged the then Conservative leader to move on to other topics.

The civil service are there during elections not just to keep you company but to ensure that you don't overstep the mark by using the Department's press office to secure political advantage. You forebear telling them you are there to stop some dozy official publishing something that has been lurking in the bureaucratic undergrowth for months and could cause an electoral ruckus. Sitting in Richmond House it felt as though Labour would win – more because of the inadequacies of the other two parties than because the electorate were that enthusiastic about giving us another go. The Conservatives were on their third leader since the previous election and were still trying to convince the electorate that they were likeable. Tony Blair and Gordon Brown had patched up their differences and were seen eating ice-creams in a comradely manner. Before the election I had told No. 10, when asked, that I would be willing to take on NHS reform as a Minister of State. This may have percolated through to the mandarins because they gave off vibes that they expected me still to be around. The DH top brass began to talk to me about their area of the greatest concern, Labour's commitment to streamline the NHS and save £250million by 2007. They were unaware that I was no fan of the 2002 NHS reorganisation but they did know what I had done to ALBs.

My steer to Nigel Crisp and his deputy John Bacon was that they should reduce the number of SHAs significantly and align their areas with the 9 Government regions. I told them I considered there were far too many PCTs for a world in which we would see more FTs and the development of GP commissioning. I wanted to see fewer PCTs who were capable of commissioning more effectively from the powerful acute sector, protecting community services and public health budgets and no longer running community health services. I doubted whether this advice went down well with these two veterans of the acute hospital sector, with many colleagues in the soon to be reduced SHAs.

After a low turn out and some casualties Labour claimed its historic third election victory on 12 May 2005. John Reid had secured his release from DH and was piped aboard as Defence Secretary in the building next door; and Patricia Hewitt became Health Secretary with three new Ministers. The gender balance of the Health Ministerial team switched from 4:2 in favour of men to 4:2 in favour of women. (At the Labour Party Conference in September the women were all on stage like Girls Aloud receiving the Party's acclaim, while Liam Byrne and I kept below the platform like a Boy Band warm-up!). I was promoted to Minister of State and inherited a mixture of NHS delivery and reform issues from John Hutton.

My portfolio required me to increase patient choice, implement a new tariff system for paying hospitals; ensure existing targets were met and implement the new commitment of no-one waiting more than 18 weeks from GP referral to hospital treatment by 2008; establish a better system for commissioning NHS services; implement the National Programme for IT; improve access to primary care and produce a new White Paper for services outside hospitals; deal with all workforce issues (including pay and pensions); monitor NHS and DH financial performance, including PFI schemes and the capital programmes; and expand the role of the private sector in diagnostics and elective surgery to increase NHS capacity and competition with NHS providers. Appropriately enough I took my wife to see "The Cosmonaut's Last Message" at the Donmar Theatre on the night of my appointment.

No-one reading the upbeat civil service briefings for in-coming Ministers would have thought there were any serious clouds in the sky. The Annual Report by the NHS Chief Executive at the end of May 2005 was totally reassuring. The NHS was improving its performance steadily with the prospect of more to come from five years of 7% real terms annual growth. The NHS workforce was continuing to grow and there were 300,000 more NHS staff than in 1997 who were better paid, with good recruitment and retention figures. There seemed few problems with the National Programme for IT. I was aware that the 18 weeks' target was challenging; that expansion of the private sector would be controversial; and that delivering a quality White Paper on services outside hospitals as quickly as the Prime Minister wanted would be difficult. What I didn't realise was how weak the DH policy capability was on NHS reform and how Panglossian was the briefing on money, workforce issues and IT. Only as Ministers went round the NHS and better understood the frailty of the DH management structure did we realise that there was a Darth Vader darker side.

In 2005 the expectation was that the new Ministerial team would pick up the threads quickly and start delivering the Manifesto. That was certainly the view of an impatient Prime Minister, now rashly committed to leaving before the next Election. What most of the new Health team had uppermost in their minds was getting through unscathed to the summer recess with a Tory opposition in disarray as they prepared to select yet another new leader. It looked as though we would make it as I chose to start work on the new White Paper, the 18 weeks target and the Manifesto commitment to streamline the NHS.

Streamlining the NHS

'Streamlining' was the softer term chosen to avoid saying we were going to reorganise the NHS again only three years after the last reorganisation. I am not sure that we fooled anybody. The NHS knew it meant reducing the number of SHAs and PCTs and I saw little point in pretending otherwise. The DH senior management had taken some notice of my pre-election steer on streamlining but were still in a very different place to me in the briefing they provided for incoming ministers. They seemed ever hopeful of saving some of their chums from the Ministerial axe. This briefing said there were 304 PCTs in England but they were looking to reduce this number to around 200 by April 2006; and that there were 28 SHAs with "plans to significantly reduce this number by April 2007."

The first 'streamlining' paper in May was proposing "an orderly 'fit for purpose' process which identifies weakness in organisation and puts in place changes – some of which could be mergers – and development". I was being handled by a bureaucracy that wanted to suck Ministers into a process of slow evolutionary change with little connection to what was required for commissioning and PBC. In part this was because there was little Departmental understanding that if PBC increased you needed fewer PCTs. There was little evidence that DH top management understood what a commissioning-led NHS involved. The appetite for a purchaser/provider split in PCTs seemed non-existent. I was supposed to be reassured that everything would be all right because there was a draft 'Strategy Risk Review Plan' – written in a unique form of English known only in DH/NHS management circles. Translated this said over the next three years the 28 SHAs (who were going in any case to be reduced significantly) would project manage everything and would be held to account. The time had come to turn the Ministerial screw on the bureaucracy – a necessity for all governments periodically.

In a series of meetings over the next few weeks involving Ministers, special advisers, No. 10 and civil servants we moved by early July to a completely new position. During June officials moved to halving the number of SHAs and saving £70million instead of the original £40million and completing the changes by 2007. A reduction to150 PCTs was beginning to be contemplated but 200 was still the front runner. The rest of the savings were coming from the PCTs' commissioning functions, despite the fact that we wanted the PCTs to strengthen commissioning! Under continuing Ministerial pressure there was some policy analysis on the role of PCTs with them concentrating on commissioning and hiving off their provider functions being contemplated. Early in July I was continuing to push officials towards larger PCTs of at least half a million population so that PBC could flourish and be implemented everywhere by the end of 2006. I was urging the separation of provider services with PCTs commissioning community services and primary care and only having a default responsibility to provide satisfactory community services where they could not be commissioned from elsewhere.

A clearer set of functions for SHAs was emerging. I was making progress on acceptance of SHA boundaries being based on Government Office regions. By the time of the NHS birthday (5 July) the issues of commissioning, PBC, streamlining PCTs and SHAs and the impact of more FTs, were now being linked together in the thinking and drafting by officials. To encourage momentum I decided to publish on 30 June the National Ambulance Adviser's review of ambulance services which brought ambulance trusts into the streamlining exercise with its proposal to halve their number.[8]

To close the debate I told Nigel Crisp in early July that we needed an agreed set of "givens" to communicate to the NHS by the summer recess (then set for 21 July); and that we should complete all the organisational changes – PCTs, SHAs and ambulance trusts by April 2007. Patricia Hewitt supported the idea of bringing closure on the streamlining topic but we both realised that presentation would be important. What neither of us could have foreseen was that getting the presentation right would not be helped by the decision of some British Islamic terrorists to blow up parts of the London transport system and kill 50 people on 7 and 21 July 2005. This was hardly the best time to be finalising our streamlining document as Ministers turned their attention to this and the work of the emergency services. We had to support and thank NHS staff for what they did, especially the London ambulance service who were first on the scene deep in the underground stations.

The letter of 28 July 2005

There was a frenetic burst of activity to produce a document to go out to the NHS before the end of July explaining what was to happen on streamlining and within what timetable. The result was an unassuming-looking but radical document entitled "Commissioning a Patient-led NHS" with seven pages, thirty eight paragraphs and a one-page timetable.[9] This was sent out on 28 July 2005 by Sir Nigel Crisp with a covering letter and what turned out to be an explosive charge. The document made it clear that practice-based commissioning was to be rolled out everywhere by the end of 2006; asked SHAs to conduct an exercise locally by mid-October on the right number of PCTs in their area against certain criteria; explained that there would be a later White Paper on services outside hospitals that was likely to produce new models of care; and indicated that PCTs would become commissioning-led organisations with their role in provision reduced to a minimum by the end of 2008. It announced a rigorous development programme for hospital trusts with the aim of getting them to FT status by April 2008. SHAs were told that they would have to make the case for not being aligned with Government Office regions. The letter also said that ambulance trusts would be reduced substantially in number following Peter Bradley's Review.

There was to be public consultation later in the year on proposals for PCT changes; but the timetable for reorganisation was brisk. Organisational changes were to be completed by April 2007; and changes to PCT service provision by the end of 2008. The document also said "there will be a progressive move towards greater use of other providers, including those from the independent sector."[10] I had achieved most of what I wanted except a much greater reduction in PCTs. Jane Kennedy, who was the Minister for London, declined to reduce the number of PCTs in London at all; and I had no political support for imposing a ceiling on the number of PCTs. This London decision turned out to be a particular mistake from which London still suffers.

Virtually all of the 28 July document was consistent with the 2005 Election Manifesto. It was the correct strategy but three things went wrong. It took too long to settle the policy so drafting was rushed, much of this delay arising from the lack of DH analytical capacity. The second mistake was down to political error and oversight. Somewhere very near the end the wording on PCTs divesting themselves of their provider services became more dirigiste than certainly I intended. Between the last draft I agreed and the letter's published version the wording moved from wanting PCTs to concentrate on commissioning and moving to separate out their provider services to compelling them to do so by the end of 2008. The result was we de-stabilised 250,000 community staff who thought their jobs would be at risk in the period up to the end of 2008. Mentioning greater use of the independent sector only inflamed matters and convinced the trades unions that they had a privatisation stick with which to beat us. The third error was DH management ignoring Ministerial requests for a proper communications plan before the letter was issued to the NHS. Nigel Crisp decided to brief the 75-strong NHS Leadership Forum in confidence which inevitably led to the story being leaked to the media who were happy to write about Labour splits over privatisation.

The result was that a sound policy implementing a recent election manifesto became a political and public relations disaster. Our policy for separating commissioning from service provision was absolutely right and will have to happen at some stage. As Niall Dixon, then Chief Executive of the King's Fund, said in the Health Services Journal on 12 July 2007:

> "The strategy itself ...had much to commend it. The PCTs and strategic health authorities created by Alan Milburn were too small and numerous to be effective or to attract the quality of senior management required.
>
> Commissioning was clearly not working as it should, or as it would need to do in a reformed system, and it made sense for PCTs to concentrate on that rather than be distracted by the conflicting demands of being a significant provider of community services.
>
> It was the timing and manner of implementation that were all wrong."[11]

Niall was absolutely spot on.

Patricia Hewitt recanted on the compulsory divesting by PCTs of their provider services and reassured the NHS that it was for PCTs locally to decide whether they wanted to do this. Not surprisingly few did. Patricia tried to reclaim ground when she spoke to NHS Chairs on 20 September by making it clear that PCT provider functions were unlikely to stay unchanged:

> "The enhanced focus we are placing on getting commissioning right and our desire to provide patients with choice in primary and community services naturally gives rise to changes in the PCT's role in providing services... It is difficult for PCTs to facilitate innovation and choice in community services if they continue to be the monopoly suppliers of those services. It is also difficult for a PCT Board with a large provider function to worry about giving the necessary focus to its commissioning responsibilities."[12]

A Labour Government had moved on from its 1997 opposition to an internal market for health care. We might be retreating from the compulsory divesting of PCT provider functions within a given timetable but the greater focus on commissioning and choice would require PCT's to change eventually. However not sticking to our guns and pushing PCTs to divest themselves of their community provider services was a major mistake, along with retraining so many PCTs.

Reducing the number of NHS organisations

During the summer, led by Unison and the Royal College of Nursing, opposition to compulsory PCT provider change grew. MPs were brought into the squabble as they returned from holidays to prepare for the Party Conference season and the return of Parliament in October. The campaign was broadened to opposition to any further NHS organisational change. As Ministers we did not retreat further and insisted on completing the SHA-led provision of local plans for PCT changes by mid October based on the criteria in the 28 July document. At the end of September I established an Expert Panel to look at SHA plans and help produce a set of options for PCT change in each SHA area as a basis for statutory consultation. This independent element in the process helped reduce the temperature a bit. SHAs were encouraged to involve MPs in devising their local plans and MPs calmed down. Most of the Parliamentary noise was in Labour constituencies where much of the dispute was really about cutting jobs. The Conservatives seemed rather uninterested in the whole issue.

On 14 December a set of proposals for the re-configuration (and reduction) of SHAs and PCTs was published for a 14 week statutory local consultation. The commitment was given that no decisions would be taken by Ministers on re-configurations until the local consultations had been completed; and the SHA recommendations had been considered by the Expert Panel. Strong guidance was given to SHAs about holding public meetings and continuing to involve local MPs. On the same day I launched a consultation document[13] setting out proposals for reducing the number of ambulance trusts from 31 to 11 (including London which remained unchanged). This followed the review of ambulance services published in June but I went much further with trust reductions than the review proposed. Most ambulance areas would be the same as those for SHAs and much larger than the existing ambulance areas. The consultation period would be 14 weeks to coincide with that for SHAs and PCTs.

Throughout the consultation period I met frequently with officials to monitor progress and to ensure assistance was given in any hotspots of unrest. For the most part – whether from the reassurance of a double consultation or sheer exhaustion – the consultation on SHAs and PCTs went smoothly with a modest amount of Ministerial involvement with MPs. With one exception the consultation on ambulance trust mergers was reasonably peaceful, in contrast with the Home Office attempt to merge small police forces for similar efficiency/value for money reasons. The exception was the West Midlands where a large ambulance service based on Birmingham was to merge with three smaller services. The resistance was led by Staffordshire and its Chief Ambulance Officer, Roger Thayne. The massive opposition campaign mounted by Staffordshire and the less than distinguished performance of the then West Midlands ambulance service caused the other two small services to stiffen their resistance. Threats were made to stand against MPs (nearly all Labour) who supported merger at the next Election and write-in campaigns by constituents made some of these MPs nervous.

The colourful Roger Thayne campaigned openly in opposition to the merger in the media including going head to head with me on the Today programme. Unfortunately for him he got involved in an accident when personally driving an ambulance that he was not authorised to do and collided with a car driven by the wife of a police officer. He resigned to go and advise the Welsh Assembly on their ambulance services but left that position early. The Staffordshire saga was time-consuming but not without its entertaining dimensions. I negotiated a settlement that satisfied the local Labour MPs, with Staffordshire remaining as a separate trust for a while but working in partnership with the new enlarged West Midlands Ambulance Service and with a commitment to merge later.

The tortuous process of 'streamlining' was brought to a conclusion in April 2006 when Patricia Hewitt announced that the number of SHAs would be reduced to 10 on the 1 July; 302 PCTs would be reduced to 152 on the 1 October and the 31 ambulance trusts would be reduced to 12 on the 1 July with a later reduction to 11 when Staffordshire merged with West Midlands.[14] We had eliminated 190 unnecessary NHS bodies and with a bit more political steel could have abolished another 80 or more.

This exercise was never going to be popular but the mistakes of the 2002 reorganisation had to be rectified and there was an Election promise to streamline the NHS. The Audit Commission later found that £90million was saved in 2006/7 with a one-off cost of a £192million in redundancy and severance payments but with increased savings to follow in 2007/8 and subsequent years.[15] New boards and management teams were for the most part recruited and in post in 2006. The new SHAs were a considerable improvement on their predecessors; and the larger ambulance services meant they were better able to plan and to cope with serious emergencies, a change long overdue. I succeeded with ambulance trust mergers while the Home Office abandoned their plans for reducing the number of police forces because of opposition by Chief Constables and their police authorities.

The 'streamlining' exercise was messy and brutal. It used up a lot of political credit with MPs, the unions and the NHS; but it rectified most of the botched 2002 reorganisation and placed the NHS in a better position to deliver reform. I regret that I did not argue more vociferously with my political colleagues about reducing the number of PCTs to around 50-60: I now believe 40-50 commissioners was the number we needed and were capable of staffing with competent commissioning skills. We were wrong to beat a retreat so hastily on separating commissioning from provision in PCTs. Our policy was right and the Labour Government has wasted 5 years not bringing about this change. The underperformance of PCTs as commissioners was described in the previous chapter but as community service providers they were little better, as I discuss in Chapter 12. Unfortunately Hewitt and Warner's Ministerial successors have been unwilling to tackle the problems now inherent in PCTs, seemingly keener on appeasing public sector unions over jobs.

In mid-2005 the Department of Health seemed capable of playing only two tunes – targets and reorganisation. The rest of 2005 and 2006 were spent getting senior personnel in the Department to learn some new music involving commissioning, PBC, a 'payments by results' tariff, choice, competition and regulation. This required creating an operational framework so that we could operationalise reform rather than simply talking about it. To do this in 2005 we had to establish a new Strategy and Policy Directorate to provide the capacity to deliver change. Delivering change in an operational form is the biggest challenge that all reforming Ministers face, as the Coalition Government will discover. In the NHS this is even more difficult because of the large number of people involved, a number that had been greatly increased by Labour as I discuss in the next chapter.

6

The people business – or where
the money went

The NHS is a people business employing over 1.3million people, accounting for nearly two-thirds of NHS spend. A lot of Ministerial time is spent on workforce issues: pay, pensions, recruitment and retention, new national contracts, education and training and a whole range of obscure terms and conditions of service issues producing industrial disputes. The NHS is highly unionised with over 60% of staff being members of trades unions (which include the BMA);[1] and many of these unions are important Labour Party funders, which brings its own dimension. NHS industrial relations are theoretically decided by negotiation between staff interests and NHS Employers but when significant sums of money are involved or there are wider issues of public sector pay and pensions, then Ministerial agreement is required. To complicate matters further there are independent pay review bodies for doctors and dentists and for nurses and most other professional staff.

The result is that some unfortunate Health Minister gets caught in a labyrinth of negotiations, usually pretending they are not interfering. In reality they are trying to reconcile a raft of individual decisions for different staff with the overall money available for the NHS and the prevailing public sector pay policy being run from the Treasury. This task is easier when there is plenty of money to lubricate the negotiations but when money is short the discussions get nastier. NHS Employers and unions invariably want to reach a deal that suits the NHS; but DH Ministers have a collective Government responsibility with the Treasury breathing down their necks. History suggests that most of the new contract deals done in the NHS cost more than was estimated. Ministers are birds of passage so there is a good chance that an incumbent Health Minister will be sorting out the legacies he or she has inherited. That was certainly the case for Patricia Hewitt and me.

In May 2005 we inherited a new consultant contract, a new GP contract (nGMS) and Agenda for Change which brought nursing and other NHS staff into a new system of grading and harmonisation of terms and conditions of service that took 5 years to implement. There was also a major upheaval in the training of doctors – Modernising Medical Careers (MMC). Negotiations on most of the pay contracts started under Alan Milburn but were concluded and implemented after his departure in 2003. They were intended to benefit staff and the NHS and were for the most part well-intentioned. They all turned out to be more expensive than expected and were important contributors to the financial meltdown of 2005/6 described in Chapter 9.

Contracts for paying doctors

The new GP contract was part of a more complex process of changing the way GPs worked in the NHS and is considered further in the next chapter. It is sufficient to say here that it cost much more than anticipated. NHS finances took a further knock from the new consultants contract that came into effect in 2005/6. In negotiating that contract Alan Milburn had been trying to secure a greater transparency in identifying the NHS work done by consultants and paying more precisely for what they actually did. An impasse over productivity had been reached in the negotiations with the BMA when Alan left in June 2003. It was left to John Reid as the new Health Secretary to head off a major conflict by agreeing a new deal that left productivity improvements to be settled locally between hospital trusts and consultants.

This outcome inevitably depended on the skill and robustness of local managers for delivering efficiency gains under the new contract. Equally inevitably they were extremely variable in their success with local medical colleagues. In practice the new contract's potential gains were too rarely realised. Instead a clock-watching culture was encouraged in some specialties that disadvantaged the NHS. Some specialties with little scope for private practice secured unexpectedly large increases. What happened in reality was that the new consultants' contract cost the NHS over £100million a year more than had been estimated, with the full financial implications not being realised until 2006. There was little evidence that the new contract led to hospital consultants working more than 50 hours a week on average or doing more evening or weekend sessions.

As with the GP contract, the extra cost was to lead to new grievances with the BMA. We staged the Doctors and Dentists Review Body's (DDRB) pay award for consultants for 2006/7, although by the year end they were being paid the full award. Unpalatable evidence was given to the DDRB on hospital consultants pay for 2007/8 which explained that there were no recruitment and retention problems because the 3-month vacancy rate for consultants had dropped between 2004 and 2006. When I gave oral evidence in December 2006 I told the DDRB that we had 117,000 doctors working in the NHS which was over 27,000 more than in 1997. We had record numbers in training in UK medical schools and we no longer had to rely on overseas doctors as much as we had in the past. I could show that for 2006/7 the average earnings of consultants had increased by about 4.3%, compared with the whole economy which was averaging around 4%.

I explained to the DDRB in oral evidence that NHS pay awards had to be affordable and that if an unaffordable pay award was made by the DDRB there would be NHS job losses. On these grounds I considered NHS consultants should only receive a 1.5% increase in 2007/8. The BMA did not like my arguments and members of the DDRB were clearly uncomfortable at being asked to take account of affordability and the threat of job losses. I took the view that it was time for a dose of financial reality.

The financial problems with the consultants' contract were less serious than those relating to GPs and the dispute did less damage to our relationship with the BMA, even though they did not like the Treasury screwing down public sector pay. The difficulties were also less serious than those over Agenda for Change, where there were a lot more unions involved.

Agenda for Change

Alongside the two new doctors' contracts, negotiations had been proceeding over several years with nurses, physiotherapists, ambulance officers and other NHS staff, on what was intended to be a landmark deal to achieve greater fairness in pay and relativities. Under these 'Agenda for Change' negotiations – largely overseen by John (now Lord) Hutton – a new national pay structure was to provide for individuals to be slotted into the right point on pay spines through local union/employer job evaluation. A complex harmonisation process was to take place on local conditions of service. Sceptics would say these local arrangements were often what are described as "Spanish practices", although this may be unfair to our EU partners.

I was to learn gradually over the coming months in 2005 that the reality on Agenda for Change was somewhat different from the benign civil service briefings I had received on taking up the job. There are always winners and losers in job evaluation exercises; the winners stay silent and losers make a lot of noise. I learned more about arcane aspects of local ambulance trusts' meal break policies than I wished as disputes and strikes threats surfaced nationally. Implementation of Agenda for Change had occupied much more local management time than expected so implementation was slow and so was the arrival of the extra money in staff pockets. As local negotiations and disputes were settled across the NHS it was usually by levelling up than the reverse.

As we grappled with the NHS financial crisis of 2005/6 I learned how the myriad of local negotiations on Agenda for Change had made their own contribution to that crisis. Although Agenda for Change had produced a warm trade union glow in the run up to the 2005 Election, by the end of 2005 it was clear that this new deal was going to cost £300million a year more than anticipated. That had to be factored into the evidence given to the nurses' pay review body for the 2006/7 pay round; and was to play its part in the cutback in NHS recruitment in 2006 that caused so much NHS noise (see below). When things got rougher in the autumn of 2006 on NHS recruitment and redundancies I agreed with the Home Office that we should remove nursing posts at Agenda for Change bands 5 and 6 from the shortage occupation lists that justified work permits for overseas nurses. This reduced competition for jobs to UK nurses from overseas nurses. Trades unions found it difficult to accept any link between the extra cost of Agenda for Change and the cutback in new jobs.

The burgeoning NHS pay bill

The financial problems over these new contracts were part of a wider malaise over workforce planning and control of the pay bill, both nationally and locally. The proliferation of centrally-driven targets turned out to be toxic for the NHS pay bill. Not only were many more permanent staff employed but use of agency staff expanded significantly. The latter staff were often paid more than NHS rates and there was usually also a 15% mark-up on top for the agency. Agency staff numbers were not shown in NHS headcounts either. The relentless rise in NHS staff together with increased agency staff and costs was unaffordable without unprecedented improvements in NHS productivity.

Between 1996 and 2006 the total number of NHS staff (full-time equivalents, FTEs) increased from 1.057million to 1.339million or 2.5% each year. As many staff worked part-time the absolute numbers employed were greater. The annual increase for nurses alone – the largest section of the NHS workforce at about 400,000 in 2006 – went up by only 2.3% a year but this does not include the significant number of agency staff.[2] At any one time the NHS might be employing 10% of nursing staff through agencies; and I discovered in 2005/6 the NHS was spending about £1billion a year on agency staff who never appeared in NHS head counts.

The highest increases in staff numbers were those relating to doctors, scientific, therapeutic and technical staff and managerial and central functions staff. The increase in the number of doctors employed in the NHS in ten years is staggering. From a base of about 86,600 doctors in 1996 the numbers increased to 126,250 in 2006 – a nearly 50% increase. Consultant numbers increased by some 60% at an annual rate of about 5%, as did hospital registrars. The GP increases were more modest at a little over 20% or about 2% a year.[3] It was the highest earning professionals who were increasing the most rapidly and impacting significantly on the pay bill. As their pay was also increasing as a result of new contracts this was a double whammy for the NHS pay bill.

Doctors were not the only group increasing rapidly in number. The scientists, therapists and technical staff employed by the NHS zoomed up from 94,300 FTEs in 1996 to about 134,500 in 2006, an annual rate of increase of 3.8%. This group also have a large number of agency staff not included in these numbers. Support to all these clinical staff also increased by about 25% in the ten years to nearly 360,000 in 2006.[4]

Most of these staffing increases were never criticised in the media and were accepted by virtually everybody as a good thing. Indeed Ministers – including me – continued to brag about the staff increases as part of the mantra on the improvements Labour had made to the NHS, although we kept quiet about the increase in managers. To listen to the Conservatives and much of the media in 2005 and 2006 it was managers that were bringing the NHS to its knees. To some extent this was poetic justice for Labour after their ill-advised pre-1997 onslaught on "men in grey suits" – unfortunately sexist as well because the NHS has many female managers.

The reality differed from the media coverage in that the total numbers working on NHS infrastructure increased only from about 174,200 to 209,400 in ten years or just under 2% per year.[5] Within this number were only some 36,800 managers and senior managers – about 3% of the total NHS workforce. Admittedly their number had increased by about 15,500 since 1996, or about 5.6% a year but the NHS budget had trebled in cash terms. A more legitimate criticism could be levelled at the big increase resulting from the misguided 2002 NHS reorganisation: the numbers of managers and senior managers jumped by 8,000 between 2001 and 2003.[6] Without that fiasco the rate of increase in managers would have been unexceptional. The cost of managers has little impact on the NHS pay bill and no political party can cut the NHS pay bill by much simply by slashing the number of managers, however good it makes them feel. Despite the inefficiencies in back office services NHS administrative costs are relatively low at around 5% of the budget, which as a Minister I constantly tried to tell anybody who would listen, which was never that many.

The NHS has the more serious problem of a shortage of high quality managers – especially in its financial and human resources directorates – for the complexity of services managed. Too few doctors become managers and there is a lack of leadership in many NHS trusts – issues I return to later. This message on NHS managers unfortunately does not suit the gut prejudices of most of the public and media and many politicians, doctors and nurses. None of this is to deny the surfeit of quangos and bureaucratic processes which needed tackling, as described in Chapter 5.

This large increase in NHS staff was concentrated in the years 2000 to 2005 when the number of NHS staff increased by 250,000. In the early years of that period the numbers were going up by a totally unsustainable 50,000 to 60,000 a year. This was an unprecedented level of continuing increase that was well beyond the capability of the NHS to cope with, both financially and in terms of sensible deployment. It was clear to me in mid-2005 that large parts of the NHS – Boards, management and clinicians – had no idea of the financial hole they had dug for themselves through their recruitment policies. At that time the DH management was incapable of relating their workforce data to financial data, much like the rest of the NHS, or to fully understand the damage being done to NHS finances by a combination of rapid staff expansion and inadequately costed pay deals.

Controlling the pay bill

It was not until Ministers began tightening the financial screw in early 2006 that the burgeoning NHS pay bill started to be brought under control. In part this was through a policy of pay restraint but also because Ministerial curbing of expenditure inevitably led to slowing recruitment. For the first time in nearly ten years NHS staff numbers reduced between September 2005 and September 2006 by about 30,000.[7]

This change of direction brought a chorus of complaints and warnings of doom from staff interests. There was little sympathy or understanding from Labour's trade union comrades, with the years of rapid staff growth conveniently forgotten. As Ministers tried to bring NHS finances under control there was little appreciation that excessive recruitment and unaffordable pay deals had contributed to the financial chaos. Life on the sunny NHS uplands was thought by the public sector unions as something that would go on for ever. Little attention was paid to earnings data coming out of people like Income Data Services (leading analysts of public and private sector pay). This showed in the Spring of 2006 that gross earnings for full-time staff averaged about £514 a week in the private sector compared with £531 in the public sector: for women the gap was even wider - £406 a week in the private sector and £480 in the public sector.[8]

As financial retrenchment to balance the books increased in 2006, the trade unions campaigned against job cuts and redundancies. In June 2006 the Royal College of Nursing issued a dossier claiming that "15,000 NHS jobs now at risk." I had already tried to calm MPs' nerves in May by writing to them to refute allegations of widespread job cuts. In July I had another go at explaining that the NHS had to balance its books and the fact that some trusts had announced job cuts did not "translate as some reports have claimed, into widespread compulsory redundancies." I pointed out that the NHS Jobs electronic recruitment service advertised over 8,000 vacancies in May which suggested that there were still many jobs available.[9]

What the public sector unions wanted was no change – the same number of posts in existing locations, new jobs in new locations, inflation-proofed pay and pensions, no challenge from outside providers and continuing increases in education and training budgets (which had increased substantially over the past 3 years). Instead they chose to see NHS privatisation, especially ISTCs, as the primary cause of their woes. As public sector pay restraint was pursued by the Treasury, the NHS was chosen as a battleground by the unions.

A pivotal moment in this change of mood occurred with Patricia Hewitt's appearance at the Royal College of Nursing's Annual Conference on 26 April. I was due to speak at the Conference but Patricia became nervous about a non-elected Minister speaking so she took over the slot. The RCN leadership failed to control a jeering, slow-handclapping rebellion from the conference floor which forced Patricia to bring her speech to a conclusion, although she continued with questions. Unfortunately this was televised and the image of nurses booing a Labour Health Secretary did huge political damage. The Conservatives could not believe their luck. Despite subsequent apologies from the RCN – which I found less than convincing – the damage was done. Our relationship with the RCN never really recovered under their then General Secretary, an American nurse, Beverley Malone. Subsequently I had a one-to-one meeting with her to explain in words of one syllable that it was difficult to have a relationship of trust with trades unions if the trust came in only one direction – from Ministers.

This episode damaged not only Patricia Hewitt but the Government as well. It was a mistake not letting me keep the speaking engagement because it almost certainly would not have been televised. When I spoke at the BMA's GP conference six weeks later in July, catcalls and boos started so I asked them to do it a bit louder as I couldn't hear them. This prompted the Chair to call the gathering to order and asked them to let the Minister speak even if people disagreed with him. We continued with some good humoured banter and I completed a perfectly satisfactory question and answer session. Despite all my many disagreements with the BMA I continued throughout my time to have a reasonable working relationship with the BMA Chairman, Jim Johnson, and the GP Chairman, Hamish Meldrum. We could discuss matters privately without confidences being broken.

While all these jobs and pay arguments were going on we were also dealing with the issue of NHS pensions. My difficulties with the BMA over GP pensions are described in Chapter 7; but strangely enough we made good progress over the pensions for other NHS staff in terms of curbing the cost of the growing pensions bill to the NHS. We did this in the wider context of curbing the growth in costs of public sector pensions.

Several issues were in play – retirement age, final salary schemes and employers' contributions. Departmental Ministers were trying to negotiate changes in these areas in local government, teachers, Civil Service and the NHS. (The police unfortunately and unfairly were given a special exemption.)

In the NHS working through some able staff in DH and NHS Employers we reached agreement with the unions on a new NHS Pension Scheme that would start in April 2008. Under the scheme the normal retirement age would increase to 65 from 60; employee contributions from 5% or 6% to 5% to 8% depending on pay level, with the employers' contributions frozen at 14%; and there would continue to be a final salary scheme based on an average of the best 3 consecutive years in the final 10 years of work. With help from the TUC and goodwill on both sides the deal was done that stopped the growth of NHS employers' contribution without too much bad blood. Employer liabilities in public sector pension schemes had to be curbed. However public sector staff , particularly the lower paid, did not deserve to be punished for the demise of final salary pension schemes in the private sector; and I considered it right to protect final salary schemes for NHS staff provided the retirement age was raised substantially and the higher paid contributed more to their pensions. This we achieved.

2006 was the year in which public sector pay restraint was the order of the day and the NHS – because of its size – was very much in the firing line. After staging pay awards for 2006/7 the Chancellor wanted to keep public sector pay increases for the 2007/2008 pay round to 2% despite the rapid rise in fuel prices in early 2006. The Treasury insisted that the Consumer Price Index would fall to 2% in the second half of 2007 so DH evidence to all pay review bodies reflected this. We proposed a headline figure of 2% for nurses and other staff and 1.5% for hospital medical staff. We pointed out to the review bodies that NHS staff benefited from considerable 'wage drift' which meant that earnings always went up by much more than the headline pay increase through increments and supplementary payments like overtime.

I explained again to all the review bodies that there was no separate pot of money for NHS pay costs. For NHS employers unaffordable pay increases would mean hard choices between cutting services and jobs. The large staff and increases meant the NHS had good staffing levels across virtually all pay groups. There had to be pay restraint and higher productivity for all the extra staff and money pumped into the NHS. This was an unpopular message for review bodies and unions. At the end of 2006 the good times for NHS staff looked to be ceasing to roll. Little did we know then that the Iron Chancellor, awaiting his party's call to higher office, would continue to pump extra money into the NHS when he got there.

The row over staff cuts

The row over staff cuts and redundancies continued throughout 2006. In the summer I set up better data collection on jobs and redundancies from the new SHAs in order to refute the increasingly wild stories about slashing NHS job cuts and redundancies. The RCN, Unison and other unions had continued campaigning on these issues as the Party conference season approached. The campaign under the title of NHS Together (which included the BMA) issued documents that blamed privatisation and the government for the cuts in jobs. There was no recognition of the huge growth in NHS jobs that had already taken place. Not filling vacancies was casually equated with redundancies. There was no acceptance that the NHS had to balance its books and that staff costs had to be included in the exercise. Whatever mistakes Ministers had made – and we had made some – it was almost impossible in the summer and autumn of 2006 to engage in any rational discussion of these issues with NHS staff interests. A group hysteria and paranoia had taken over, with many Labour MPs getting into a funk over Labour losing NHS support.

To try to calm things down I wrote a five-page letter to MPs of all parties on 30 October and placed copies and supporting documents in the House of Commons library. This letter pointed out that in the normal course of events about 10% of NHS staff – 130,000 people – left their jobs each year, moving around the NHS or retiring, working outside the NHS, or taking maternity leave. Some of these vacancies were often not filled immediately. Claiming there were huge numbers of redundancies was simply untrue. The evidence I had collected from SHAs showed 900 redundancies in the six months to September 2000, virtually all of which were voluntary. This was many fewer than the 20,000 people being claimed as being put out of NHS jobs.[10] I tried to convince MPs and the public that the jobs slowdown had to be seen in the context of the extra 300,000 extra NHS jobs Labour had created, including 85,000 extra nursing posts. Supply and demand were now in better balance in the NHS job market; and "we should not be apologetic about asking the NHS to offer better value for money to the taxpayer".[11] I explained what we were doing with NHS Employers and SHAs to help displaced people find jobs and to place newly qualified staff, including working with the private sector and local government. I refuted all the hugely bogus figures put out by the 'NHS Together' campaign about ISTCs and the National Programme for IT, who were said to have spent NHS money that should have gone on more staff. This was simply not true and deliberately muddled up capital and revenue expenditure.

The most extraordinary feature of this campaign was the total unwillingness by the unions to recognise the huge increase in NHS staff that had taken place and their seeming belief that expansion could continue indefinitely. Things cooled a little after my 30 October letter, but discontent continued to rumble on. What the events of 2006 show is that Ministers interested in managing the NHS efficiently will get little support from public sector unions if they try to curb the rise in jobs, constrain pay to affordable levels or drive efficiency and productivity. Union leaders were quite prepared to mislead the public and to campaign against an elected government doing what it said it would do on competition in its election Manifesto. As an ex-public sector manager I was unsurprised and unmoved by this union behaviour but my elected colleagues were less phlegmatic, particularly when the Conservatives overindulged themselves. Suddenly the Conservatives were the new best friend of NHS staff; and David Cameron promised undying commitment to the NHS and its doctors and nurses.

While the row on jobs and staff cuts was in progress I tried to cut the NHS spend on agency staff. This seemed a no-brainer given the need to preserve NHS jobs. The shift nature of NHS work and the peaks and troughs of activity make it essential to have some 'bank' staff (a cost effective way of using NHS staff outside their normal jobs) and agency staff (a more expensive way of plugging workforce gaps). But by 2005 the NHS was spending over £1billion a year on agency staff and was finding it difficult to kick this addiction.

The DH had set up an arm's-length body – NHS Professionals – to try to reduce the cost of agency staff by competing with agencies; but the body still needed a considerable DH subsidy to make ends meet. As part of the ALB review (see Chapter 5) I had tried to float it as a commercial going concern on the grounds that if it was really meeting NHS needs then it should not require a subsidy. I reduced both the subsidy and the spend on nursing agency staff. I made speeches on the subject and found NHS people who had reduced agency spend to share conference platforms. The progress made on reducing nursing agency spend was not matched by medical and scientific/technical staff where agency spend continued at far too high a level. This is an area where a more commercial approach is needed to drive down payments to agencies and reduce the usage. NHS Professionals should be made subsidy-free and turned into a fully commercial operation. An answer to a Parliamentary Question I put down in July 2009 reveals that the DH was still grant aiding NHS Professionals.[12] I note that the Coalition Government is minded to pursue a more commercial approach in this area and I hope it will.

Pay bargaining and productivity

What the rows over pay and workforce numbers in 2005 and 2006 brought home to me were the weaknesses of a centralised pay bargaining system.

As a Director of Social Services in the 1980s in Kent I had seen the advantages of coming out of national pay bargaining and the flexibility in grading and pay-setting it offered. This is an issue that needs to be addressed with more urgency because the NHS is simply too large to settle all its pay, grading and related issues nationally. Central settlement of NHS pay, grading and conditions of service divorces a high proportion of NHS costs from the accountability of local trusts for running their health services efficiently and effectively within the resources available to them. Too many costs 'givens' are handed down to them from the centre and too much responsibility and scope for driving efficiency and productivity is removed from them. National pay bargaining also takes insufficient account of the variability of pay in local labour markets.

This view is anathema to public sector unions and in particular their paid officers. Their power is greater under central bargaining, particularly with a Labour Government, where they contribute to both party funds and the constituency expenses of some MPs and have considerable influence over the election of the Party leader. However they would still have a role to play regionally and locally and there would still be a few issues to be dealt with nationally such as pensions. But if one looks at the productivity performance of the NHS – as well as that of other public services – some major questions need to be asked and answered about whether centralisation of pay bargaining is really benefiting taxpayers and patients. At the heart of this debate are the issues of efficiency and productivity in a labour-intensive and costly industry like healthcare.

There is much academic debate about how best to measure productivity in healthcare and indeed more generally in the public services. Measuring quality of services and the cost of best practice are themselves issues of some complexity and disagreement. There has been a long running argument between DH and the Office of National Statistics (ONS) about the measurement of quality in health care and how to factor this into measurements of NHS productivity. I contributed to this debate as a Minister on the side of DH saying that current productivity measures of the NHS do not adequately reflect the improvements in quality such as shorter waiting times and improved access and better patient outcomes. These issues are still unresolved to a great extent because it takes time to establish the qualitative improvements and measures for a given level of inputs. However despite any acknowledged limitations we cannot ignore the present data on inputs and outputs produced by ONS.

For some time ONS through the UK Centre for the Measurement of Government Activity has been measuring productivity in public services and showing how healthcare compares with other public services.

Essentially they calculate the growth in the index of inputs and the same for outputs and take the former from the latter. Their latest paper on this was published in June 2009 covering the period from 1997 to 2007 and does not reveal a very convincing picture on UK healthcare productivity.[13] The ONS data shows healthcare inputs going up from 100 in 1997 to 157.3 in 2007; but productivity dropping from 100 to 95.7 in the same period. In each year outputs were less than inputs – over 60% of which are likely to be accounted for by the pay bill. The decline in productivity increased in every year to 2005. Only in 2006 and 2007, after the tougher approach to pay and the curb on jobs' growth described in this chapter, did productivity start to improve, although inputs still exceeded outputs by some margin. There were improvements in healthcare quality which ONS acknowledges are not captured by their input/output analysis. Nevertheless ONS data showing nearly a 60% increase in inputs over 10 years producing a 4% reduction in outputs presents a very sobering picture on NHS productivity under Labour. The gap is unlikely to be convincingly filled by quality improvements. Centralised pay bargaining and the NHS approach to creating jobs are likely to have contributed significantly to this poor performance, as is the reluctance to change business processes and patterns of care delivery.

In 2009 I asked a Parliamentary Question on NHS expenditure, finished hospital consultant episodes and health care productivity. The answer I received on 16 July 2009 showed similar grounds for concern. NHS expenditure increased between 1996/97 and 2007/8 by 63% in cash terms and 52% in real terms. In the same period finished consultant episodes increased by 28%. There has been some slight improvement since the new consultant contract but the annual improvements in recent years do little more than match some of those in the mid-1990s under the old consultant contract. The UK Health Care Productivity Index figures shown in the Parliamentary Answer reveal a similar pattern to the figures already cited, again with the only improvement in productivity in 2006 and 2007, apart from a blip in 2001.[14]

The big surge in NHS numbers and pay between 2002 and 2005 seems only to have driven down NHS labour productivity, however much they pleased staff. The improvements in waiting times, better access and improvements in killer diseases have been achieved at the price of substantial and probably excessive increases in labour costs. The trajectory shown by the NHS on productivity is a poor one and poses a real problem for the NHS as we approach a period of greater financial austerity. It needs to be tackled as I discuss in the final chapter. However there is one workforce issue that impacts considerably on productivity and that will continue to tax Health Ministers, as it did me. This is ensuring a pipeline of doctors of the right quality and quantity.

The medical pipeline and the European
Working Time Directive (EWTD)

When I took on responsibility for NHS workforce issues in May 2005 I little understood that this included the tangled and sometimes fraught issues of medical education, numbers of medical schools, use of overseas doctors and changes in the training of specialists. I was preoccupied by other contentious NHS reform and organisational issues and these medical topics did not seem an area of concern. A major programme for revamping medical education called "Modernising Medical Careers" (MMC) was in progress but it was being supervised by the four UK Chief Medical Officers and a professional secretariat. It looked to be a professional matter that a lay politician would be criticised for interfering in. Separately a lot of work was also going on relating to professional revalidation through the General Medical Council and again the CMO was in charge of this within DH.

The UK was opening more medical schools to produce more doctors so that the NHS would be less reliant on overseas doctors in the way it had been since its inception. This seemed a creditable and ethical thing to do and we appeared to have the money to do it. There were a number of initiatives for training nurses and other health care professionals to take on the more routine tasks from doctors and this seemed to be making some progress, if a little slowly. We were appointing more and more consultants and GPs and the period for which vacancies were left unfilled was reducing overall. On the medical supply side the only serious cloud on the horizon was the 1993 European Working Time Directive which was reducing the hours doctors worked. This meant that junior doctors would work fewer and fewer hours, thereby impacting on their time for training and for dealing with patients. A reduction to 52 hours by August 2007 was in progress with a further reduction to 48 hours a week due to be made by August 2009. Problems had been created by two rulings by the European Court of Justice – the SIMAP and Jaeger cases – which effectively deemed doctors to be working if they were resident on call and sleeping in the curtilage of the hospital. These rulings were creating a real rostering problem in many hospitals and specialties and were leading towards the UK needing many more consultants.

The SIMAP/Jaeger judgements were in many ways a pyrrhic victory for junior doctors. By counting sleeping time as paid duty time they effectively stopped junior doctors getting as much training time as they would have got as well as costing their employers much more. Combined with the overall reduction in hours for all doctors they produced convoluted rostering that had to be trialled across the NHS. The impact of the changes was different in different specialties and different locations.

Lifestyle improvements for junior doctors would mean more of their senior colleagues being available as cover. This would not only upset consultants but would cost more. Change was inevitable and all I could do was to try to buy more time for transition – to 2012 – and exploit any legal loopholes in the Directive.

I was to learn that my attempts to get the Prime Minister at EU summits to argue for UK dispensations on SIMAP/Jaeger and slower progress on reducing doctors' hours was intimately tied up in the minds of other EU heads with the UK's obstinacy over the opt-out from the Social Chapter provisions for shorter working weeks for all employees. More leniency for the NHS would cause more trouble with the CBI and industry over compulsory shorter working weeks for everyone else. I worked with the Attorney General, Peter Goldsmith, to see if we could use patient safety and training arguments to secure exemption for particular specialties like obstetrics and for particular, more sparsely populated, areas. The legal eagles on EU law made it clear that if we wanted a derogation from the 2009 deadline for a 48-hours maximum working week for doctors then we would have to agree this on a case by case basis. This would mean a major data collection and monitoring exercise, which we started to put in place. It also meant a huge amount of local trialling of different medical rosters, specialty by specialty. The BMA junior doctors had refused to rule out legal action against any hospital trust that did not apply the letter of the SIMAP/Jaeger rulings. So now doctors became shift workers in the best traditions of factory life. Anxiety about whether juniors would receive enough training was constantly expressed to me but was insufficient to cause BMA negotiators to adopt a more flexible position.

The DH had little choice but to accept considerable extra cost – approaching £0.5billion a year – and to exhort the NHS to find more creative solutions while we worked out the best case possible on derogation. This is where we were when I left at the end of 2006 but the saga continued. The DH came clean at the end of 2008 and accepted that the NHS could not achieve the 48-hour maximum working week for doctors in training by August 2009. It secured a derogation under Article 17 (5) of the EWTD for doctors in training working in particular services: some hospitals delivering 24-hour services, immediate patient care, some supra-specialist services and some small remote and rural units. However DH had to admit that it still did not have sufficient information to identify with confidence all the specific services that would be affected and would fail to meet the August 2009 deadline. Instead it limited the derogation to a further 3 years (i.e. to August 2012) to try to achieve the 48-hour maximum working week for junior doctors throughout the NHS. To aid this process the Government pumped in over £300million extra into the

NHS in 2009/10. Effectively the NHS has paid the cost for holding out on the UK implementing the EU Social Chapter.

The saga of the maximum working week for junior doctors has lasted nearly two decades – since 1991 when they secured a "New Deal" to limit their hours. No parties come out of this well. A data-light DH and NHS have struggled to manage the whole process effectively. A recalcitrant BMA junior doctors' committee, uncontrolled by the rest of the BMA hierarchy, seemed not to recognize when they were damaging themselves over their own training and career progression. Worst of all the European Court rulings showed a complete lack of understanding of the variable needs of diverse healthcare systems across the EU. Individual Health Ministers occupying the workforce seat in DH were largely confined to damage limitation as the saga unfolded, with healthcare funders ultimately footing a substantial bill for improving the quality of life – but not the training – of junior doctors. Alongside the juniors another group of doctors were complicating the working of the medical pipeline – NHS doctors from outside the EU.

Overseas doctors and modernising medical careers (MMC)

Labour had the praiseworthy aspiration of reducing dependence on overseas doctors which had produced a steady flow of doctors from poor countries to bolster the NHS's shortage of home grown doctors. Many of these overseas doctors had propped up services in unglamorous places like Grimsby, Rochdale, and Hartlepool, with a significant proportion coming from the Indian sub-continent. The respectable reason for their coming to the UK was that this enabled them to extend their training and experience before returning to their own country. The reality was different in that few did return – until near retirement – and many were unable to secure the specialist training that would enable them to secure consultant posts. Some remained in a no-man's medical land doing a valuable local job without the pay and status of consultant. Some turned to general practice. Some left for the US where the money and status was better in a healthcare economy spending twice that of the UK.

In 2005 there were a lot of non-EU overseas doctors working in the NHS in different circumstances. Some were in permanent non-training posts either as GPs or hospital doctors: they usually had UK citizenship or the right to remain here. Others were here as junior hospital doctors completing training and seeking to achieve a post-graduate qualification. The BMA estimated that there were some 9,000 of these doctors in short-term junior and senior house officer posts. These doctors had traditionally been allowed to come here to complete this training without work permits. Several events conspired to produce a major political explosion.

On the medical front the MMC programme was moving towards the point of transition from the old system to the new. This meant that after completing medical school, medical graduates would do two Foundation years involving post rotation (in place of the old junior and senior house officer jobs) before applying for specialist training posts. When this training was completed and the specialist qualifications obtained doctors could apply for consultant posts. The more I learned of this new arrangement – which would produce doctors faster and introduce more competition for specialist training posts – the more I realised there was a problem with the flow through this new pipeline.

Once the increasing number of graduates from expanded UK medical schools had been funnelled into Foundation years 1 and 2 then you had to have enough specialist training posts to absorb the extra throughput. Given that the inflow seemed to be increasing faster than the expansion of specialist training posts – which the NHS had to find the funds for – this would cause difficulties for some young doctors unable to secure specialty training of their preference when they completed Foundation year 2. If you added into the equation the large number of overseas doctors in training in the UK the specialty training problem got worse. If the established overseas hospital doctors outside training grades were allowed to compete for specialist training slots – as many wished to - the problem became seriously difficult. It was far from clear to me that the senior doctors master-minding MMC had considered these consequences.

This was a classic case of uncoordinated DH policy initiatives – expansion of medical schools and the introduction of MMC, linked to changes in immigration rules and the increasing number of non-EU doctors, especially from India. There were virtually no arrangements for modelling how these other factors fitted with MMC. The growing public concerns over increasing immigration resulted in the Government changing the immigration rules first in 2004 and again in 2005, which added to my problems. The changes reduced the number of people coming into the UK without work permits, unless they came in under a new Highly Skilled Migrants Programme aimed at attracting people with qualifications and skills that the UK economy was short of. These changes impacted on all those overseas doctors – mainly Indian – who traditionally trained here without work permits.

The first MMC Foundation year 1 intake began in August 2005 so they would complete their Foundation years in August 2007. I needed to start turning off the tap of overseas doctors coming into the country for training as soon as possible. The best way - or more accurately the least bad way - to do this was to use the new immigration rules to require work permits for overseas doctors coming here to train. However we had to ensure there were some transitional arrangements so that doctors in training already in the UK could complete that training. There was no way to do this without a political row and it required DH, the Home office and the Treasury to agree on what should be done, never something easy to achieve.

I was bound to be accused of betraying overseas doctors, especially those from India, who had helped the NHS over many years. For decades now these overseas doctors had been allowed to come here to complete training in junior doctor posts without work permits. Some of these posts had been reserved for overseas doctors. Many of these doctors stayed on after completing their training, working in general practice, as locums or in sub-Consultant hospital posts. In some parts of the country these doctors had been critical to the local NHS, sometimes comprising two-thirds of all the NHS doctors in a particular area. The Government was going to be very unpopular for changing these long-established arrangements now that we were producing more UK-trained doctors.

It took some time to negotiate transitional arrangements and to agree new immigration rules across Whitehall. News leaked of what we intended and this produced some unforeseen consequences for the Highly Skilled Migrants Programme (see below). In April 2006 we published the new immigration rules and details of the transitional arrangements. Predictably the balloon went up. Overseas doctors could no longer automatically seek training placements. Hospitals had to prove that they could not recruit a junior from Britain or the EU before they could shortlist candidates from other countries. Cries of betrayal rang out. The British Association of Physicians of Indian Origin (BAPIO) claimed at least 15,000 doctors might have to leave Britain heavily in debt without completing their qualifications. The BMA were more moderate saying 9,000 might be affected; and accepted we required a new system in which the numbers of doctors coming to the UK should be based on the needs of the NHS. Hundreds of overseas doctors protested around Richmond House and lobbied MPs, with BAPIO in the lead.

I went on the Today programme to explain that as we were becoming more self-sufficient in training our own doctors we had to reduce the flow of doctors from overseas. I pointed out that we had increased the medical school intake by 70% over seven or eight years so we had to have sufficient post-graduate specialist training posts for that higher output. The public for the most part seemed to accept my explanations. MP lobbying was modest, concentrated on areas with high numbers of Indian doctors. The Indian Ambassador came to see me and was extremely courteous. He accepted something had to change but sought improved transitional arrangements. These we undertook to try to achieve, together with some protection for long-standing medical training schemes set up between particular UK and overseas institutions. In June he kindly sent me, with just a trace of irony, a copy of Amartya Sen's 'The Argumentative Indian'. Some noise continued to rumble on over the summer but by the time of the summer recess it looked publicly as though things had calmed down.

The MMC specialist training debacle

Back at Richmond House civil servants brought me more bad news. A growing number of overseas doctors were applying successfully to the Highly Skilled Migrant Programme (HSMP). Until February 2006 on average about 200 overseas doctors a month had come into the UK under this programme. It then started to rise rapidly, apparently as a result of our moves on work permits. By April/May the numbers were around 600 a month and looked to be rising. What appeared to be happening was that many overseas doctors – some living in the UK – who had completed their training and had gained Royal College medical qualifications were using the HSMP to secure NHS positions, I suspect with the collusion of NHS employers. By the autumn it looked as though we were facing a situation of as many as 10,000 overseas doctors putting themselves in a position to compete for specialist training posts in August 2007, after the first group of UK graduates of MMC Foundation years 1 and 2 competed for the places available. This was seriously bad news, as huge numbers of doctors – UK and overseas – would fail to get specialist training positions.

The civil servants and I began an assertive campaign across Whitehall to close what was obviously an HSMP loophole. Eventually we got the Home Office on side with the then Immigration Minister, Liam Byrne, taking a constructive approach to introducing new immigration rules. However despite my conducting a robust correspondence and several highly-charged telephone calls with Treasury Ministers they were adamant that no changes to the HSMP should be made. I was treated to the extraordinary explanation by one Treasury Minister that they thought more overseas doctors coming into the UK by this route would produce more competition for consultant posts and thereby moderate pay rates for NHS doctors. When I taxed the Treasury with the Government's policy of greater UK medical self-sufficiency through expansion of medical schools, an investment policy supported by the Treasury, I received no coherent response. Politically and officially the Treasury declared itself unconnected to the rest of government on this issue and thwarted curbing the HSMP.

I launched an internal exercise though the SHAs to establish how many specialist training posts the NHS was likely to be able to afford in August 2007 so that we could compare this with the likely output from Foundation years 1 and 2. By the end of September 2006 it looked as though we would be able to offer between 22,000 and 23,000 specialist training posts in the NHS in 2007. Viewed from the perspective of UK candidates this was a reasonable position to be in. There would be competition and some applicants would not get posts. Some juniors would take a career break and try again; some would stay longer in a training grade. Some would be found not capable of progressing to specialist training. However if we injected between 5,000 and 10,000 overseas doctors into this competitive process I knew that we would have an even bigger row than earlier in the year, particularly as some would be better candidates than their UK-trained counterparts, whose failure rate would be much higher.

News that there could be a problem of insufficient specialist training jobs began to seep into the public arena. The BMA junior doctors started campaigning in September 2006 that over 11,000 doctors would be unemployed because of MMC. Some were claiming that junior doctors would be left unregistered and would not be able to perform life-saving procedures. Distinguished doctors whose offspring were in medical training took to the media. Hysteria was whipped up. I tried to calm things down with media interviews and interventions.

To make matters worse the testing of the new IT and selection process for specialist training under MMC was not going well. The new Medical Training Application Service (MTAS) introduced by those masterminding MMC had two features that were radically different from the past. There was to be a standard application form and the application was to be made online. The selection of those for interview was to be made on the basis of anonymity. This was intended to tackle some of the criticism of racism of the old paper-based system where research in the mid-1990s – published in the British Medical Journal – had shown British-trained doctors with Asian names were less likely to be short-listed than those with English names. Since the short-listing was being done by hospital consultants – their members - this posed a discrimination problem for the BMA. The standardisation and anonymity of the MTAS system had been designed and trialled with the medical profession and the medical deaneries. It was intended to tackle a problem acknowledged by professional leaders, with their full support and agreed by the 4 Chief Medical Officers. This was not a position these medical leaders were keen to acknowledge publicly when things went wrong.

Unfortunately there were serious problems with the IT when it went live which damaged the reputation of MTAS. But many of the other criticisms of the form itself were for the most part misguided. When the scions of eminent doctors failed to get their expected choices this was more to do with their own shortcomings than those of the application form. What had not been allowed for adequately however was that with an online application process, pressing the "send" key could transmit multiple applications to large numbers of hospital trusts which made short-listing a nightmare. But what caused the real crisis was the unwillingness of Treasury Ministers to close legally the HSMP loophole in a timely way and reduce the number of people applying.

Before my departure as a Minister I had gone on the Today programme yet again and used other media opportunities to try to reassure an increasingly angry cadre of junior doctors and the BMA that the NHS would have enough specialist training posts to accommodate most of the output of Foundation years 1 and 2. Collective Ministerial responsibility prevented me from explaining the true position on the HSMP loophole but judging by some of the numbers the BMA was starting to use they seemed to know what was going on. Their position was that the Government should have made the right number of places available; they wisely did not get into the clinical merits of people in the HSMP versus those coming out of MMC Foundation Years.

After my planned Ministerial resignation the plane crashed. The MTAS system was swamped. The IT failed and the online MTAS system was abandoned in the spring of 2007. Angry applicants and their parents attacked the Government over insufficiency of specialist training posts. More than 13,000 doctors from UK medical schools did not get specialist training posts. The media was full of stories of young British-trained doctors emigrating. The medical establishment rose up in arms against MMC even though they had been fully involved in its development and supported a system agreed by the 4 UK Chief Medical Officers.

The DH issued guidance saying that overseas doctors (including those in HSMP) could only be considered for specialist training posts if there were not suitable graduates from the UK and EU. BAPIO challenged the legality of this guidance saying that thousands of doctors came to the UK under the HSMP with the prospect of permanent residence after four years but the DH had changed this retrospectively through guidance. In November 2007 the Court of Appeal ruled in favour of BAPIO saying that overseas doctors should be allowed to compete for specialist training posts. Before this Patricia Hewitt decided in April 2007 to set up an independent inquiry into the MMC framework and processes under the Chairmanship of Sir John Tooke, Dean of the Peninsula Medical School. The inquiry was to make recommendations for improvements to MMC for 2008 and beyond. It produced interim proposals for consultation in October 2007 and a final report in January 2008.[15] Although the report made many detailed recommendations, it did not fundamentally change the structure of MMC.

Meanwhile, far too late, the Treasury capitulated and the HSMP loophole was closed. So when in April 2008 the Law Lords dismissed the DH appeal against BAPIO's November 2007 victory in the Court of Appeal their victory was a limited one. The ruling meant that only some

4,000 to 5,000 overseas-trained doctors already in Britain would be able to compete for specialist training posts. Meanwhile Alan Johnson implemented some of the Tooke recommendations but deferred action on others, so the MMC saga is limping to a conclusion.

Mistakes were undoubtedly made over MMC and MTAS but they were mistakes more of implementation and management than concept. It was medical leaders who had agreed MMC and then tried to disown it when things went awry. The Treasury, not DH, prevented the closure of the HSMP loophole that caused taxpayer's money to be invested inappropriately in specialist training for HSMP doctors instead of UK medical graduates. More significantly MMC, implementing the EWTD and new national schemes and contracts for large and expensive pay groups, all exposed serious weaknesses in the DH/NHS workforce planning and delivery system.

Workforce planning and delivery

Getting the right NHS workforce in place at the right time is a complex and difficult job. It involves activity – and coordinated activity at that – at the local, regional and national levels and across government. It requires good information; good modelling; and knowledgeable professionals at all levels. Good negotiating skills and strategies are required. There is a complex web of relativities between staff groups to be considered and a national production line of health care professionals to be maintained – especially doctors, nurses, therapists, scientists and technicians. All this has to be fitted into a structure of public sector pay and pensions and for a service where technological change means almost continual variations in the roles and training of professional groups. Alongside this, EU legislation and changing immigration rules can complicate matters further, particularly as the market for skilled health professionals is a global one.

My time as the NHS workforce Minister suggested to me that at all levels – DH, SHA and trust level – we have not invested in the skills needed to do the job well. MMC was not fundamentally flawed but its policy work and management were under-resourced for such a complex and sensitive change. Often the huge growth in NHS personnel over the past decade or so has been a random collection of disparate local decisions unconnected to financial management or productivity. The NHS human resources function is under-skilled and under-resourced for the organisational development the NHS needs. DH and the NHS invest in the development of new health personnel such as nurse prescribers, physician aides and paramedics but there are no mechanisms for ensuring their widespread use after proof of concept. Too often the NHS lacks the leaders and managers (especially medical managers) to dynamically lead change. Too many decisions on workforce pay and grading issues are taken nationally that impose obligations on local management that undermine their local budgetary and performance accountability.

The result is a system of nominal political accountability under which Ministerial birds of passage pick up disparate issues, usually when the cards have already been dealt, and do the best they can. Often all they can do is minimise damage on individual items without regard to any whole system strategy.

A classic example of this was the delay in providing me with a long-sought submission on the evidence for the further medical school expansion favoured by the CMO and the medical hierarchy. It arrived shortly before my departure during the chaos over MMC, MTAS and overseas doctors. There was little evidence in this Ministerial submission to support the case for expanding medical school outputs significantly in the way being proposed. I declined to approve any further expansion and said this should be reviewed in two or three years' time when a better modelling system was in place. Whether this will turn out to be a good decision I do not know but it was the only responsible decision to take at the time on the evidence available.

These problems with NHS workforce planning have long been recognised. The Health Select Committee produced a report on Workforce Planning in 2007 that identified serious failings in the way that the NHS planned its policies on recruitment and retention of staff.[16] In 2008 it produced a report on Modernising Medical Careers and criticised DH and the medical Royal Colleges.[17] Ara Darzi's Next Stage Review report acknowledged the failings of workforce planning in DH and made two recommendations for improving matters. These were an independent body, Medical Education England (MEE), to advise DH on the education and training of doctors, dentists, pharmacists and healthcare scientists; and a Centre for Excellence to provide "objective long-term horizon – scanning, capability and capacity development for workforce planning functions", for the entire NHS workforce, not just doctors.[18]

These changes are certainly an improvement on what was available to me when I was wrestling with NHS workforce issues. Whether they are sufficient in an increasingly devolved NHS is doubtful. As the Health Select Committee said in the conclusions to its March 2009 report on the NHS Next Stage Review:

> "We welcome the Department's increased focus on improving its workforce planning in the NHS. However we note concerns that planning will be concentrated in the Department. In our recent report on Workforce Planning we recommended that SHAs have a key role in this area. The Department should ensure that regional NHS employers are given a role in identifying future workforce requirements."[19]

It was always my intention when creating the new ten SHAs, as described in Chapter 5, that there should be a strong workforce planning element in their role, linked to coterminous medical deaneries. The Coalition Government's decision to abolish SHAs from 2012 now removes that option but it will still need to find a better workforce planning and delivery system within both DH and the NHS if it wishes to secure the NHS efficiency and productivity improvements it seeks. The people's health service requires better people business processes.

7

GPs – gate keepers or change agents?

GPs in our society

Over 90% of the annual public contacts with the NHS are with GP surgeries. GPs and their staff are the portal into the NHS for most people. Compared with other healthcare systems the NHS is unusual in offering people registration with a GP of their choice as a way of guaranteeing access to free healthcare. However this means that usually you can only access specialist care via your GP unless you pay for that privilege outside the NHS. The views of most people about the NHS are shaped therefore by their experiences in the GP surgery.

GPs are part of the British way of life. They have been around in some form since before the NHS. They feature in literature, films and television. They have been the subject of soap operas. They are emblematic of the NHS for both people in UK and those overseas who have heard about the NHS. They attract high levels of trust in the British population, regularly featuring at or near the top of most surveys of groups people trust. The deeds of Dr Harold Shipman seem not to have dented their trust. In today's more secular society some see GPs as replacing priests as personal confidants.

There are myths and contradictions about GPs. Most members of the public – including some MPs – do not realise that GP practices are, usually, small businesses, with a profit and loss account. Although GPs are not employees of the NHS they have managed to persuade successive governments to regard them as such for inclusion in the NHS pension scheme. Their remuneration and pension are negotiated with government on their behalf by a trade union – the BMA - which is an unusual arrangement to say the least for small businesses. That union drove a hard bargain on their behalf at the inception of the NHS and has on occasion threatened to withdraw its members from the NHS, collecting undated signatures for withdrawal. Those of us who have negotiated with the BMA over the years know that GP negotiators play hardball as well as any industrial trade union. Yet in the public mind the aura of Dr Finlay's Casebook and trusted confidant persists even though GP magazines devote almost as much space to business affairs as to medicine.

Against this background it is not surprising that most Health Ministers develop a certain ambivalence about GPs as a collectivity and treat them with caution and even suspicion. Yet because they are businesses as well as doctors GPs also present an opportunity. They understand money and how to use it and make a profit. They can be enterprising in the way they run their businesses: GPs were the pioneers of IT in the NHS. They will set up new services if they are paid to do so. They will, if it suits them, borrow money to develop their premises and practices. But they can be highly individualistic and reluctant to participate in wider collective enterprises. They are also shrewd negotiators when it comes to pay deals, usually outsmarting the DH negotiators as happened with the 2003 contract negotiations.

In today's NHS GPs remain gatekeepers for their patients, but their role is changing. Under the Conservatives in the 1980s and 1990s GPs showed that they could hold budgets and commission services for their patients. For a while GP fundholding changed the relationship between GPs and hospital specialist doctors by putting GPs more in the driving seat on the way services were delivered to their patients. This offered the prospect of wider reform of acute hospitals once some of the problems with fundholding were ironed out. Foolishly Labour abandoned the fundholding experiment until I applied across England a version of it as practice-based commissioning (PBC) in 2006. However neither GP fundholding nor PBC have been allowed to achieve their full potential for reshaping service delivery.

Nevertheless important changes took place under Labour in the GP workforce and its organisation and remuneration arrangements. These changes offer scope for GPs to become more than gatekeepers to specialist services. The Darzi model of polyclinics is one new route that GPs could take, although many GPs have expressed opposition to it. The Royal College of General Practitioners came up with an alternative model of grouping practices into federations. Changes in the organisation and pattern of general practice seem inevitable as its workforce changes, with more women, more part-timers and more salaried GPs. The 2003 new GP contract offered more opportunities and services that encourage scaling up practices. This contract may pave the way for significant change even though it proved an expensive deal for the NHS. Unfortunately clawing back some of its financial excesses soured relations with the BMA and some GPs. Understanding the history of that contract and its aftermath is important because some of its changes offer the possibility of taking general practice and primary care in new directions.

The new GP contract

It has been easy to criticise the new GP contract and overlook its potential benefits. When it was negotiated in 2003 there was thought to be a shortage of GPs. Between 1997 and 2003 their number had increased by little more than 1,000 and the BMA could show that about 3.4% of GP posts had been vacant for over three months, equivalent to a shortage of 1,000 doctors. There was continuing public concern about access to GPs; and GPs wanted to change their 24hour/7 days a week responsibility for their patients - a part of their service terms and conditions since the start of the NHS. The rise in the number women going into general practice meant more part-time working and a growing number of practices were reluctant to take on out-of-hours work. Health Ministers wanted a new contract that rewarded clinical interventions that improved health outcomes. Change in the old contract was inevitable therefore but past experience of changing the GP contract suggested it could prove expensive.

The new contract undoubtedly cost a lot more than expected. GPs were allowed to opt out of providing out-of-hours services from 6.30pm to 8am on weekdays and all weekends, public and bank holidays. Most did so because the income they sacrificed was on average only about £6,000 a year. Yet according to a 2006 National Audit Office report it cost PCTs well over £300million a year in total – about twice as much - to cover those responsibilities with contracts for new providers.[1] Many of these PCT contracts went to the same GP cooperatives and private companies providing out of hours services before, but at higher rates. The out-of-hours changes alone left a considerable hole in many PCT budgets. A later report by the Public Accounts Committee (PAC) in October 2008 estimated that allowing practices to opt out of 24 hour responsibility eventually cost £182million a year more than expected.[2] The change also brought in more overseas doctors for out-of-hours work, some of whom had English language difficulties. There have been a small number of high profile serious cases where patients died which has raised questions about PCT quality assurance of these contracts.

For the first time the GP remuneration system included a productivity provision - a new Quality Outcomes Framework (QOF) which paid about 25% of a GP's income on the basis of achieving certain indicators. QOF ensured that patients benefited from a more consistent approach by their GPs to many basic procedures and chronic conditions. Many commentators thought that the bar was set too low for the achievement of the payments to be made. In the first year, 2004/5, the median achievement rate for those indicators – which remained the same for 3 years - was already 85%. The rate had increased only by about 6% by the third year, 2006/7. QOF was a good idea but it has to be driven much harder by more demanding clinical indicators if patient care is to be improved significantly for the extra money. The 2008 PAC report estimated that the new QOF system cost £332million more than planned because GPs performed at a much higher level than expected.[3] In other words the initial indicators were too easy.

Although GP pay may have been too low before the new contract, that was not the case after its introduction. A generous inflation factor, more scope for local contracts and a generous minimum income guarantee for small practices (MPIG) all combined to push up average GP earnings significantly. MPIG alone cost well over £300million a year without any performance requirements. According to the NHS Information Centre between 2003/4 and 2005/6 the average pay of a GMS GP partner increased from £77,152 to £106,312.[4] Alongside an attractive pension scheme and the freedom to determine their own working hours and outside activities GPs seemed to become the new elite of the NHS workforce in pay terms and with the average working week for GPs dropping by about 15% since the early 1990s.

It was to be some time before the full financial impact of the new contract became apparent but by mid-2005 it was already clear that it had contributed significantly to the poor state of the NHS finances. I was also to discover that only about 60% of GP partners worked fulltime in their practices. Many had other sources of income including hospital contracts, non-NHS work, other local contracts with PCTs, and profits from practice-based commissioning. How they spend their time is up to them because they are self-employed and they choose how to run their businesses. (I had to explain this to one or two members of the Health Select Committee when I gave evidence to them.) Because GPs can control the skill mix they use in their businesses this gives them considerable flexibility over the way they run their businesses and sustain or increase profits.

By the end of 2005, as we entered the next round of pay negotiations with the BMA, it was clear that the new contract had rewarded GPs far too generously for what patients and taxpayers received in return. Needless to say the BMA's GP negotiators, led by Hamish Meldrum, a Yorkshire GP in a small practice, did not agree. I reminded them that GPs had now moved from being possibly the lowest paid in Europe to the highest – much better paid than their French or German counterparts – and that their pensions were extremely generous. There was no meeting of minds on these issues especially when I set out in the public arena how well paid GPs were. I was not surprised subsequently to see the GP magazine's front page story in October 2007 with the headline "UK GPs happiest in Europe on pay" following a French survey of French, German, Italian, Spanish and British GPs.[5]

My negotiating position was efficiency gains in the QOF points together with improvements in patient access through more flexible opening times and better telephone services. I wanted to reduce the amount spent on MPIG, which basically just paid GPs for being there and created a disincentive to take on more patients; and to achieve faster take-up of the Choose and Book system. We managed to come to a deal for the financial year 2006/7 in which there was no inflation increase, a modest set of changes to the QOF system and a few other improvements that attracted modest extra payments. All this did was to postpone a bigger row about increased productivity under the new contract until the following year.

More stories appeared in the media about how well paid GPs were as journalists obtained the data on their earnings. Front page stories started to appear of Mercedes-driving GPs earning £250,000 a year although when I looked more closely at the Daily Mail GP picture the Mercedes, was about 10 years old! None of this pleased the BMA. What annoyed them more was my insistence that we introduce a new system of patient surveys to measure patient satisfaction with practices which they realised I intended to use to influence their pay. Ipsos/MORI trialled a survey system for introduction in 2007/8, which I had to impose because the BMA negotiators would not agree to the trial.

Relations continued to deteriorate through 2006 as I authorised work on trying to phase out MPIG. The BMA would only agree to this if a further huge sum of money was injected into the Global Sum available for all general practices so that you could float protected practices off MPIG without worsening the position of anyone. This would have been a total waste of public money, and was not something the Treasury would ever have agreed. I wanted to go for a two or three year phase out with some financial losses; but I could make no progress with the BMA. They reminded me endlessly that DH negotiators had created MPIG in order to stop so many practices losing money under the new contract and possibly ceasing to practice. This may have well been true but it did not alter the fact that the new contract had overpaid GPs and MPIG was one of the least defensible parts of it. It cosseted small practices that needed to merge, discouraged taking on new patients and roles and effectively deprived patients of a wider range of services.

MPIG was a classic example of a last minute contract negotiating fudge that went on paying out over £300million a year for virtually no taxpayer or patient benefit. It was to take Ara Darzi's 'Next Steps Review' and a 2% increase in the Global Sum by Alan Johnson for the 2009/10 pay deal with GPs to start reducing the number of GPs receiving MPIG. Johnson said in October 2008 that it was likely to remain for another 5 years and even then there would still be some practices left on MPIG.[6] MPIG remains a highly questionable way of spending public money and restricts changes to practices and new entrants to the market.

In 2006 pay negotiations with the BMA were at stalemate. Matters were made worse by my unwillingness to retrospectively dynamise GP pensions by the amount to which the BMA claimed they were entitled.

Given the wider negotiations on public sector pensions, agreeing to a 3-year dynamisation of well over 50% for GP pensions seemed to me outrageous. My position was complicated by the fact that the BMA had persuaded successive governments that despite being self-employed businessmen running profit and loss accounts, GPs were entitled to a pension scheme in which they were treated as though they were salaried NHS employees. Because their NHS earnings were only known in retrospect, the uplifting of pension entitlements – dynamisation – had to take place retrospectively.

Dynamisation was applied to earnings, not inflation, another questionable proposition. Because the new 2003 contract had pushed up earnings so much the impact on GP pensions was huge. I took legal advice on whether I could dynamise at a lower figure of about 35% over three years. I was told that I had a good case but there might be a legal challenge. The Treasury in any case would not agree the BMA's figure so I imposed the lower figure and effectively told the BMA we would see them in court. Just after I departed as a Minister the BMA won their legal challenge which did not help Patricia Hewitt's position or the NHS bank balance. The issue of expensive GP pensions remains a controversial issue for the new government.

Facing an effective pay freeze for GPs the BMA decided that they were fed up with DH Ministers and would do better appealing to the Doctors and Dentists Review Body (DDRB). I took the view, after seeking legal advice, that the new GMS contract meant they could not do this. Prior to the 2003 contract the DDRB applied its mind to what was the "Intended Average Net Income" for a GP, collected evidence and ruled accordingly. However as I explained to the BMA the new GP contract that they had agreed was a contract with a group practice not individual doctors so the concept of an "Intended Average Net Income" for individual doctors no longer applied. The new contract provided practices with a level of investment for taking on responsibility for delivering services to patients and gave practices considerable flexibility about the way groups of GPs did this. These practice organisations now contained a range of professions, not just GPs, all of whom either draw pay or a share of the profits from a practice's earnings. The different earnings have different uplifts applied to them, many well outside the remit of the DDRB. I considered that the DDRB had no role in setting individual GP pay and wrote to the DDRB's chairman saying that the Government would not be giving any evidence on this issue to the Review Body for their 2007/8 pay ruling.

This interpretation of the 2003 contract seriously upset the BMA who claimed that the Government was removing their "recourse to an independent body" over pay and that it was for the DDRB to determine the levels of investment within the GMS contract. I wrote a 5-page letter to the Chairman of the BMA Council on the 20 November 2006 on behalf of all the UK Health Departments refuting their position and making clear that we would not give evidence for any GP pay increase for 2007/8. This letter pointed out that we had underpinned the 2003 contract by a guaranteed 36% increase in resources over the 3-year period 2003/4 to 2005/6. In practice the increase totalled over 50% and at that time practice profits were forecast to rise by over 70% in that 3-year period. I made it clear that on grounds of fairness to other NHS staff there could be no significant further increase in pay for GPs. My only peace offering was possible cooperation with a one-off review by the DDRB of the GMS contract for the 2008/9 pay round but this would have to look at the totality of resources invested in general practice over the 5 year period 2003/4 and 2007/8 (including GP's profits) compared with investment in other parts of the NHS. This remained my position when I gave oral evidence to the DDRB on the 4 December 2006.

Despite their huffing and puffing and threat of judicial review the BMA, for the second year running, achieved no pay increase for GPs in 2007/8. By hard bargaining and facing down the BMA, I managed to claw back some of the over-generosity of the 2003 contract. I knew that the over-payment was substantial and in October 2008 the PAC estimated that the over-spend on the 2003 GPs contract between 2003/4 and 2005/6 (i.e. 3 years) was £1.8billion, although the NHS Chief Executive claimed it was less.[7] However this clawing back money from GPs was at a cost of a deteriorating relationship with the BMA and the profession. GPs found their public image taking a beating. Some of the criticism was unfair to many GPs but the profession's leaders had brought it on themselves, with a little help from me over the damage done to the NHS's finances by the generosity of the 2003 deal.

The tough negotiating stance on GP pay continued after I left. The DH evidence to the DDRB for the pay settlement for 2008/9 argued that no uplift in pay should be considered for GPs unless they accepted tougher QOF targets, promised to reinvest a greater proportion of their profits back into their surgeries, make efficiency gains or agree to movement on the phasing out of MPIG. The 2003 contract ended up being something of a pyrrhic victory for the BMA but a costly change for the NHS. GP profits for 2006/7 and 2007/8 were estimated to be down by 7% in each year. But by then some GP negotiators had given the game away when in trying to protect the 2003 contract they were saying that its whole purpose was to enable GPs to control their workload with any extra work depending on the size of the pay rise. This over-generous deal did wonders for GP recruitment because the number of GPs rose from about 29,200 to nearly 33,400 between 2002 and 2007.

Despite its cost the 2003 GP contract did produce some structural changes to the way GPs are paid that help modernise primary care. By introducing QOF it has made it possible to incentivise change and clinical improvement through the remuneration system. By moving away from a system that settled individual doctor remuneration to rewarding a whole practice it has made the contract a basis for changing the way practices operate and makes it easier to bring in new providers and change the pattern of general practice, as discussed in the next section.

Changing GP and primary care capacity

There are now about 36,000 GPs in England; and the number of GPs rose by about 26% between 1999 and 2009. The traditional position of GPs being independent contractors and male has changed considerably and continues to change. Women doctors have increased from nearly a third of the GP workforce in 1999 to nearly 44% in 2009. Nearly 62% of GP registrars – the next generation of GPs – are now women. This change in the gender balance is reflected in the dramatic rise in salaried GPs in the past decade from under 800 in 1999 to about 7,300 in 2009, with annual increases of over 10% a year. The fulltime equivalent of the number of GPs is about 32,000, so many are working part-time.[8]

The number of GP partners has been fairly static over the past decade, rising only by about 3%. They are working in practice groups whose size is bigger on average. The number of GP practices fell from 9,034 in 1999 to 8,228 in 2009, with an increase in the average number of patients per practice from about 5,600 to about 6,600. The number of single-handed practitioners has reduced by about a third in a decade and is now down to under 1,300. The GP workforce is however an ageing one with the proportion aged 45 and over rising from about 49% to nearly 57% between 1999 and 2009. Over 20% of current GPs qualified overseas. However in 2009 the number of doctors joining general practice was about double the number leaving – nearly 3,700 compared with nearly 1,800.[9]

Despite the growth in the number of GPs by over a quarter in a decade the number of practice staff they employ directly has increased much less. Overall the number of staff went up from nearly 106,000 to just over 114,000 in ten years – a little over 63,000 (FTEs) to just over 72,000 (FTEs). The numbers have declined since a peak of nearly 120,000 in 2006. Over 70% of the practice staff are administrative and clerical staff (including practice managers); and only about 19% are practice nurses (about 13,000 FTEs in 2009), with another 7% (just over 5,000 FTEs) shown as 'direct patient care'. Although practices have grown in size these numbers suggest that GPs as a whole seem not to have increased significantly their investment in directly-employed staff. That may be because the number of patients per GP has fallen gradually from 1,788 in 1999 to 1,520 in 2009; and there are now 70 GPs per 100,000 population compared with 58 in 1999.[10] Patient pressure on GPs seems to have reduced under Labour.

Much has changed in the way GPs are paid. Prior to the 2003 contract there was little alternative to GPs being paid largely on a per capita basis under a GMS contract negotiated nationally between the DH and the BMA. The GPs had individual lists of patients and were individually responsible for them under their terms and conditions of service for 24-hours a day, 7 days a week. It was for the GP to make their own deputising arrangements and if these broke down the individual GP would still be liable for the patients' care and treatment. All this changed when the new GMS contract (nGMS) was introduced; and the 2005/6 average net profit (after expenses) of GPs under GMS went up to £106,312, a 10% increase on 2004/5. This was more than a doubling in real terms of their net income under the old system 20 years previously.[11] No wonder they were happier over their pay than their European counterparts.

Perhaps more significantly many GPs have switched from a GMS contract to more lucrative alternatives. Over 40% of GP practices held Personal Medical Service (PMS) contracts in 2009. These contracts allow practices to negotiate a local agreement with PCTs for the particular services they provide, having regard to local healthcare needs. The average net income of GPs on PMS contracts in 2005/6 was even higher than for GMS at £120,272, which represented a real terms increase of a third compared with 2002/3. These averages concealed some very large increases for particular GPs and practices under the new contract. Nearly 15% of GPs in contract with PCTs (i.e. not salaried GPs) had net profits in excess of £150,000 in 2005/6, with about 1% having profits in excess of £250,000. It was this sharp increase in profits that prompted my attempts to claw back some of them in the tetchy discussions with the BMA already described. So when the 2006/7 earnings were analysed the average net income (after expenses) for GPs had decreased slightly compared with 2005/6: by 2.6% for GMS contractors and by 1.5% for PMS contractors.[12]

Even after this claw back GP contractors are now much better paid than before the 2003 contract and they can now enter into a wider set of income-generating arrangements with PCTs. Little of the extra profits seem to have been invested in directly-employed staff. GPs' responsibilities are less with the transfer of out-of-hours work to PCTs and the reduction in the average number of patients on GP lists. GP contractors have been able to secure extra income by handing over responsibilities to the rising number of salaried GPs – often women – whose income is usually substantially less than the average net income for contractors. The average income (before tax) for salaried GPs was between £50,000 and £60,000 a year, with fewer than 5% earning over £100,000.[13]

A Parliamentary answer to me revealed that between 1997/8 and 2008/9 the expenditure on GP medical services doubled from about £4billion to £8billion a year in real terms. (It had risen to £8.5billion in 2005/6 until I began clawing back some of the excessive generosity of the 2003 contract.)[14] In these circumstances it is unsurprising that new entrants have entered the market under new contracts. These entrants fall into two groups: Alternative Provider Medical Services (APMS) contracts and Primary Care Trust Medical Services (PCTMS). The latter are where PCTs employ staff directly and manage the provision of services themselves. APMS allow contracts to be bid for by the private, voluntary or public sectors. 2009 information from the Information Centre shows 173 practices holding APMS contracts of which 35% are administered by private companies. There are another 23 practices where the contract seems to be a PMS contract run by a limited company.[15] There has been an expansion in the services offered through GP surgeries, as more nurses (especially specialist nurses), midwives, health visitors, physiotherapists and other professionals employed by PCTs and others are based in or linked with GP practices.

The GP model has served the NHS well and is still popular with the public, despite its limitations and the case of Dr Harold Shipman murdering 300 or so of his patients. GPs continue to secure high ratings in public trust surveys, especially compared with Ministers, MPs and journalists. The annual patient surveys of GPs that I established show continuing public satisfaction even if the response rates are a bit low. In the 2008/9 survey, with a 38% response rate, 70% of the public found it easy to get through on the telephone; and over 80% could see the GP on the same day or within two days. Of those who tried to book ahead, three-quarters could do so. Only 6% waited more than 30 minutes past their appointment time; there were high satisfaction rates with premises and practice nurses; and 90% were pleased overall with the care they received.[16]

Although there is plenty of room for improvement on opening hours and booking appointments, general practice provides a respectable platform for GPs to take on wider roles and be change-agents as well as gatekeepers. Much depends on whether a critical mass of GPs are willing to invest the time, effort and money to do so and if they can secure greater access for their patients to specialist services outside hospitals – as happened to some extent under GP fundholding and more recently with PBC. There remains a problem about the ability of many GPs to exert influence over the capacity and effectiveness of community-based services outside their direct control and their ability to commission specialist and other services from budgets that they control. GPs can be critical of the vision of transferring more work outside hospitals but if this is to happen, other changes are also necessary because GPs cannot do this on their own.

First we need to incentivise a higher growth rate for people qualifying as GPs and health professionals working in the community. Second we need the facilities and support staff that will coax specialists out of their hospitals to undertake more sessions in the community. Third we need to continue expanding the number of GPs with special interests. And lastly we need to expand the work started at bringing more private companies with the necessary scale and management capacity to provide NHS primary and community services. For all these things to happen the infrastructure for services being provided outside hospitals – facilities, equipment, technology, IT and transport – need to be strengthened either through public capital or by incentivising GPs or the private sector to invest more in this sphere. Above all the community health services need to significantly improve their management and productivity, expand capacity and become better integrated with general practice.

Community health services

Historically investment in community facilities and staff has been modest but it improved under
Labour. Community health services now account for about 10% of NHS expenditure but have virtually no performance measures. Indeed DH admitted following the Darzi Review that these services lack robust data, tariffs or metrics. Between PCT areas there is a large variation in quality, care pathways and costs. Much of the infrastructure, technology and buildings are outdated as DH have acknowledged. Yet these community services are critical with an ageing population, with nearly 60% of those over 85 in contact with district nurses: stroke, continence issues and wound care are three of the main areas of work for these nurses.

More than 250,000 nurses, health visitors, pharmacists, midwives, therapists and other health professionals work in NHS community health services. These PCT- managed staff do not include the 114,000 staff (72,000 WTEs) in GP practices mentioned above; but only about a quarter of GP staff are practice nurses or other 'direct patient care' staff. So alongside GPs there are about 300,000 clinical staff working in the community. In a 2009 Parliamentary answer I was told that between 1997/1998 and 2008/2009 community health services annual expenditure had increased in real terms from about £2.8billion to £7billion.[17] A significant part of that increase would have gone on staff costs – either more staff, better pay or a combination of the two. However from evidence I acquired in early 2009 when chairing the London SHA Provider Agency it would be safe to assume considerable variability in the efficiency and productivity of these community staff.

A London study by external consultants looked at the performance of district nurses and health visitors and in particular the percentage of time they spent with a patient. For district nursing across London the average observed face time (including travel time) was around 25% with no PCT achieving 50%. A desirable and plausible target was 70% and the consultants had observed this and an average over 50% in some areas outside London. For health visitors the figures were much better with an average of 47%, nearly double that for district nurses. If the 70% target had been reached the consultants estimated that the NHS in London could either have saved between £25million - £30million a year or achieved well over an extra million visits a year to patients from London's district nurse and health visitors' workforce.[18] However much one wants to critique the consultants' methodology there was a message that better organisation and management of community health services would deliver significant productivity gains. There is no reason to believe London is an exception because the DH has admitted that community health services have the potential for a 10%-20% improvement in their productivity and efficiency.[19]

In summary Labour has funded a substantial expansion of community health staff and GP capacity but done little to ensure a good return from this investment in terms of efficiency or productivity. The evidence suggests considerable scope for improvement if these primary and community services were organised and managed more effectively. These organisational and management issues include the facilities in which people are housed, co-location of services with social care and other agencies, administrative support and networked IT and management capability. Inevitably the issue arises of whether a substantial injection of new providers and competition would not transform services outside hospital and their ability to take on wider roles.

Infrastructure, management capacity and competition in community services

Increasing the capability of community health and primary care services requires a credible physical infrastructure and management capacity that could cope with a major shift of work from hospitals and expand GP commissioning. Labour's extra money has not done a great deal to improve infrastructure and management capacity. This was recognised by

Ara Darzi in his London Review with his proposed new model of polyclinics as a base for shifting care outside hospitals but which was opposed by many GPs. Progress on providing new facilities is inevitably slow and relies heavily on local management – PCTs and GPs - to bring about change. Transforming Community Services – a DH initiative - had a budget of £4million in 2009/10, a drop in the ocean for what needs to be done.

A longer-term programme was launched by Alan Johnson to provide 100-150 GP-led health centres in PCT areas with the greatest shortage of GPs, and a few polyclinics are in the pipeline. The backlog of maintenance in GP premises is considerable and the upgrading of these premises depends a great deal on groups of GPs using their profits to expand capacity. There are still far too many small practices, with one or two partners, who lack the resources or will (or both) to expand their facilities or services or to join with other GPs to do so. The fantasy of the virtues of single-handed general practice is still alive and well in the minds of BMA negotiators and some parts of the public, especially older patients. The lack of investment in management capability and the fragility of some GP consortia have limited the scope for GP commissioning; but

facilities and technology have improved under Labour. Chapter 8 describes the expansion of the community health and GP IT programmes such as the electronic transfer of patient records, Choose and Book for health appointments, access to confidential NHS email and electronic prescribing. As the Connecting for Health programme is more fully implemented the connectivity of GP and community health services will improve further. Yet telecare and assistive technologies remain hugely under-exploited in NHS primary and community services. New community and GP facilities have been built on a greater scale than in the parsimonious Conservative years, especially through the LIFT schemes, but the investment has been modest compared with that in hospitals. In few areas are there credible plans stretching into the future for an expansion of well-managed and integrated primary and community health services linked to social care and accommodated in appropriate facilities that could provide for patient treatment and care closer to home.

New service providers can more easily enter poorer areas where the NHS has failed those communities but there has been a reluctance at the heart of government to use market-testing to replace the many inadequate primary care and community services with new investment, new service models and new management. The Darzi polyclinic model has struggled to make progress. Instead more recently we have seen DH Ministers pursuing haltingly a programme that separates the service provider arms into autonomous provider organisations (APOs) within the PCT so that the NHS jigsaw can be rearranged without letting in many outsiders through market-testing. Just prior to the 2010 Election these APOs were on the threshold of SHA overseen reconfigurations that fit into four main models: standing alone as Direct Provider Organisations; mergers with each other; the conversion of some into Community Foundation Trusts; and vertical integration of APOs into a hospital trust. This would be another NHS reorganisation with little emphasis on either competition or integration with primary or social care.

In March 2010 the DH quietly but complacently announced that good progress was being made with developing and assuring PCT proposals for the future provision of their directly-provided community services. Eight proposals (often involving several PCTs) were approved to go forward to apply to Monitor to become Community Foundation Trusts: Norfolk; Hertfordshire; Cambridgeshire; South Birmingham; East and Coastal Kent; Central London; Liverpool; Ashton Leigh and Wigan with Warrington. Six were approved in principle to continue as Direct Provider Organisation: Tower Hamlets, Cumbria, Knowsley, Wirral, Isle of Wight, Stoke on Trent.[20] Some APOs were seeking to convince the Competition and Collaboration Panel that they could merge with each other or vertically integrate with an acute trust. Virtually all these proposals avoided outside challenge. They show the NHS doing what it does so well, complacently creating new monopolies when old ones fail, rather than put services out to tender and let new providers enter the fray in the public interest. Their actions are often encouraged covertly by Ministers, and sometimes openly.

Just before the 2010 Election was called the East of England SHA did try to use competitive processes for the future of its PCT community services and was prevented from doing so by the then Health Secretary, Andy Burnham. The Competition and Collaboration Panel had to cease consideration of a case involving one PCT where the voluntary and private sector had complained. I raised in Parliament the issue of what was going on in the East of England because I considered that the DH action might be in breach of EU competition law and I thought that the Health Secretary might well have ignored legal advice that his new 'NHS as preferred provider' policy could be illegal.[21] The challenges led to unconvincing new DH guidance on PCT procurement rules being issued just before the Election, which hopefully will not survive too long with a change of government.

Despite the extra resources invested in community health services, the weak management, lack of performance regimes, inadequate infrastructure and lack of competition, mean that serious doubts remain about whether these services can deliver a step increase in care closer to home. In too many areas these services are not integrated properly with primary care or adult social care. Too few GPs have taken positive steps to link their own services with community health services in shared common facilities, although I did open a few model centres which housed GPs, community health, mental health and social care on a single site. In many areas GPs have not been drivers for change and improvement in the way community services are run. Many GPs were decidedly frosty towards Ara Darzi's polyclinics proposal and have been reluctant to use the LIFT programme for more ambitious schemes. Too many GPs have preferred relaxing into the financial comfort zone provided by the 2003 new contract.

Commissioning and GPs

There are undoubtedly many reform-minded GPs with an appetite for change in the way services are delivered in the community. I worked with some of them in the development of PBC as described in Chapter 4. Many of these change agents had been GP fundholders who were willing to take on new roles and challenge established practices in local hospitals. Since the days of fundholding there have been some helpful changes in general practice as I have outlined: larger groups of GPs; a wider range of contracts; new private providers with stronger infrastructure and investment capability; and increased GP capacity, with more GPs pursuing special interests.

Yet both GP fundholding and PBC have been limited in their achievements. Much GP fundholder attention was focussed on outpatients' elective surgery rather than the full range of hospital activity. Their activities were confined to some 20% of the NHS budget. Only about half of GPs at the time took part in fundholding, with many parts of the country untouched by it (especially inner-cities with 1 or 2 doctor practices). The extra management and clerical costs of handling transactions could cost more than the benefits achieved. This mixed record has been brought out in a 1996 Audit Commission report and other studies described in a recent Nuffield Trust briefing.[22]

PBC was hard work to get going as I have shown. Far too many PCT commissioners felt threatened by PBC and failed to work cooperatively with GP commissioners. Budgeting and service information was too often not provided at all or in a timely fashion. Too often GPs lost heart at the lack of interest in PBC shown by their PCTs. As with GP fundholding, PBC has not been able to achieve a transformational shift in the way services traditionally provided in hospital are delivered or check rising expenditure by PCTs on acute hospital services. PBC has not provided the range and volume of new models of care delivered in the community that I and other supporters of GP commissioning would have expected to see. This lack of progress with PBC was identified in a Health Select Committee report published just before the 2010 Election.[23]

To date neither GP fundholding nor PBC have been able to effectively challenge the might of the acute hospital sector and produce large-scale changes in the way services are delivered outside of hospitals. The weakness of many PCT commissioners has undoubtedly been a contributory factor but there are also limitations within general practice itself. Too many GPs are reluctant to expand their range of responsibilities to achieve an enterprise of sufficient scale to justify the investment needed. The average size of GP practices at under 7000 patients is simply too small for effective commissioning or to provide a large range of community-based services. So far insufficient larger-scale independent sector GP organisations have entered the market – or been allowed to do so – to compensate for reluctant GP incumbents who prefer more traditional gate-keeping roles and forms of practice organisation. This is unlikely to change much while there are 150 PCTs whose very existence is threatened by a more dynamic commissioning role for GPs.

The new Coalition Government clearly believe that GPs can be change agents through commissioning despite the limited success of both fund holding and PBC. The White Paper they published in July 2010 makes it clear that GPs and other primary care professionals will be put in charge of redesigning patient care pathways through commissioning. Local consortia of GP practices will have the responsibility for commissioning services and hold the budgets for doing so.[24] This is an extremely bold gamble and assumes that you can scale up successful, entrepreneurial clinical businesses to a much larger scale. It also assumes there is a critical mass of able and supportive GPs to tow many of their more reluctant colleagues into a brave new world.

The decision now seems to have been made for GPs. They are to become change agents as well as gate keepers; and will work in new configurations, with people with different skill sets. The financial responsibilities they will collectively assume will increase substantially. Some GPs will support these changes more than others; and some will be highly uncomfortable about the new roles envisaged for them. The enthusiasts will end up in a leadership role, towing the rest into a new world for general practice unless there is overwhelming resistance from the mass of GPs. The extra GP capacity, extra community and primary care investment and the new GP contract provided by Labour will all help with the changing and expanded role envisaged for GPs. However the community services infrastructure and management do not match the Coalition Government's vision and need considerable enhancement. How this will all work out in practice remains to be seen but weak community services efficiency and productivity remains an important issue for attention.

8

Computer games – connecting for health

Creating a national programme

The National Programme for IT (NPfIT) was probably the most frustrating item in my Ministerial portfolio. It was a complex ten-year programme supposedly ending in 2013/14 and estimated to cost over £12billion without the local NHS costs of implementation. Its main aims were to provide a single transferable electronic patient record for all NHS patients; and connect up over 30,000 GPs with over 300 hospital trusts and thousands of pharmacies. This programme was said to be the largest civil IT project in the world. It was at the heart of the Labour Government's attempts to bring e-Government to public services often reluctant to embrace IT. It aroused considerable passion – for and against – within the NHS which had no real experience of networked IT. It provoked civil libertarians opposed to giant government databases holding personal data. It was a ready target for those who doubted any government's ability to both contract for and implement large-scale computer programmes and to safeguard the privacy of personal data held on these databases. It was not the kind of project for which Ministers rushed to be responsible.

One of my first Ministerial actions was to remove my desktop computer which was a distraction. I was certainly not a computer buff looking to roll an IT steamroller over the NHS. However I value data and easy access to it and I assumed clinicians did too. To achieve this meant supporting technology that could transfer data swiftly in line with the needs of modern medicine. If patients were to exercise choice they needed information readily available. Patients move around so information about them needs to be mobile. The NHS paper-based information systems were cumbersome, often unreliable and increasingly costly to operate. The Government had rightly tried to tackle these problems through NPfIT which began in October 2002. By the time I arrived in 2005 its opponents were beginning to build up the noise level. Many of the criticisms were unfair; some were politically opportunistic; but equally the DH marketing of NPfIT was weak and implementation was too slow, particularly of the electronic patient record. Evidence of clinical benefit was in short supply. A rose-tinted view of the pre-IT NHS was developing, alongside a rewriting of NPfIT's history – or Connecting for Health as it was re-branded in April 2005.

Origins of NPfIT

Prior to the Labour Government the NHS had been working to a 1992 NHS Information Strategy which tried to create a new infrastructure for IT based on national standards which in theory would enable local systems to operate with each other. The reality was lots of local initiatives but little inter-operability. Although in 1997 the NHS was spending some money on computer systems – particularly in general practice – a common feature of these systems was their incompatibility and their inability to pass information from site to site. To move information from one place to another the NHS relied on paper or word of mouth. When patients changed GP their (usually bulky) paper records went by Royal Mail to the new GPs – earlier in the NHS's history via a clearing house in Southport. Most arrived with the new GP many weeks later but some were lost on the way. Unkind but largely accurate critics have described the pre-1997 NHS as one of the last bastions of garage-built computer systems and paper.

In 1998 Labour launched a new national strategy to support the development and implementation of electronic patient records but relying on each health authority to create their own local implementation strategies.[1] This resulted in an electronic record pilot programme known as ERDIP which produced a few successful but small-scale local installations. This programme failed to be taken up nationally for three main reasons. There was a lack of local funding for IT because these budgets were not ring-fenced and were used for other purposes. A high degree of variability in local standards operated, with most hospitals continuing to work with separate unintegrated departmental clinical systems because hospital consultants could not agree on an integrated system. Thirdly there were considerable cost inefficiencies from buying one-off separate local systems which made this approach unaffordable nationally.

The ERDIP programme only lasted three years and led to a new DH strategy group being set up under the chairmanship of Sir John Pattison, then the DH Director of Research, Analysis and Information. This group produced in 2002 a report which became the genesis of NPfIT, with four key strands.[2] These were the idea of a lifelong patient record with details held locally and a summary record available nationally; a system to deliver prescriptions electronically between GP practices and pharmacies; and another one to enable electronic booking between GPs and hospitals. The fourth would be an NHS broadband infrastructure - later to be called N3. Despite later rewriting of history by critics that there had been little consultation with NHS users, the 2002 strategy was the result of learning from the ERDIP pilots; and an extensive consultation with NHS users by the then NHS Information Authority. Hundreds of frontline users were consulted about their experiences with the regional procurements which had suffered major affordability problems. Conservative politicians who weighed into NPfIT conveniently forgot the considerable difficulties that their Government had experienced with devising NHS computer systems that went live at an affordable price and were inter-operable. One of the achievements of NPfIT was that it did learn from NHS experience of previous mistaken approaches.

Indeed it was the consultation with the NHS that led to two significant additions to NPfIT that were not in the 2002 strategy document. The first and most significant of these was Picture Archiving and Communications Systems (PACS) which arose from the NHS's wish to move to film-less hospital diagnostic imaging departments. For the previous hundred years film had been almost the exclusive medium for capturing, storing and displaying radiographic images of patients. Much like a digital camera PACS captures X-rays and scans and stores them electronically. Images became more quickly available because they did not need to be transported by hand – often from hospital basements; and they could be studied at different locations. Lost X-rays – up to 12% of the total – became a thing of the past; and the NHS no longer had to give over space storing X-rays. The second addition was an online GP payment system, following the 2003 GP contract, which was implemented by NPfIT in six months.

By the time I arrived as the responsible Minister in 2005 the shape and scale of the NPfIT had been largely settled, with a complex set of inter-related programmes. Each element had its own purpose but most contributed to a common goal of moving patient clinical information around a complex and dispersed healthcare system spread over thousands of outlets. Some projects such as implementing a new broadband system for the whole NHS provided the foundation for other parts of the system to operate. Many of these 'foundation' type projects had to be delivered first which meant that the clinical advantages of NPfIT took longer to show. A wholly transferable electronic patient record was not possible without a functioning spine containing a Personal Demographic System (PDS). The sheer scale and complexity of what was being attempted was rarely acknowledged by many of the critics of the NPfIT.

In May 2005 the NPfIT had eight core projects to complete:

- N3 – the new secure broadband national network for the NHS.
- The NHS Care Record Service (CRS) which was at the core of the new system with a PDS which stored basic demographic information about each patient and their NHS number as an identifier. When complete the CRS would enable patient information from different parts of the NHS to be linked electronically with detailed records

kept locally and a Summary Care Record that would be available across all NHS organisations in England to meet the needs of out of hours and emergency care. (Scotland, Wales and Northern Ireland had declined to be part of this system.)

- Picture Archiving Communications Systems (PACS) which would replace film-based systems with digital X-rays and scans.
- Electronic Transfer of Prescriptions (ETP) which would enable prescriptions to be sent electronically from GP prescribers to the pharmacy to reduce errors and costs and increase patient convenience.
- Choose and Book (CAB) which was a new electronic booking system enabling GPs and patients to book first outpatient specialist hospital appointments so that patients could choose the most convenient available appointment from different hospitals.
- Support for general practice IT, including several programmes: choice of GP systems; GP2GP which transferred patient records electronically when people changed GP; and QMAS a new system for paying GPs under their new contract.
- NHS mail (or Contact as it was re-named) which provided a secure e-mail and directory service for the NHS.
- Secondary User Services (SUS) which provided the NHS with high quality data to enable investigation of trends and emerging health needs that could inform health policy. SUS was of particular benefit to researchers and had a capacity to anonymise individual patient data for the benefit of research.

These core projects were demanding enough in themselves but NPfIT had accumulated other "must do" projects. Depending on whom you talked to the reason for this 'mission creep' was either empire building by the programme or political/top management pressure on the programme director. Choose and Book and QMAS were definitely the result of political pressure and PACS resulted from NHS pressure, but many other programme elements arose from opportunistic interventions by DH and the local NHS. The NPfIT project I inherited had many additional elements from those originally intended, whatever their source. These included Single Assessment Process systems for care of the elderly; the Map of Medicine which provided electronic support to prescribers; radiology, A & E and theatre systems; and replacement of patient administration systems (PAS) because so many were on the verge of collapse. There were also new ambulance communication systems; community, clinical and child health systems (for immunisation and vaccination programmes); and systems to support care in prisons. There were also systems to support processes such as data-mining and placing orders, as well as the new 'Smart Card' registration system to ensure access security for NPfIT.

It is not difficult to justify the addition of these individual items and there may well be others before the programme is completed. But together they increased substantially the complexity of NPfIT's management, the scope for things to go wrong and the ability of the programme's critics to mount attacks. As an incoming Minister there was little I could do about the programme's scope and scale. The hand had been dealt, as it had been with NPfIT's contracts.

Contracts, contractors and momentum

Public sector IT contracts – including earlier NHS experiences – have been bedevilled by substantial cost overruns and non-delivery by contractors within agreed timescales. Government departments had been - and continue to be - criticised for agreeing contracts which placed all the risk with them rather than the contractors. Protecting the taxpayer in NPfIT contracts had been taken to heart by Richard Grainger who had taken up the post of DH's Director-General of NHS IT in October 2002. Richard had been involved with large scale IT programmes including the London congestion charging scheme and was said to be the highest paid civil servant, earning more than the Prime Minister - which attracted regular media attention. Richard was the architect of the contract system for purchasing and running NPfIT.

The contract architecture Grainger had devised was divided between national and local programmes. For the local programmes England was divided originally into five "clusters" – Southern, London, East and East Midlands, North West and West Midlands and North East. A Local Service Provider (LSP) was contracted to deliver NPfIT in each of those areas. This structure avoided dependence on a single supplier and introduced a measure of competition. The benefits of this approach became apparent later when two LSPs – Accenture and Fujitsu - withdrew (see below). The original five LSPs were CSC for North West and West Midlands; BT for London; Accenture for both the North East and East Anglia/East Midlands; and Fujitsu for the South. In addition National Application Service providers were contracted for services common to all users like Choose and Book and the Care Record Service (CRS). BT took on responsibility for the CRS and the new national broadband network (N3). ATOS were chosen for Choose and Book and EDS for NHS E-mail. Underneath these main contractors were a series of subcontractors, the most significant of which were those chosen to produce the software for the CRS which continues to be the programme's biggest problem.

When the NPfIT contracts were let in 2003 they were seen as a model for government IT procurement with their transfer of risk to the private sector. Giving evidence later to the Public Accounts Committee, the then Chief Executive of the Office of Government Commerce, John Oughton said: "I think the procurement process for Connecting for Health was an exemplary example of procurement. It was run to a very tight and rapid timescale; it started when it was intended and completed when it was intended; and it produced a very good result. I do not think any of the suppliers were disadvantaged in that process."[3]

Whatever revisionist views developed subsequently Richard Grainger was the golden boy of government IT contracting when I became responsible for NPfIT in 2005. When I went to Cabinet Committee meetings, other government departments struggling with their IT programmes were encouraged to look at the DH experience. Contractors were paid only when they delivered and that was that. They had gone into the contracts with their eyes open and were global companies with armies of lawyers and accountants who were unlikely to be bamboozled by Richard Grainger and DH civil servants. It was clear to me from my meetings with senior personnel from the main contractors that they knew what the score was with NPfIT contracts. The difference for them from some other government contracts was that Warner and Grainger stuck to the NPfIT contracts when things started to wrong. We paid only for what had been delivered.

Some things had gone awry before my arrival. In March 2004 EDS had their ten year contract to supply NHS Mail terminated and they were replaced in July by Cable and Wireless. In 2005 IDX Systems Corporation were starting to fail to meet deadlines in the Southern Cluster. In August 2005 Fujitsu cancelled the IDX contract and replaced them in September with Cerner Corporation. Shortly after I arrived there were problems for CSC CoM Medical's contract for supplying PACS in the North West and West Midlands. In early 2006 CoM Medicare were replaced by GE Healthcare. All these instances however showed the strength of the NPfIT contracting methodology. If main contractors were being let down by subcontractors and didn't get paid they replaced the subcontractors with no financial consequences for the taxpayer. The former Chief Executive of BT, Ben Verwaayen, told the Sunday Times in May 2006: "Richard Grainger is doing a good job. He's one of our most difficult, demanding and therefore capable customers." Verwaayen said Grainger's critics had got the scale of NPfIT's problems out of perspective and needed to understand the extent of the changes being implemented.[4] Few critics took much notice of this experienced Chief Executive's view.

These contractor failures provided some warning signs: it took time to replace contractors and deadlines for implementation slipped. We were two years into the contracts and there were few frontline systems in operation which did not help NHS support for the project. In Spring 2005 there were well under 100 local systems installed and working, nearly all of which were relatively small – Choose and Book, GP systems and Single Assessment Process systems for the elderly. No new PASs had been implemented and the NHS frontline had little to show for the national programme. GPs were being restricted on the IT systems they could choose and might be required to relinquish systems they had developed personally. Local people were waiting for NPfIT to replace systems that were falling apart, sometimes believing misguidedly that NPfIT would pay for all the transition to new systems. The gloss was wearing off and main contractors were struggling to implement too secure payment. We might be saving taxpayers' money by not paying for work not done but we were not transforming the NHS electronically either.

By the autumn of 2005 NPfIT was heading for a big under-spend. This was helpful in terms of the DH budget overspend (see Chapter 9) but not in terms of progressing Connecting for Health. I accelerated the take-up of Choose and Book systems as part of the choice agenda and I encouraged more action on the electronic transfer of prescriptions and PACS at my regular meetings with the NPfIT team. Some local patient administration systems were on the verge of collapse and more effort was needed on these. There was growing unrest among GPs about the rigidity of NPfIT over the replacement of their systems. After a lot of pressure and some difficult negotiations, I persuaded Richard Grainger to give GPs a wider choice and to use some existing suppliers to GPs, providing there was compatibility with the NPfIT systems' architecture.

These efforts led to an increase in the number of local systems installed in 2005/6 despite the financial problems in the NHS. Between April 2005 and March 2006 over 5000 local systems were installed, over 4000 of them Choose and Book systems. About 60 PASs and over 300 GP systems were installed but unfortunately few of them were in big acute hospitals where they were badly needed. Nevertheless this frontline system activity was a major improvement on the previous year.[5]

Problems increased with the software for electronic patient records. IDX was in difficulties financially and concerns were being expressed about the business practices of Isoft, the software company working in the North. Isoft issued a huge profits warning in mid-2006 and revised their previous year's accounts. The value of their shares dropped by 90%, leading to the sale of the company and a Financial Services Authority inquiry, only recently ended. The Isoft solution for the patient record, Lorenzo, was popular with doctors, but has remained a major cause for concern in terms of successful implementation in hospitals. The timetable for most of the core projects was slipping and people were beginning to notice.

The National Audit Office started an enquiry. Complaints over lack of payments were starting to be heard from main contractors as we moved into early 2006. My growing suspicion was that with the expanding global demand for IT skills, many of the contractors were struggling to attract talent. I thought we might also have too narrow a range of sub-contractors but Grainger's team did not agree. The financial year 2006/7 brought both greater progress through increased pressure on contractors and the greatest contract challenges. The big event was the demise of Accenture.

In Spring 2006 Accenture made public that it was making a provision in its accounts of $450million (£237million) for losses on NPfIT because of delays in delivering software by Isoft (i.e. the Lorenzo system). I knew things were getting serious when at one of my meetings with the main contractors, Accenture's UK representative was accompanied by a colleague from US headquarters who looked as though he was auditioning for The Sopranos. The Accenture situation continued to deteriorate. Driving back from Scotland from a break with my family I had to pull off the road to take a call from Richard Grainger saying that unless we coughed up more money by their next Board Meeting then Accenture might well walk away from the project. I thought this a rather crude blackmail and I told Grainger to hold them to the contract and only pay for what had been delivered.

The crunch came in August when Accenture said they wished to withdraw from their contract. We could have said 'See you in Court' which would have led to a lengthy hiatus in delivering the NPfIT or tried to negotiate new terms. This would have involved giving them more money when their delivery record was poor and would have encouraged others to pull the same stunt. There was also an option of transferring the hospital work to CSC, leaving Accenture to deliver the primary care element. This would have lost economies of scale and pushed up the total programme cost over 10 years by well over £0.5billion. I did not fancy any of these options. My preferred approach was to transfer the whole contract to CSC for 9 years at the same price as we would have paid Accenture – nearly £2billion – and pay Accenture just for the work they had done – about £50million. This enabled CSC to continue supporting Isoft – a British company – and those NHS organisations using Isoft. These were my negotiating instructions to Richard Grainger and this was the deal that was done with CSC, with Accenture allowed to keep implementation of PACS which they were doing effectively.

The temptation to go after Accenture in public was enormous. They had let us down badly and subsequently I found out that Sainsbury's and

Centrica had had difficult experiences with them. However NPfIT's monitoring had not picked up that the software supplier's description of progress was so removed from reality. (Isoft's product, Lorenzo, has continued to be a major problem both for CSC and the NHS.) There was the bigger agenda of trying to make progress with NHS implementation which a lengthy virility contest with Accenture would not help. There were external critics who argued that if a knowledgeable firm like Accenture could see no future in the programme then that boded ill for NPfIT. We found ourselves with a PAC enquiry to handle and a growing row over the security and confidentiality of the system (see below), as well as maintaining implementation momentum. I was relieved to get some media support for our approach. Michael Cross in The Guardian said "Congratulations to the NHS for facing down Accenture" and added correctly that Accenture "should have known that the NHS faced a technical challenge of unprecedented complexity". In a slightly backhanded way he even congratulated Ministers on holding their nerve.[6]

Despite all this brouhaha we maintained momentum on frontline implementation. I somewhat confounded Jeremy Paxman on Newsnight by saying I would resign if we had not implemented Choose and Book by March 2007. By the end of 2006/7 about 9,000 frontline systems had been installed. Nearly 8,000 of these were in the Electronic Prescriptions Service and Choose and Book systems. But there were also another 300 GP systems installed and the GP2GP patient record transfers were beginning to take place on some scale. Another 50 PASs were installed; and virtually all the local programme projects had some progress to show. Connecting for Health had momentum when I departed and was well on the way to 15,000 local project installations in total.[7] However progress was slow on implementing PASs in acute hospitals where only about 25 systems had been installed.

The contracting system had stood up to failure by contractors without the cost of failure being transferred to the public purse. In its 2006 report on NPfIT the National Audit Office said the programme was much needed; well managed; based on good contracts; had made substantial progress; and the central expenditure was being managed within budget. The NAO study had taken 18 months to complete but I was satisfied that it gave a fair picture of NPfIT. It said rightly that the programme had the potential to deliver substantial financial, safety and service benefits for patients and the NHS. The NAO drew attention to the fact that the programme had strong Ministerial and senior management support and was an example of best practice arrangements and structures for delivering the programme. Savings had been achieved by using NHS centralised buying power (e.g. some of the lowest Microsoft costs in the world) that provided estimated savings of £860million. The tough contract negotiations at the outset had lowered prices from bidders by £6.8billion.[8] Despite this strong endorsement the critics continued to swarm. Why all this hostility?

NHS 'buy-in' and uncertainty over costs and benefits

Although the NPfIT contracting processes were superior to previous attempts to bring the benefits of IT to the NHS they were only part of the ingredients for success. Such a centrally-managed contracting process could become a problem itself because NPfIT had at its heart massive changes to the working practices of doctors and nurses and the systems they had relied on for decades. Such IT systems as the NHS possessed had been largely designed and implemented by groups of local clinicians in GP practices and hospitals. Grainger and the Connecting for Health enthusiasts were trampling over these beloved creations with a networked system that demanded architectural compatibility. To see through this level of change successfully required a clinically-focussed marketing effort of unprecedented proportions over many years.

To move from where they were to a fully networked IT system GPs and practice managers, hospital consultants and managers and commercial pharmacies all had to invest a lot of time, effort and money. They had to replace their paper-based, film-based and unnetworked (and often obsolete) IT with new kit. Moreover the nature of the kit was to a great extent going to be dictated by people at the centre, or contractors on their behalf. The fact that these arrangements might save money and improve efficiency and benefits for patients did not always convince them of the merits of change. Then there was the matter of who paid for all the local transition work of changing processes, training staff and absorbing this centrally-driven kit and software. How was the time to be found to handle this transition with all the other NHS reforms going on?

By 2006 I knew that the DH attempts to sell and manage this transition were inadequate. Looking back now I think we got this completely wrong and I wish I had been more challenging about it then. The main problem was that the DH Management Board never really owned the project, despite a paper trail pretending it did, because the Board saw NPfIT as Grainger's project and responsibility. NPfIT was never integrated into the narrative on NHS reform and was never incorporated operationally into the priorities of SHAs and local trusts. By the time his successor attempted to do this there was a lot of ground to be made up. As Ministers we must take some responsibility for this failure but it was certainly shared with DH top management.

I found it difficult to persuade the Chief Medical Officer, Liam Donaldson, to become a strong personal advocate for the programme to the medical profession, despite the programme's potential to improve patient safety. Early on he had appointed one of his deputies, Dr Aidan Halligan, to work alongside Richard Grainger but Halligan left DH and was never really replaced. Able clinical leads for parts of the programme were appointed who I met periodically; but their efforts would have been aided enormously by a CMO willing to go on the stump for Connecting for Health with the BMA and the medical Royal Colleges and to feature the programme prominently in his annual reports. It was not to be.

At the local level the absence of clear messages over the priority NPfIT was to receive was a significant problem, made worse by the lack of clarity about what resources the local NHS had to find for implementation. This problem was exacerbated by the low base the NHS started from in terms of IT expenditure In the US the equivalent of the average well-run acute trust would be spending 4% or more on IT and would secure a lot of clinical benefit and management efficiency in return. In the UK in 2005 it was probably less than 2%. To run an IT system that secured the benefits of Connecting for Health the NHS would have to spend much more annually on IT to achieve the efficiency gains and patient benefits. At the point of transition, with staff training and moving data into new systems, the annual cost would be more before the benefits were achieved. The management effort for the transition would be considerable. None of this was properly explained to the local NHS or built into their annual operating plans and priorities.

When the rows over NPfIT hotted up in the spring of 2006 its critics kicked up a lot of dust over the programme's costs, claiming that costs were out of control and the ten-year programme would cost £30billion. The true published figures – accepted by the NAO – were £6.8billion for core national contracts; £2.2billion for national implementation activity and new projects; and £3.4billion of local expenditure on NHS implementation of CRS and PACS. This was a total of £12.4billion at 2004/5 prices over a ten-year period. I had always thought that this understated the true cost of implementation locally but nothing like as high as £30billion over ten years.

With the help of officials I tried to construct a better estimate of what the total cost of implementing this programme would be over its duration. I considered that the NHS might well be expected to spend an average of £1billion a year or so on IT as more and more of the programme came on stream alongside the central contracts. The more reasonable total cost seemed to me to be likely to be about £20billion in total, although there would be unmeasured but considerable offsetting benefits/savings, some of which would come on stream before the programme's full implementation. To counter the flow of stories about NPfIT costing £30billion I gave an interview to Nick Timmins of the Financial Times to get across my views on costs and explain why the electronic patient's record was going to be delayed.[9]

This did little to quieten the critics who were quite unwilling to accept that it had always been the case that the central contracts were only part of the cost story or that the NHS simply spent too little on IT for a modern healthcare system. The local NHS declined to accept that they would be wise to spend more on IT while extra money was available in order to secure the future benefits. We were too slow in producing an effective narrative for the NHS on the benefits of Connecting for Health and this was one of the few criticisms made by the NAO.

I tried to prod the DH into action on explaining NPfIT's benefits but without much success. It was to be long after my departure that in early 2008 DH published the first coherent "Benefits Statement" for NPfIT, covering the period to the end of 2006/7. This revealed that over 14,000 frontline systems had been installed under the programme by the end of March 2007. For the first time the DH was able to show the actual and recurring savings on the money spent so far. There were cash-releasing savings of over £200million at the end of March 2007, which in the seven remaining years of the contracts (i.e. to the end of March 2014) would produce over £1.1billion of NHS savings, with the recurring savings stretching into the future.[10] This was the return on the £2.4billion spent so far by NPfIT on the systems delivering these benefits. It took no account of the benefits that would accrue from an electronic patient record; or what the NHS would have had to spend to keep old, outdated systems going. In other words, by early 2007 Connecting for Health was representing good value for money despite its critics but the story had not been told publicly.

It was not until August 2006 that action was taken to operationalise NHS responsibility for implementing NPfIT by David Nicholson. He made clear that responsibility for the implementation and benefits realisation rested with the SHA and PCT Chief Executives under a new NPfIT Local Ownership Programme (NLOP).[11] nfortunately it took until July 2007 to transfer responsibility for management and the associated resources to the SHAs so there was further delay while SHAs negotiated with the programme's central staff.

The critics

By the second half of 2006 the absence of a clear narrative on costs and benefits, contractor failure and delays and the lack of clinical and NHS buy-in was providing fertile grounds for a growing band of critics. The lack of progress on the electronic patient record and the increasing noise about the confidentiality and privacy issues relating to the record only encouraged persistent sniping at NPfIT. Much of this came from a group of information technologists and Conservative Party supporters, with Computer Weekly as their vehicle of choice. Some of this was good old-fashioned Opposition politics which I didn't take too seriously. Some of it was IT people deeply suspicious of any big government IT programme with large databases and networked systems. Some of these critics seemed to hate the idea of any government IT project ever being successful or well managed. There was a strong civil libertarian strand to this criticism which thought giving personal data to government IT systems was inherently bad because it was bound to be misused and would not be secure. Any facts or arguments on patient benefits, true costs, realistic implementation timescales and security systems were simply disbelieved or ignored. It was a dialogue with the deaf.

As a Government Minister it is difficult to complain about an orchestrated campaign against a government programme like NPfIT without appearing paranoid and over-sensitive - Richard Grainger and his team were more convinced that the criticism was orchestrated than I was but they had some evidence to support their views and many of the critics were unfair, unpleasant and difficult to expose. Grainger was a strong contracts manager but he was not the person to sell Connecting for Health to the outside world. He became, unfairly, a personal focus for the critics; and his naturally combative style only attracted more gunfire. As a Minister I needed to defend him and the programme but lacked a Departmental capability to mount an effective counterattack to the critics.

It was only after my resignation as a Minister that the extent of an orchestrated campaign against NPfIT became apparent to me from a large volume of emails sent to me anonymously covering the period of 2006 and 2007. I was able to draw on these in a House of Lords debate on 21 June 2007 on Public Sector IT projects. It is worth quoting verbatim from Hansard what I said in that debate.[12]

> "Some of my puzzlement over hostility to the programme has been removed, since leaving office, by discovering people working together to campaign against this programme. The campaign seems to be made up of the Foundation for Information Policy Research, the Big Opt Out organisation, the Conservative Technology Forum, Computer Weekly, Medix surveys and the Worshipful Company of Information Technologies, which I only recently discovered. An energetic presence in this network is a Cambridge professor called Ross Anderson. Some interesting e-mails of his have found their way to me. One e-mail of 27 November 2006 says:
>
> "The Big Opt Out Org will be a separate campaign (which many of those help). The principle organiser is Helen Wilkinson" – who I believe is a Conservative Councillor. Another e-mail of 13 February, talks about "how we might put the IC on the spot".

"The IC is, of course the Information Commissioner. Another e-mail of 8 March, after Professor Anderson had been asked to be an adviser to the Health Select Committee, says: *"Well I said yes on the grounds that I can probably do more on the inside than on the outside."*

"Another e-mail which I particularly like is of 24 May 2007 sent after a lunch with Conservative front bench spokesmen Damien Green MP who is quoted as saying: *"The Tories had taken an uncharacteristically principled line on the ID card and now felt exposed."*

"Ross was asked to provide some other arguments – a little less principled, I assume. Finally in a quote from an e-mail of 20 December 2006 we have something a little closer to home: *"After speaking to Andrew Lansley, Tim Loughton, Malcolm Harbour and Lord Lucas I may be starting to get the message across."*

"I have insufficient time to entertain the House with more extracts. I am willing to let them be seen on a private basis by my honourable friend in the other place who chairs the Health Select Committee. In a spirit of bipartisanship, I would encourage Conservative parliamentarians to look closely and sceptically at some of the sources of advice they appear to be using. The Connecting for Health IT programme should not be a political football. Too much is at stake for patients and the NHS."

So it appears that some paranoia was in order as 'they really were out to get us.' I noticed that after this debate and a robust defence of the NPfIT in the House of Commons on 6 June 2007 some of the more rancorous criticism abated. The slow progress on the electronic patient record continued, rightly, to be attacked.

The electronic patient record: delays and disputes

The jewel in the crown of NPfIT was an electronic patient record (EPR). This detailed patient record would be available to locally networked services, with the national system able to transfer around the country a summary record of an individual patient's key details if there was an emergency. Such a system required a large measure of national agreement on the information to go in the EPR. For all this to work the local NHS hospitals needed to have modernised PASs. Sadly many hospital PASs were not fit for purpose and needed to be replaced; and some were on the verge of collapse, the so-called "burning platforms" in NPfIT jargon. Outside hospitals most community and mental health systems simply did not have a PAS that could easily move patient details around electronically.

Before significant benefits from an EPR could be realised it was always going to be necessary to re-equip the NHS with better local patient systems. We failed utterly to explain effectively to the NHS and the public that there was a massive modernisation of NHS local IT to be accomplished before people could have an electronic NHS Care Records Service. We have still not resolved the problem of moving the large NHS acute hospital sector to a modernised and more standardised set of PASs from one where it has a range of home-grown systems with bits added to over the years. NPfIT was never going to be able to make this happen in 3 or 4 years without a massive clinical engagement and marketing effort, together with generous local financial incentives. Even then it would have needed most NHS clinicians to be convinced that there was a working EPR that was going to meet their clinical needs at the end of the process. The failure to incentivise and persuade the acute hospital sector to transform its IT still holds back modernisation of the NHS.

Matters are further complicated by the wider challenges that programmes like NPfIT pose for public, professionals and politicians. Is there sufficient public trust of governmental agencies to place vast quantities of personal data on central databases, in order to improve the efficiency and quality of public services? The whole of the former Government's "Transformational Government" programme had this fundamental question at its heart, with different people holding fundamentally different views. Some believed that large networked databases were major threats to civil liberty, no matter what safeguards were put in place. Civil service carelessness in losing discs with huge amounts of personal data merely confirmed that these big databases should not be allowed. Individual cases of illicit entry – particularly to the personal data of celebrities – seemed to offer further proof. For these critics, records of individuals using public services should be kept locally, not networked. Transferring data between different organisations should be blocked unless personal approval has been given so that individual patients can limit the flow of their personal data around the NHS, whatever the potential benefits to their care. Some doctors are fearful of data moving outside their surgery without their patients' permission. Many of NPfIT's critics held these views and still do.

There are many other people – and I include myself amongst them – who regard it as inevitable that the great majority of the individual citizen's personal transactions with the state and public agencies are going to be electronic and digital in the future. The public services including the NHS cannot be insulated from a digital electronic revolution that is going on in society. Tax returns, benefit claims and payments, information on health issues, securing and renewing various licences, a wide range of tax payments, hospital appointments are all going electronic. These are just some of the services that are already a long way down this track. The UK public sector spends about £16billion a year on IT and this will increase further. We cannot, as a country, afford to go back to public services that ignore new technology, just as the private sector cannot. There is no turning the clock back for the NHS or other public services.

Persuading NHS professionals that a networked system of patient records will both work and benefit patients remains difficult. Most doctors want systems designed around their own circumstances and working practices. This is what GPs have done in the past and why I had to make the NPfIT more flexible about the systems on offer to them. The more standardised hospital systems offered by NPfIT tended not to provide all the bells and whistles of current local systems that clinicians wanted to retain. Until recently there were few examples of hospital-wide locally networked systems being implemented.

To make matters worse the chosen subcontractors for PAS/EPR in the NPfIT, were hardly making a great job of convincing the NHS to use their products. Cerner's anglicised version of an American system, Millennium, had significant problems with its deployment in London and the South. In the Midlands and the North the problems were even worse. I was endlessly told how positive clinicians were about Isoft's Lorenzo product and how they preferred it to Millennium. Just be patient Minister it will come right in the end. Release after release was postponed but contractually it was difficult to dump the Lorenzo product, particularly when CSC the LSP main contractor effectively took responsibility for it. You wouldn't want to dump a British company would you Minister? Well actually with hindsight I should have done so because we seem still to be waiting for the first acute trust-wide deployment of Lorenzo.

There was also the problem of the NHS's own unrealistic assessment of the effort they had to put in with staff to successfully deploy and implement these new systems. Contractors were concerned not to bankrupt themselves by picking up costs they regarded as not covered in their contracts. The scope for dispute between NHS, LSPs and software subcontractors was considerable. Amongst the subcontractors there was an absence of specialist deployers of systems who were permitted to choose alternative software systems if the main suppliers could not deliver. To convince myself that it was possible to make a networked EPR work in a major healthcare system I went to look at the US Veterans Administration (VA). When I lived in the US in the 1970s the VA had been a byword for inefficiency and lack of accountability that was always able to extract more money from Congress because veterans were involved. In the late 1990s the VA had transformed itself and at the heart of that transformation was implementation of an Electronic Health Record (EHR) networked across all the VA outlets in the US with over 200,000 employees. The EHR operated across all inpatient and outpatient environments and I saw how a patient's information follows them in all clinical situations wherever a US veteran happens to be.

Lessons from the US Veterans Administration

In Washington I met the Under Secretary for Health in the Department of Veterans' Affairs and many doctors. It had taken the VA ten years to design and implement their system and to secure the clinician "buy-in" to use it. I spoke to doctors who had been opposed to the whole idea – very similar to their English counterparts - but who now supported the EHR including its summary version. This was because whenever and wherever they saw a patient they could retrieve up-to-date data. I also discovered that the VA's EHR was also a mechanism for optimising and standardising clinical practice – a particularly threatening issue for doctors in the UK. It provides real-time error checking, clinical support and is the primary means for generating corporate and individual provider performance data. The EHR had been the main basis for improving the safety, quality and efficiency of care within the VA. A good example of this was the simple measure of what they called "patient chart availability". In 1995 patient charts had been available in only about 60% of patient/clinician encounters; ten years later it was virtually 100%.[13]

The efficiency gains of the EHR were considerable. In the US one in five lab tests are repeated; and one in seven hospitalisations occur because previous records are not available: I suspect something similar happens in the UK. Yet the VA's EHR costs about $80 a year per patient to operate, the equivalent of not repeating a moderately inexpensive lab test. I returned to the UK with the absolute conviction – which I still retain – that the VA is the best example of a live large-scale networked EPR with clinical buy-in that is able to show sceptics how such a system improves patient care and healthcare efficiency. On my return I discussed with officials, especially Harry Cayton, the DH's National Director for Patients and the Public, how we might expose the BMA and other sceptics to the VA experience. I agreed that Harry should lead a group of clinicians to see the VA system in action and learn from their experience. While this did not solve all our problems the visit did quieten down some of the noise and did change some attitudes.

Privacy and consent

I decided in June 2006 to make another attempt to gain agreement with the medical profession on the EPR. There were disagreements between GPs and hospital doctors and within each group, all of which had compounded the problems of delay. Some GPs argued that patients should be consulted before any of their information was uploaded to the network and wanted to restrict severely the amount of information recorded nationally. I asked Harry Cayton to chair a new taskforce that would develop by the end of 2006 "a detailed action plan" for speeding up implementation. Alongside this I pressed the Department to produce the long-promised information campaign that would explain the benefits of the EPR to the public. I decided to speak at the annual conference of local medical committees to announce this to GPs together with a firm date for a new set of pilots to test the uploading of personal data to the national system. I asked them to exercise more clinical leadership to ensure that patients received the benefits that an EPR could bring.

This new initiative built on work that had been started in 2005 when we had set up a Care Record Development Board to ensure that ethical issues were properly addressed. This Board represented the users of the care record, including patients, and provided independent oversight of how the care record was to be used. An NHS Care Record Guarantee had set out the rules governing use of patient information and what control patients had over it. The Guarantee had provided some reassurance to patients but there were continuing calls in the media to give patients a clear right to opt out of the Care Record Service. Critics wanted doctors to secure formal consent from all individual patients to having their medical records uploaded on to the national database. This would be time-consuming and so far the government had resisted it. However it was clear to me that we would have to give ground, particularly when The Guardian ran a write-in campaign to enable people to opt out of uploading their data nationally. I asked the Care Records Board for advice and they recommended giving people the opt-out of national uploading providing that it was explained to them that this could have adverse consequences for them in accessing appropriate healthcare.

I was determined to make progress on uploading summary patient data on to the national spine as this was the only way to progress the new Care Record Service. After publishing the Board's recommendations I decided to make concessions and start a pilot scheme in several areas. In December 2006 I gave an interview to John Carvel of The Guardian saying that we had changed our policy: "Minister admits U-turn on NHS database amid privacy fears" as The Guardian headlined it![14] I said I thought the fears of unauthorised disclosure of medical histories were groundless but if patients didn't want their data uploaded they could stop it. However I made it clear – and the Guardian printed it - that campaigners who were in the minority did not have the right to stop the scheme or prevent the majority of people having their information shared or uploaded because of the protests of a minority. I pointed out that in

Scotland where they had created an Emergency Care Record with uploaded data, only 250 people out of 6 million patients had asked for their data to be withheld. People would not have to give reasons for stopping uploading but they could not delete all their GP's data from his or her computer unless they could demonstrate mental distress. I made clear that patient control over their medical records was not absolute. Just before my departure I launched trials of uploading data in Bolton, Bury, Bradford, South Birmingham and Dorset. NPfIT wrote to nearly 650,000 patients in the five trial areas and we ran public information campaigns there on people's right to protect their data. When the trials ended two years later about 2,500 people opted out and 500 said their records could be uploaded on condition that NHS staff asked their approval on every occasion they accessed their file.

My compromise approach and the pilots enabled progress to be made after my departure. At the end of the pilots 635,000 patient records in the pilot areas were uploaded to the national database and my successors decided to start uploading the summary records in other area. New rules were agreed by the Care Records Board that required NHS staff to seek prior approval of all patients fit to give it when they access a record. The practicality of this latter proposal remains to be tested and it is not one that I would have been inclined to accept if I had still been the responsible Minister. By the beginning of 2007 the Care Record Service was progressing through a compromise on patient confidentiality that had been accepted by doctors and most critics. I had also set in train before I left a strengthening of the Care Record Board by linking it initially with the Patient Information Advisory Group, on its way to becoming part of a new statutory National Information Governance Board when a legislative opportunity presented itself. This was done in the Health and Social Care Act 2008; and the new statutory Board came into operation in January 2009 with Harry Cayton moving seamlessly to becoming the new Board's Chair.

There were still rumblings (and probably always will be) about security around access to patient records but the NPfIT's "Smart card" security system with graduated access to patient clinical information is probably as good as it is possible to achieve. Offending against it is a dismissible offence but with such a large workforce in the NHS it is almost impossible to prevent some individual blunders and malpractices – just as there had been with paper records but now with stronger sanctions.

The aftermath

On my departure from DH, NPfIT had made considerable progress despite a continuing barrage of criticism. Nearly 14,000 frontline systems had been installed. The National Spine and a secure e-mail and directory for the NHS were operating. The new system was highly reliable with system availability scores of consistently over 99.9% - equivalent to 167.9 of each week's 168 hours of operating without unplanned breakdowns. Choose and Book was fully operational although sometimes thwarted for patients by poor hospital PASs and uncooperative hospital management rather than by GPs. Nearly 100 PACS systems had been installed to give the NHS digital imaging instead of film and these were clinically popular. With about 4000 pharmacies and GP practices covered, the electronic prescription service was making steady if unspectacular progress. The row over patient confidentiality and opting out of the national database had been largely defused; and the governance structure around a Care Record Service was being strengthened. The central contracting system had been endorsed by the NAO and had coped with the failure of one of the four original Local Service Providers, Accenture.

The biggest outstanding problem was the absence of a credible plan for completing acute hospital PAS/EPR implementation. This has caused the programme to fall behind schedule despite the progress made on all the other projects. In June 2008 the NAO estimated that the care record system was 4 years behind schedule; and said bluntly that the original timetable was "unachievable, raised unrealistic expectations and put confidence in the programme at risk". It identified particular problems over deployment of the Lorenzo system; and said that delays meant only £3.6billion has been spent on new IT services under the NPfIT.[15]

NPfIT's inability to produce convincing PAS/EPR products has made it difficult to persuade NHS acute hospitals to make the effort to replace their antiquated systems. NPfIT struggled to respond effectively to Fujitsu's decision in May 2008 to walk away from their £1.1billion contract for the South of England covering three SHA areas. This created an outstanding legal dispute, possible costs for the programme and loss of momentum on new systems installation that has lasted over 2 years. When Fujitsu jumped ship the new central team at DH (after Richard Grainger's departure) and the SHAs were unable to agree with Ministers an alternative implementation strategy. The Northern SHAs and hospital trusts have been unwilling to abandon Isoft's Lorenzo product despite its problems. There has been no credible plan for replacing Fujitsu in three SHA areas. BT has struggled in London with financial problems in its Global Services Division and slowness to fix problems with Cerner installations. The uncertainty about what will happen to NPfIT in the acute hospital sector remains unresolved.

Outside the acute hospital sector progress has been maintained. An answer to a Parliamentary Question I was given on 6 January 2010 revealed that nearly 7000 GP practices would have Electronic Prescription

Service by March 2010 and over 9000 pharmacies would. Over 7500 Choose and Book systems have been installed and over 1100 modernised GP systems. Over 5000 GP practices now have GP2GP medical record transfer systems. There are over 400 new clinical specialist systems in A and E, mental health trusts, community services, operating theatres, radiology departments and child health services. PACs are in over 300 hospitals, virtually completing the programme. Even PASs have now been installed in over 60 acute trusts.[16]

What NPfIT badly needs is a credible plan to bring programme implementation to a conclusion in the next few years and the leadership – political and managerial – to make this happen. That leadership needs to ensure also that the NHS will commit itself to maintaining and developing its IT infrastructure for the benefit of patients and NHS efficiency, with dedicated IT budgets. What it does not need is any reckless throw of the dice such as the suggestion in July 2009 to transfer confidential medical records to internet servers such as Google and Microsoft. The original contracting model for NPfIT has protected the interests of taxpayers in terms of cost but has proved too inflexible for such a large, diverse and sometimes cantankerous organisation like the NHS. A wider range of software and service providers are required with more local choice on which ones to use in order to finish the job of creating a networked EPR and modern patient administration systems in our acute hospitals. Only then will the NHS and its patients reap the benefits that the US Veterans' Administration has shown can be produced by a networked EPR.

The Coalition Government wants to see an information revolution in the way patients, clinicians and managers access and use information. This is a worthy aspiration and the revolution is long overdue when one considers how behind the times the NHS is in its use of information and IT compared with the private service sector. But it will require a huge cultural change by the NHS - management and staff who suffer few consequences for failing to change their ways.

9

Financial meltdown and recovery

Throughout my time as a Minister I remained unimpressed by the NHS's approach to money – and I still do. One might have thought that after being kept on short rations by the Conservatives the NHS would take more seriously than it did the safeguarding of money, curbing waste and fraud and improving systems of financial control. But my continuing sense was that the NHS culture meant that one had to keep on people's backs over money both at DH and within the NHS. These concerns came to a head in 2005/6 when the NHS approached financial meltdown and the prospect of literally running out of cash.

Chapter 5 described the work done to cut quangos and bureaucracy where too much growth money had gone on activities of little benefit to patients. In that first Ministerial job I was responsible for the NHS Counter Fraud Management Service (CFMS) set up in 1998 because of growing concern about abuse of taxpayers' money by contractors, staff and patients. The Conservative Party talked a lot about tackling waste and abuse but they had done little to tackle NHS fraud when in office. By the time we reached the 2005 Election I was able to say that CFMS had reduced key areas of fraud by over 40% saving £670million. This was the equivalent of several new hospitals. It had stopped many of those providing services to the NHS from swindling it and deterred others through some 500 successful prosecutions and civil and disciplinary sanctions against individuals and companies. In mid-2005 the CFMS had over 450 doctors, dentists, nurses, pharmacists, companies and others under investigation.[1] I remain far from convinced that left to their own devices the local NHS will pursue counter-fraud measures vigorously.

In 1997 patient fraud was running at about £170million a year and this had been halved by 2005. There was still a significant problem of foreign visitors receiving NHS treatment to which they were not entitled without paying locally. In one celebrated case in 2004 I authorised freezing the world-wide assets of a wealthy Egyptian national and non-UK resident and caused him to surrender his passport until he paid the NHS the £30,000 he owed. An anti-competitive cartel conducted by some generic drug companies had cost the NHS tens of millions of pounds. We retrieved £4.5million from one company but the Serious Fraud Office managed, after long delays, to fail with its prosecution of other companies, despite having the accused's own notes of their meeting at a hotel near Heathrow Airport.

The NHS reduced fraud through pressure from the centre; but too many trusts lacked good financial management systems and expertise.

Before the 2005 Election the Conservatives had mounted some effective attacks on money being wasted on bureaucracy but neither they nor Labour Ministers realised the scale of financial commitments stacking up without the money to pay for them. The DH financial systems could not forecast effectively the unfunded commitments building up: the three new pay deals; the rapid growth of NHS staff and their pay and pension costs; and the increasing NHS management and overhead costs. These issues have been discussed earlier. The unfunded financial overhang in 2005/6 was well over £1billion but fortunately for Labour this did not become apparent until after the 2005 Election.

The gathering financial storm

At no time during the 2005 Election campaign did the DH top brass raise with me any financial concerns. Their main preoccupation was the NHS organisational streamlining described in Chapter 5. The post-Election briefing that the new Ministerial team received was reassuring on finance although it was now apparent that officials expected that there would be an overspend in the financial year – 2004/5 – just ended. I realised that overspending money in one year meant that you started the new financial year having to pay it back. Being of a sceptical nature I started, with the help of my private office, to probe the financial aspects of my new Ministerial portfolio. On 17 May 2005 I sent Patricia Hewitt and Sir Nigel Crisp a five page memorandum on my 'Week One' first thoughts, with an opening section on finance and productivity that included the following passage:

"2.There are some serious issues of concern about how the extra money we have pumped into the NHS is being managed:

- The failure of Bradford Foundation Trust a few months after getting FT status may signal a wider malaise: inadequate attention to reconfiguration of services; poor management of costs; faulty income projections.
- The 2004/05 overspend (currently estimated at £150million - £200million) may mask higher overspends in the South East offset by balanced/under-spent budgets in the North and Midlands. There are some chronic budget problems in the South East stretching back in time and they may have been worsened by the current 3-year PCT allocations. (This is marginal seats territory!).
- We have little provision for contingencies as things stand.
- Destabilisation is likely to occur in 2006/07 and 2007/08 if we complete implementation of payment by results in that

timetable. I have yet to see a convincing narrative on how we will handle the shake out of failing departments/hospitals from payment by results.

- We have Manifesto commitments that are likely to add at least £250million to the NHS budget."[2]

With hindsight my warnings should have been stronger. I had restricted circulation to just Patricia, Nigel Crisp and the special adviser Matthew Swindells. Crisp who only a few months previously had been a candidate for the Cabinet Secretary post never engaged with me on the memorandum, preferring to reassure a new Secretary of State that everything would be alright in their one-to-one meetings. His position seemed to be that we would not have the final figures for 2004/5 until later in the year and that in any case the NHS always delivered and would produce financial balance in 2005/6.

As we moved into the summer it became increasingly clear that we lacked reliable monthly data on NHS expenditure and what we did have could not be triangulated with data on workforce growth or activity levels to test the reliability of the financial figures. We were told that the figures for the first few months of the financial year were not meaningful. It took a month after the end of each monthly accounting period for the NHS figures to be collected and validated to be sufficiently reliable to be put to Ministers. In motoring terms, we were driving a car with a highly unreliable speedometer and as we were to discover later we didn't know much about its braking system either!

In my memorandum of 17 May I suggested that "we need by the summer recess to look urgently at several areas", including:

- The build-up of a contingency reserve that can be used to help with the service reconfigurations/PbR and to implement Manifesto commitments.

- Drive the existing efficiency agenda harder – Gershon; ALB Review (settled budgets for 2006/07 and 2007/08); purchasing improvements through the Commercial Directorate; and regulation/inspection cost reductions.

- Develop a strategy and delivery mechanism for increasing significantly NHS productivity. Our political opponents are going to concentrate on this issue and we need to raise our game especially re Agenda for Change, consultants' contract, GP contract and increasing use of agency staff. All these are driving up costs without clear evidence that they will increase output measured by either quality or volume. The NHS also has a reputation for being slow overall to accept innovation and change in the way services are delivered."[3]

DH management did virtually nothing on these issues in the summer of 2005 while much of my time was devoted to starting work on a new White Paper the Prime Minister wanted on primary care and services outside hospitals; the Manifesto commitment on 18 weeks; and tackling the organisational consequences of the Manifesto commitment to save £250million a year from streamlining the NHS (see Chapter 5). Only when people returned from their holiday in September did it become clear to more people that the NHS finances were heading over a cliff.

The Private Finance Initiative

Before tackling the 2005/6 expenditure crisis I had started to wrestle with another NHS financial problem – the Private Finance Initiative (PFI) for building new hospitals. Labour had come to power in 1997 determined to show it could run the public finances prudently. At the heart of this prudence was Gordon Brown's 'Golden Rule' under which over the economic cycle the government would borrow only to invest with the net public debt being a "stable and prudent" proportion of GDP – taken to be 40%. This earlier Brown approach to the public finances meant that there was a limited amount of public capital for investment in improved public sector infrastructure. To deal with the conundrum this posed and a public sector hungry for new hospitals and schools, Labour embraced with enthusiasm a PFI system initiated by the Conservatives. The Iron Chancellor and his close advisers at the Treasury saw the hire purchase approach of off-balance sheet PFI as the way the NHS could have the new hospitals it craved for after four decades of underinvestment whilst at the same time preserving the Golden Rule.

Local people deprived of new hospitals suddenly had a once in a lifetime chance to get one on the 'never-never.'

Many of the local assessments of an organisation's ability to meet the repayments for the new hospital from their annual income were extremely optimistic. The DH and the Treasury allowed the early PFI enthusiasts to sign up for financial deals that were too financially one-sided in favour of the financiers rather than the somewhat naïve NHS boards and managers. The so-called risk transfer to the private sector looked to me as though it was permanently stuck in reverse. The large increases in NHS revenue only fuelled over-optimism on the part of the public sector clients. Too many NHS clients were committed to long-life and inflexible buildings and a traditional district general hospital model at a time when the medical technology was changing so fast that shorter life, more flexible buildings were called for. The first generation of PFI hospitals often turned out to be too expensive for trusts to easily meet the revenue payments, particularly given the rigidity of the contracts. Built more efficiently by private contractors to time and price they came on stream quicker but so did the "hire purchase" payments. By 2005/6 this was beginning to become an issue for the NHS because the number of future commitment to PFI schemes was building up fast.

During the first half of 2005/6 I was still responsible for the PFI programme and I became increasingly concerned about whether the NHS could afford the long list of prospective PFI schemes. I asked officials for a list of these schemes and their costs. I found that on the estimates available in mid-2005 we were on a trajectory to build a further £12billion worth of PFI hospitals. However looking at the DH revenue income projections to 2012 the NHS would be lucky if it could afford a shopping list of more than £7-8billion.

I decided to cut the PFI programme significantly, even though it included some very high-profile projects such as a rebuilding of the Barts and Royal London hospitals estimated to cost over £1billion and a totally unaffordable PFI project for Leicester hospitals in Patricia Hewitt's constituency. At the same time a total fantasy scheme was developing in Westminster for rebuilding the Royal Brompton, St Mary's and Hammersmith hospitals and a new academic medical campus at Paddington Basin. Leaving aside the planning problems - such as a bridge over the Regent's canal - the projected costs were already over £1billion and looked to me to be heading to nearer £2billion. Despite the expenditure of £13million on consultants' fees I ordered officials to kill off the Paddington Basin project through the SHA. This was eventually done much to most of the local NHS people's relief at the price of some political flak over wasting public money on consultants' fees.

The Treasury became very agitated about the effect on "the market" when they found out that I wanted to cut the PFI programme by at least a third. I held a meeting in my room with DH and Treasury officials and Gordon Brown's special adviser Shriti Vadera (now Baroness Vadera). There was a grudging acceptance that the programme had to be cut and that many of these projects would not pass HMT value for money tests. But the market I was told had to be prepared for an announcement and we needed an appraisal process for pruning the programme. After a certain amount of brouhaha there were no substantive arguments that the £12billion programme had to be slimmed down to nearer £7billion because the arithmetic on unaffordability was unambiguous.

As so often in the public sector there was a long debate over process, rather than the action that needed to be taken quickly. It was clear that the programme had to be brought back to more manageable proportions but my efforts had exposed a number of high profile projects that were likely to be axed. The most glaring of these was the Barts and Royal London scheme that became the subject of a high profile campaign by the Evening

Standard, with the parading of celebrities whose lives had allegedly been saved by the hospital. Politics intervened quickly and it became apparent that my managerial approach to the PFI programme was not the order of the day.

All this coincided with a ruckus in the Labour Party in October 2005 about my proposals for reducing the number of PCTs and removing their provider services from them. This had produced huge opposition from the unions, especially Unison, and a backlash from a growing number of Labour MPs. A Parliamentary Labour party meeting addressed by Patricia produced the view that unelected Lords Ministers should not be allowed to handle contentious issues. (Later I didn't hear them saying this to Lord Mandelson!) One of my fellow Ministers, Jane Kennedy, wanted to move into my territory and take over some of my functions. I was softened up for a change of roles but resisted a major redistribution on the grounds that I should do the job Tony Blair had asked me to do and we should not kow-tow to the prejudices of Labour backwoodsmen. However I had to concede some ground and suggested to Patricia Hewitt that Jane Kennedy should be the Minister for efficiency and productivity on a new Cabinet Committee and that I would transfer to her responsibility for productivity, service reconfigurations and the PFI programme. I insisted that I should "retain responsibility for overall NHS finances and the allocation system because these are integrally related to system reform through PbR and commissioning".[4] While I did not threaten to resign I made it clear that this was the basis on which I would continue. Patricia settled for my proposals.

This change in responsibilities did not help control either NHS finances or the PFI programme. Elected political appetite for NHS reform, difficult reconfiguration decisions or the reduction in PCTs and SHAs diminished in DH. My ability to cut the PFI programme was removed from me although eventually the unaffordability arguments reduced the scale of some schemes. However the Barts scheme went ahead without being adequately pruned and this continues to cause the trust financial problems and prevent it achieving FT status. Delivering uncomfortable messages and decisions was not Jane Kennedy's forte and she resigned under Tony Blair only to pop up again as a Minister under Gordon Brown. In the meantime the 2005/6 financial situation worsened.

Facing up to the NHS deficit

By autumn 2005 we knew that the financial accounts for 2004/5 showed a deficit of about £250million. It was no mean achievement for the NHS to produce a deficit in a year when its budget had gone up by 8% in cash terms and over 5% in real terms. This meant that the NHS started 2005/6 by having to repay that £250million from its budget. Like most people I did not think this should cause too much difficulty, given that the 2005/6 budget for the NHS was due to increase by about 10% in cash terms and over 7% in real terms. However the arcane public accounting rules, DH management ineptitude and poor NHS financial management, together with an unexpected Treasury cash raid, caused a political storm that effectively dealt a mortal blow to Patricia Hewitt's political career.

NHS Trusts were expected to break even annually on their revenue spending and they had a statutory duty to break even taking one year with another: this was interpreted as over a three-year period, or exceptionally a five-year period. (FTs were excluded from the break even duty and could retain their surpluses but they were subject to more rigorous in-year monitoring by their independent regulator – Monitor.) All this suggested a system of effective financial discipline and as Ministers we regularly trotted out these lines in Parliamentary answers and correspondence. However the reality was somewhat different. In practice if a trust overspent there was a complex system of brokerage under which the SHAs found "volunteers" who would under-spend to compensate for the over-spenders. If the worst came to the worst the DH would keep money back in the central budgets to deal with local or regional over-spends This system of 'bungs' had become a way of life for some parts of the country, particularly in the south of England. Poor performers knew that someone else in the "NHS family" would bail them out so they had little incentive to change their behaviour.

The Treasury did not really care much about these local practices: all they were concerned about was whether the DH balanced income and expenditure overall and lived within its Department Expenditure Limit. Indeed they were not above making in-year raids on Departmental budgets to sort out some other Whitehall expenditure problem. In 2005/6 they were to do just this and make the NHS position much worse by seeking at different times to have £800million cash repatriated to them from the DH because of esoteric aspects of the Chancellor's Golden Rule involving what was known as 'near cash' problems. As an example of collective loyalty DH ministers never briefed any journalists on these Treasury raids and took all the political heat themselves. Gordon Brown's Golden Rule was preserved at the expense of NHS finances and Patricia Hewitt's political reputation.

This cosy NHS system had been in force for a long time and rewarded poor financial management but it started to fall apart in 2005/6. First the DH had to repay the 2004/5 over-spend and cover the £800million raid by the Treasury. Second there was the unrecognised financial overhang of at least £1billion, as mentioned above, from higher staffing costs not budgeted for. And third the DH central budgets were over committed as described below. To tackle these problems DH had to start enforcing repayment of local debt through SHAs. This exposed the fact that at the local level, in increasing numbers, debt was being rolled forward by deduction from the new year's budget and that there was a growing number of hospital trusts who were becoming incapable of repaying accumulated historic debt. This was the so-called double whammy of a forced reduction of income within a financial year and a need to repay accumulated debts from a reduced income. Larger historic debts were building up across the NHS - and in many places are still there today. Those who were managing efficiently and had become "voluntary" lenders were becoming extremely fed up with the unfairness of a system that allowed the financially incompetent to permanently live on 'tick'.

I discovered that there was no systematic NHS scheme of repayable loans over the longer term. Overall what was happening was making a mockery of the resource allocation system as many of the areas with the worst health needs were being forced to transfer their extra allocations back to over-spending areas with lower health needs. Essentially money was transferring from the health-needy North, who seemed to manage their finances better, to the wealthier South, with its more inept but crafty financial management. Alongside this, the new payment by results system that began to bite in 2005/6 produced new winners and losers in the acute hospital trusts together with a new set of complex smoothing mechanisms. A financial maelstrom was in progress across the NHS whose complexity was almost impossible for Ministers to understand sitting in Richmond House with little useful or timely data. The Jumbo jet we were trying to land on a postage stamp had instruments more suited to a 1940s Lancaster bomber.

The full horror of the financial situation started to become apparent in October 2005. Patricia Hewitt called what was to turn out to be a key meeting to review the first cut of the 2005/6 half year's NHS expenditure figures which showed that overall the NHS position in 2005/6 was much worse than in the previous year. The gross deficit was heading towards well over £1billion at the end of the year despite the large budget increase. Officials could not relate these figures to any workforce or activity figures or show whether or not the position was worsening significantly. I could see no grounds for the optimistic view of the NHS Chief Executive and his colleagues that the NHS would deliver financial balance at the end of the year.

At this October meeting Patricia Hewitt asked for ideas on what action might be taken. I expressed the view that I thought the situation was getting worse and that in my experience as a public sector manager there were only three areas in which you could effectively curb expenditure at this point in a financial year in a labour-intensive organisation like the

NHS. These were a recruitment freeze; undertaking only essential maintenance; and halting most training and education programmes. I recognised that winter was often a difficult time for the NHS but given how rapidly the NHS had expanded and was continuing to expand its workforce I argued for considering a recruitment freeze on selected groups of staff for the rest of the financial year.

This was strongly opposed by DH top management who said that at most such a freeze would delay the recruitment of 75,000 staff and would take time to implement. Political anxieties were skilfully played on by suggesting that this would look like a panic measure and would damage target achievement. I pressed the case for a recruitment freeze but had no support. However if we had imposed a full freeze from November (which was possible) and the average pay and on-costs of the staff affected was £30,000 a year in the remaining five months of the year nearly £1billion could have been saved. This would have more than covered the eventual deficit of just under £600million. So decisive action in October 2005 to impose a partial recruitment freeze and a package of economy measures around maintenance and training could have prevented much of what followed.

The decision was taken to improve monitoring of financial performance through the 28 SHAs, 18 of whom would disappear the following July (see Chapter 5). I thought we could not be confident about their commitment to hauling budgets back into balance but at least using the NHS Chief Executive's management line to curb expenditure would test the effectiveness of this system. Ministers and officials agreed to meet regularly to check progress and decide what else to do.

Turnaround teams were to be used to try to improve matters in the worst performing trusts. These teams were brought in from the private sector, with a DH Turnaround Director from one of the big accounting firms working to the Department's Finance Director. 175 PCTs were visited by turnaround teams and a large number of hospital trusts. What they found was a horrifying picture of poor financial management and inadequate control systems across the NHS and particularly in the PCTs. In many trusts there turned out to be poor engagement with doctors over a trust's financial problems and hopelessly optimistic planning and income projections. Some trusts seemed literally unable to stop cash going out of the door. There was a huge contrast between the financial management of FTs and those who were not FT's, as the Healthcare Commission's assessments were to reveal. The FT regulator had better and more up-to-date financial data than DH Ministers had.

Ministers made it brutally clear to senior officials at the end of 2005 that getting NHS finances back into balance was now a high political priority. All this had some impact and probably stopped further deterioration in this situation. But Patricia and I were both aware now that the DH machinery was unreliable and that alongside the PCT row and recurring problems on PFIs we were faced with serious problems over the poor usage of the extra resources the NHS had been given. But worse was to follow when I turned my attention to trimming expenditure in the DH central budgets which were supposed to be under our direct control.

Plugging the dyke

By the end of 2005 it was clear to me that the NHS deficit could well be £1billion. Patricia met with the Chancellor to try to reduce the amount of cash to be handed back to the Treasury but Gordon gave no ground and £800million was removed from DH coffers. We had boxed ourselves into a resource allocation system to PCTs for the three years 2005/6, 2006/7 and 2007/8 when before the 2005 Election John Reid had devolved 80% of the NHS budget to PCTs in accordance with the health needs formula. Our ability to claw back money from PCTs was limited to voluntary levy schemes that SHAs could put in place locally to bale out overspending hospital trusts. By continuous pressure on officials we had reached a point at the beginning of 2006 whereby a rough cut of the NHS finances was now available within ten days of the end of each month. Using this information a meeting took place on 12 January 2006 between Patricia, me and Jane Kennedy with Nigel Crisp, John Bacon, Richard Douglas and other key officials.

It was not a happy occasion. Three quarters of the way through the year the net deficit of the NHS looked to be about £1billion. I had also exposed the fact that far from being a source of comfort, the central budgets were another problem not only for the current year but for the following year as well. The DH management team had created (or allowed to happen) a system under which there were some 500 budget-holders, many of whom seemed to act like unmanaged patrons of various NHS and social care special interests. The top management seemed incapable of imposing their collective will on these budgetholders. For the next financial year (2006/7), only two months before it started, the DH central budgets were over-subscribed by about £2.5billion in relation to an allocation of £12.7billion. The Chief Medical Officer and his staff were the main culprits; and the DH Accounting Officer seemed unable to require him to adhere to budgetary constraints. The DH civil service corporate management seemed to have collapsed. It was being left to Ministers to impose financial discipline on the top management of the second highest spending government department. Effectively this is what this January 2006 Ministerial meeting did.

From then on Patricia Hewitt and I met the Permanent Secretary, Finance Director and other key officials weekly to go through a schedule of deficits and surpluses across the NHS. The approach was to interrogate them on progress on stemming the outflow of money drawing on a growing number of turnaround teams out in the NHS. The special advisers were used to help us. This relentless political scrutiny – which should not have been necessary in a well run Department – paid dividends in cutting back the eventual deficit to under £600million. This was an unlikely outcome at the end of 2005.

Alongside this I took charge, with the help of Liam Byrne, with his management consultancy background, of scrutinising and cutting the central budgets both for 2005/6 and 2006/7. All members of the Ministerial team were required to cooperate with this exercise by not approving submissions from the multitude of DH budgetholders that added new financial commitments. This was to deal with the established culture of separate submissions to individual Ministers racking up expenditure commitments with no effective corporate financial control.

At the 12 January meeting we agreed that I would work with the Finance Director to lop some £400million from the 2005/6 central budgets. Painful though it was we made considerable progress partly because I wrote to Patricia Hewitt privately the following day that I would continue – as I had pressed for at the meeting – to seek savings of £600million by cutting more of the small low priority budgets where people were holding on to money and by capitalising more of the NPfIT expenditure. Liam Byrne and I had meetings with officials and Ministers in which we crawled over spreadsheets both cutting the 2005/6 spend and starting to bring 2006/7 expenditure back into balance. Throughout the Spring of 2006 the focus of most senior officials in DH was on budgets – trying to avoid raiding parties on their own budgets and being forced into a degree of corporateness that had been lacking for too long within and under the existing senior management. Although we never achieved the saving of £600million its threat enabled us to secure close to £400million savings in the last 3 months of the 2005/6 financial year.

The position of Nigel Crisp became increasingly untenable as Ministers effectively took over the financial management of the Department. He had lost the confidence of Ministers and many in the NHS and DH and I thought it best for him to leave as soon as possible. I wrote Patricia Hewitt a personal note on 3 February 2006 expressing my concerns about Nigel staying in post.[5] These included what I regarded as one botched DH re-organisation in which he ended up with effectively only four direct reports; and difficulty with performing adequately the traditional Permanent Secretary role of supporting Ministers and working across Whitehall. I considered that the system for overseeing and managing central budgets was totally unsatisfactory with no prioritisation of new demands and no effective monitoring of commitments. The DH top team had been slow to recognize and respond to the NHS loss of financial control and had had to be forced by Ministers to take action. There was a long standing unresolved problem of an effective working relationship with a powerful CMO who effectively ran a separate fiefdom within the Department of Health. I made it clear that I had lost confidence in Nigel and did not believe he would set up and run a new DH Management Board effectively. I thought he should be replaced and his post split.

At the time I suspected that Patricia Hewitt thought I was rather harsh but rereading my letter now I regard it as an accurate if brutal indictment. I think the clincher for Patricia was my conclusion that we risked another botched Departmental reorganisation and returning to where we were in 12 to18 months time, even nearer to an Election. To her great credit Patricia Hewitt did not duck the issue and Nigel Crisp left quietly with a peerage. Thereafter a surprisingly large number of people from within the NHS came up to me privately to congratulate Ministers on biting on this particular bullet.

Through unrelenting pressure from Ministers, the DH Finance and Performance Directors and turnaround teams, the NHS, with some help from reduced central budgets, managed to keep its deficit in 2005/6 to £550million. (If the Treasury had not removed £800million there would have been a small surplus.) This deficit was less than 1% of the total budget and a smaller deficit percentage than Labour had inherited in 1997. Given the scale and complexity of the NHS and where we were in early 2006 this was no mean achievement. But the political and managerial effort involved was phenomenal and we could not go on running DH and the NHS in this way. A new corporate and financial management system was required.

Restoring financial equilibrium

The new financial year – 2006/7 – brought a new approach. McKinsey had been brought in to review and help reconstruct the DH corporate management system. The decision was taken to revert to the previous system of a separate Permanent Secretary and NHS Chief Executive. Sir Ian Carruthers, an experienced SHA Chief Executive was brought in as Acting NHS Chief Executive to steady the ship while a longer-term appointment was made. A new single DH Management Board replaced the earlier two-tier system with a wider range of personnel. Hugh Taylor acted up as Permanent Secretary and was later appointed substantively.

We accelerated the appointment of the ten Chairs and Chief Executives of the streamlined SHA structure (see Chapter 5) so these could be in place by July 2006. Patricia Hewitt and I started meeting them with the new DH Management Board on a monthly basis, with separate monthly meetings with the ten SHA Chairs on their own. A greater sense of corporateness across the Department and the new regional tier was created. Patricia did a very good job of engendering a sense that politicians and managers were engaged in a common endeavour of running the NHS – an important lesson but one lost on our successors.

The financial crisis of 2005/6 had exposed some major systemic problems with the way NHS allocated money and held recipients to account effectively for their stewardship of resources. There was not much any Health Ministers could do about the Treasury way of operating. This made it essential to create a system of contingency money, with DH acting as a shock absorber between the Treasury and the NHS; but we lacked an effective system for doing this. The Treasury system of running public expenditure meant that any over-spending in one part of the NHS had to be offset in the same year by under-spending elsewhere so that overall DH and NHS expenditure and income balanced each year. The DH capacity to exercise control was now limited by the complex financial system that had been created: a needs based resource allocation system with money handed over for the most part to PCTs; a hospital reimbursement system based on payment by result; a growing system of FT Hospitals outside Ministerial control; and increasingly, under a more marketised NHS, money following patient choice. Moreover it was proving difficult to hold to account the commissioners of services who were the primary budgetholders but could not manage demand effectively.

One thing as Ministers we decided not to do was to support the growing number of calls to write off historic NHS debt. To do this in full across the NHS in 2006/7 would mean generating the full value of the current gross deficit of the NHS – then about £1.3billion. This would have meant punishing the under-spenders and rewarding the over-spenders. Write off would have meant not repaying the under-spending NHS organisations some £600million they had loaned and raising the rest by not repaying central budgets and levying at least a further £200million from all the organisations not over-spending. This would have thrown into chaos the planned service developments of the financially well-managed parts of the NHS, undermined the resource allocation system and given those who had shown no capacity to manage their affairs prudently the opportunity to repeat their incompetence. Even writing off £1.3billion would not have dealt with the many millions of pounds of debt held under so-called SHA "planned support" arrangements across the local NHS. Instead as Ministers we took the politically more difficult decision not to reward the financially inept by writing off NHS debt and to move towards a more coherent banking system for the NHS.

Before such a system could be put in place we had to deal with a particular idiosyncrasy for the NHS of the government-wide Resource Accounting and Budgeting (RAB) system. Under this system the rigid enforcement of the statutory duty to break even over three years and rolling forward deficits year on year created a "double whammy" at NHS trust level of effectively paying off the deficit twice. This made it nearly impossible for a trust incurring a significant deficit to get back into balance. In 2006 we asked Sir Michael Lyons (then Acting Chairman of the Audit Commission and later Chairman of the BBC) to review RAB and the NHS. In June 2006 the Audit Commission published Sir Michael's report which recommended much clearer and more transparent accountability for loans and borrowing; supporting individuals to improve their financial management capacity and capability; ceasing to apply RAB at NHS trust level; and changing the nature of the capital regime for NHS trusts.[6]

During 2006/7 we implemented the Audit Commission proposals in a staged way. Over the year we replaced cash brokerage with a new formal loan arrangement. Nearly £800million of loans were issued to over 50 hospital trusts and PCTs with a requirement to pay interest and to repay the principal from surpluses that needed to be generated. The repayment periods varied from 1 to 25 years. These loans were initially funded by top slicing SHAs and PCTs (see below). For 2007/8 we agreed to change the capital regime for NHS trusts so that capital allocations for them were replaced by new borrowing regimes. Capital funding for trusts became determined solely by the affordability of proposed investments, with loans and borrowing subject to a prudential borrowing regime similar to that for FTs. This was to stop poorly managed hospital trusts 'splurging' on new facilities that they could not afford to pay for.

We accepted the Lyons proposal to remove the "double whammy" of RAB from NHS hospital trusts incurring deficits but RAB remained in place for SHAs and PCTs so that the NHS books could be balanced nationally. However we decided, as Ministers, not to implement this Lyons proposal until March 2007. We did not want to create the impression to the NHS that we were willing to remove debt just like that. For the rest of the financial year we wanted the profligate spenders to do their utmost to mend their ways and get back to in year financial balance at least. At the year end those NHS bodies that had had their income reduced as a result of incurring a deficit in 2005/6 had that income reinstated (unless they had already received the equivalent financial support) with the debt lodged with the SHAs or PCTs as a form of loan that they would need to pay off in the future from surpluses.

During 2006/7 we effectively imposed as Ministers a new way of ensuring that total resources were more likely to match demands across the NHS. There was a growth figure of £4.5billion and a 2.5% increase in productivity required. This meant that the NHS could incur new costs and pay immediate debt off the legacy of about £1.3billion from the total of just under £7billion available. Given that about £4billion was required for pay and pay reform and another £1.7billion for reducing waiting times and existing service improvements, this was a tough but fair challenge for the NHS, even with some trusts previously in balance moving into deficit.

To bring this about we handed over a large part of the central budgets to the 10 SHAs (about £7billion) but within this we held a central contingency fund of £500million: I wanted to hold £1billion but this was deemed unacceptable. This left the SHAs to make the cuts to the previous central programmes as they thought fit. Much of the expenditure reduction came from what I regarded as an inflated training programme that I had been willing to cut robustly from the centre. In addition we enabled the SHAs to build up local reserves by levying up to about 4% of allocations from their PCTs. We used the intermediate tier to constrain NHS spend locally within the resources available nationally each year because history had shown many local trusts could not or would not live within their budgets when left to their own devices. At some stage the new Coalition Government are likely to make this discovery even though they seem determined to dispense with an intermediate NHS tier.

Many aspects of these new budgetary control arrangements were unpopular especially with the trades unions who were opposed to cuts in training budgets and any recruitment slow-down or redundancies. On top of this we imposed a tougher pay policy centrally of no more than 2% a year increases. We made clear that this more robust financial regime was necessary to get the NHS back into financial balance and move to a more transparent and consistent system of loans and repayments across the NHS for the future. As Ministers we had to repeat to the point of boredom that the NHS had to take financial management more seriously; that we were not going to write off deficits; and that we intended stopping the efficient bailing out the inefficient. Labour MPs in some areas opposed the slow-down in recruitment and cut backs in services in the inefficient trusts; and did not like the forced levy on PCTs (alongside the reduction in the number of PCTs). Despite a lot of political criticism we stuck to our guns and we were supported by Tony Blair as we put the NHS back on financial track.

We pushed on with implementing a proper system of repayable loans and contingency provision as the way the NHS should run its financial affairs in the future. Before I resigned at the end of 2006 the work was well advanced on creating a system for the future that would enable an NHS Bank to oversee arrangements for repayable loans (with interest) on a consistent basis. Alongside this the SHAs could create regional contingency reserves on an agreed basis with PCTs but observing the principle that all PCT loans should be repaid so that the integrity of the resource allocation system was preserved. It had taken a totally avoidable financial crisis to improve a duff NHS financial management system that should never have been allowed to get into such a state by DH and NHS managements. Although this new system created more financial discipline in the NHS it did not fix the often lamentable financial management in PCTs and local hospital trusts.

An incomplete improvement in NHS financial management

Despite the political trauma the NHS achieved a surplus of over £500million in 2006/7, a turnaround of over £1billion in a single financial year. Nearly 80% of NHS bodies achieved financial balance in 2006/7 compared to about two-thirds in 2005/6. In their review of the NHS financial year 2006/7 the Audit Commission reported in October 2007 a significant improvement in the number of NHS bodies performing satisfactorily in the way they used and managed resources compared to the previous year, although there was still a considerable way to go before this could be said of all NHS bodies.[7]

Despite the hard work by some managers this financial turnaround was achieved primarily by an act of political will. It made Patricia Hewitt extremely unpopular politically and she left the government when Gordon Brown became Prime Minister in June 2007. Her successor Alan Johnson benefited from our work as he acknowledged. On 29 November 2007 Alan Johnson was able to tell Parliament: "financial projections at the end of September 2007 show that the NHS is forecasting a healthy £1.8billion surplus for 2007/8 with only 25 Trusts forecasting a deficit"[8]. Patricia and I had repeatedly said throughout the dark days of 2005/6 and 2006/7 that competent financial management was not inconsistent with good patient care - not a sentiment always accepted in the NHS or Parliament to this day. Too often the public is fed the notion by some politicians and doctors that the NHS can only improve with more money being thrown at it. This is not true as the Audit Commission made clear in October 2007 when commenting on the NHS's improved financial performance "Managing money well goes hand in hand with providing better patient care".[9]

The Care Quality Commission's performance ratings of NHS trusts in 2008/9 showed NHS financial management improving.[10] For the first time more than 100 (103) of the 392 trusts scored "excellent" for financial management - up from 94 in the previous year, 57 in 2006/7 and 19 in 2005/6. Those scoring "good" was 176, hugely more than in 2005/6. But 113 trusts were only "fair" or "weak" at financial management; and in 2008/9 nearly 50% of PCTs – those to whom budgets are allocated by DH

– were in this category. There is still a very considerable journey for the NHS to travel before one can be confident about its ability to spend taxpayers' money wisely.

Even with these improvements in financial performance when I asked a question in July 2009 about the number of trusts with historic deficits the answer I was given was that at the 31 March 2009 there were 45 NHS acute hospital trusts with cumulative historic deficits. The trusts with the largest deficits were mainly concentrated in London where one trust – Barking, Havering and Redbridge – had a historic deficit of over £100million that it is supposed to pay back.[11] Some of these hospitals are in a situation where it is impossible for them to pay off their deficits without major changes in the services they run and their governance. There has been little political appetite for enforcing change in these underperforming trusts; and there are still many trusts that are unable to run their affairs so that they are in recurrent in-year balance of income and expenditure. Patient choice, payment by results and a more marketised NHS means that inevitably the problems of failing hospitals and financially incompetent commissioners will have to be grappled with more energetically than has been the case in the past. The Coalition Government will discover that these local financial governance issues will only get worse as the NHS moves from feast to famine. The day of reckoning moves ever closer as I discuss later.

10

Keep taking the
tablets – pharmaceuticals and the NHS

Diseases that used to kill us no longer do so largely because of modern medicines. Infectious diseases that caused so many childhood deaths 60-70 years ago were curbed dramatically by antibiotics and other new drugs. As we create new ways of killing ourselves through bad lifestyle choices, scientists and the pharmaceutical industry come to our rescue. To fight a modern 'flu pandemic we need new vaccines and anti-retrovirals. No modern healthcare system can operate without ready access to the latest drugs if it wants to keep more of its population alive and treat conditions that reduce the quality of life. That is why the NHS spends about 10% of its budget on medicines – somewhat more with expenditure on medical devices and stockpiles of vaccines and drugs to cope with pandemics.

A significant proportion of the population relies on pills of one kind or another and increasingly believes it has a right to access those drugs irrespective of cost or personal behaviour. The latest wonder drug is paraded before a population eager for new ways of extending their lives or improving its quality. The spotlight is rarely shone on the processes for producing these lifesavers but, when it is, the public does not always like what it sees: drugs causing adverse effects; a research-based industry making hefty profits; animals being used for testing drugs before they are tried in humans. Sometimes the scientists get it in the neck – especially from the faith-based communities – for tampering with nature. Personal privacy can conflict with research needs, especially with the advances in genomic medicine: these ethical issues are discussed in Chapter 13.

Those producing the new drugs sometimes feel hard done by, despairing at the public's lack of appreciation of what is involved and its poor understanding of risk. One of Pfizer's top managers told me in early 2005 that he thought the American public regarded the US pharmaceutical industry as no better than the tobacco industry. The industry often feels misunderstood over their obligations to shareholders and the need to fund a research base that cannot produce Derby winners every time.

Equally the pharmaceutical industry can be slow to own up to mistakes and can engage in opaque practices that only fuel suspicion. Their profits from blockbuster successes are bound to attract public and political attention. These conflicting attitudes and agendas were brought home to me when in June 2003 I became the DH Minister responsible for the UK pharmaceutical and devices industries. This involved not only their regulation but also negotiating NHS drug prices and acting as the industry's sponsor Minister across government. I was expected to promote a research-based UK industry which provided high-quality, well paid jobs and supported Britain's science base but also ensure that the NHS expenditure on its products was not excessive. As I was told regularly there was a certain inherent conflict in these roles. For two years I spent an interesting and challenging time grappling with a range of complex issues, left to my own devices by a Health Secretary who had other things on his mind.

Regulating medicines - working with the MHRA

To regulate the pharmaceutical and medical devices industries a new Executive Agency of the Department of Health was established on the 1 April 2003 called the Medicines Healthcare products Regulatory Agency (MHRA). This was the result of a merger of the Medicines Control Agency and the Medical Devices Agency. The former had been established to regulate pharmaceutical products in the late 1960s as a result of the thalidomide scandal exposed by the Sunday Times. Devices were the poor relation of pharmaceuticals and were less rigorously regulated. When I arrived the MHRA was still finding its feet under its new Chairman, Sir Alasdair Breckenridge and it did not yet have a Chief Executive.

There was concern in Parliament and elsewhere that the regulator was too much in the pocket of 'Big Pharma'. The MHRA view was that you needed knowledgeable scientists to regulate the industry and inevitably many of them would have worked for large pharmaceutical companies. The claim was that poachers could become satisfactory gamekeepers. But the MHRA's predecessor bodies did not have a good reputation on transparency or involving patients in their deliberations. There was a well established group of critics rightly questioning some of the MHRA processes and judgements and arguing for more patient involvement in their affairs. It did not go down well with some MHRA personnel that I thought some of the criticism should be listened to and that the Agency should improve its communications, involve patients more in its work and look again at its systems for collecting information on untoward incidents (the yellow card scheme).

Increasingly the role of pharmaceutical regulators across Europe was being constrained and absorbed by the European Medicines Agency (EMEA) as the harmonisation of pharmaceutical regulation gained pace. The European research-based pharmaceutical industry was struggling to maintain its presence, although the UK was doing a better job of this than mainland Europe. Clinical trials for drugs were cheaper to conduct in Asia and the power of the US drugs market tended to suck research talent across the Atlantic. The US Food and Drugs Administration (FDA) was effectively the dominant regulator in pharmaceuticals; and the increasing European emphasis on controlling drug prices did not endear US 'Big Pharma' to Europe. Neither did the UK's veto on direct marketing to the public of prescription drugs.

This was a tricky time for a new Minister and a new Regulator. The MHRA's main role was assessing the safety, quality and efficacy of medicines and authorising their sale or supply in the UK for human use. It also audited the bodies that approved devices. In these roles it had to operate a post-licensing surveillance function; sample and test medicines for quality defects in their manufacture; monitor the safety of unlicensed imported products; regulate clinical trials; promote good practice in the use of medicines and control their labelling. There was plenty of scope for things to go wrong with a public hungry for new cures and an industry eager to provide them but with healthy profits. The Minister's job was to be 'hands off' on the MHRA's technical work but ensure a flourishing and safe pharmaceutical and devices industry that could generate wealth for UK plc without bankrupting the NHS. The trick was to keep well-informed, avoid detailed interference but make my presence felt with selective interventions. What was not in doubt was that if there was real trouble the Minister was going to cop it and would have to intervene however much the MHRA regarded itself as an arm's-length professional body.

I supported Alasdair Breckenridge in bedding down the new Agency, appointing a Chief Executive and developing a corporate plan for the next five years during which time the UK would hold the Presidency of the EU. A 5-year plan was published eventually in April 2004 and identified seven initiatives.[1] Among these were items I wanted to push: increasing a number of medicines available to patients without prescription; extending the prescribing rights of non-medical professions; improving the availability of medicines licensed specifically for children; improving the quality of information available to the public; and enhancing the system for reporting adverse reactions to drugs. The MHRA was under pressure from industry and government to streamline the regulatory processes to reduce costs, so this was included as well. A significant body of EU legislation was also in the pipeline on clinical trials, use of human tissue, traditional herbal remedies and medical devices. Much of this EU legislation was controversial, especially in the House of Lords.

Changing prescribing

There was much professional nervousness about taking medicines off prescription. An extensive consultation process was involved. In

November 2003 we began a 3-month consultation to allow a low dose statin, Simvastatin 10mg, to be purchased over the counter by patients. The result was a third of consultees in favour, a third against and a third not against but with some questions. The medical profession was divided with the BMA and the Royal College of GPs opposed but with other medical Royal Colleges either supportive in principle or not opposed. Some of the medical opposition had an element of restrictive practice about it but there were legitimate concerns over possible adverse reactions.

After considering all the arguments the MHRA's Committee on the Safety of Medicines advised Ministers that the 10mg Simvastatin could be made available without a prescription through pharmacies to people with a moderate risk of a heart attack (i.e. 10%-15% risk of myocardial infarction over ten years). The scientific advice to Ministers was clear but I realised that accepting it would mean we were out of line with other countries: for example the FDA would not approve any statins off prescription. Already nearly 2 million people a year in the UK were taking statins and these were thought to be saving 6,000-7,000 lives a year. By extending patient choice over access to this low dose statin through pharmacies we would empower people to take more responsibility for their health. The Royal Pharmaceutical Society of Great Britain supported the move and provided guidance to all pharmacies over the change. So on 12 May 2004 John Reid announced that the UK would be the first country to provide statins over the counter without a prescription.[2]

Controversy has continued with the statins decision in the medical journals but we continued cautiously with a case by case approach on taking some other medicines off prescription. The MHRA, after my time, also looked at some of the over-counter medicines for children with coughs and colds and recommended some should not be used for children under six. So the statins decision did not open the flood gates but it did establish the principle that there was a process, using the Committee on the Safety of Medicines and public consultation for taking medicines off prescriptions, selectively, and thereby increasing patient choice and responsibility.

Alongside this loosening of the restrictions on prescription drugs was the whole area of supplementary prescribing. This was intended to ease the burden on doctors and improve access to medicines but it had been viewed with suspicion by many doctors since initiatives in this area started in 1999. Some momentum had been injected in April 2003 when, following a public consultation, Ministers had agreed that supplementary prescribers could prescribe in accordance with a diagnosis and treatment plan agreed by a doctor. Initially I was developing a system restricted to nurses and pharmacists qualified to prescribe. Nurses were trained and restricted to a limited formulary with about 250 prescription medicines on it but slowly their range of medicines was extended. Gradually I authorised physiotherapists, chiropodists/podiatrists and radiographers to become supplementary prescribers after appropriate training. Trained nurses and pharmacists in secondary care were then allowed to prescribe controlled drugs and unlicensed drugs. Now nurses, midwives, pharmacists, podiatrists, physiotherapists, diagnostic and therapeutic radiographers and optometrists who have been through the training can become supplementary prescribers.

Over 6,000 nurses are able to prescribe a full range of drugs and about another 30,000 can prescribe from a more restricted formulary. Pharmacists are the next largest group but only about 500 are qualified for a full range of drugs. Although I managed to push the agenda along, the expansion of supplementary prescribing – especially for people with long term conditions where the diagnosis is clear – has been slow, given its potential and the willingness of Ministers and the MHRA to remove restrictions. It is a good example of how the NHS can be slow to adopt reform and take innovation to widespread application.

The Yellow Card scheme changes

The Yellow Card scheme was set up in 1964 after the Thalidomide tragedy highlighted the need for routine post-marketing surveillance of medicines. By 2003 approaching half a million reports of adverse drug reactions (ADRs) had been reported to the MHRA or their predecessor bodies. In 2003 about 18,000 ADRs were coming in under this early warning system, although a Yellow Card notification did not necessarily mean an adverse reaction was caused by the drug. But Yellow Cards could only be sent in by health professionals; and the MHRA was very reluctant to allow researchers access to the Yellow Card data on particular drugs. The limited access and restrictions on patients notifying ADRs direct were continuing sources of complaint but MHRA professionals were reluctant to change the scheme.

After several meetings and with help from the MHRA chairman I announced on the 21 July 2003 that there would be an independent review into access and use of data collected by the MHRA on suspected ADRs. This would be conducted by Dr Jeremy Metters, a former Deputy Chief Medical Officer. The review undertook some public consultation and produced a report that was published on 4 May 2004 to coincide with the 40th Anniversary of the Yellow Card scheme. The Metters report recommended improving access to data by academics and researchers and suggested that the MHRA should publish anonymised aggregated data on its website regularly.[3] These recommendations were put out for wider consultation.

Metters also recommended direct patient reporting of ADRs through the Yellow Card scheme. This caused some consternation in the MHRA, particularly when I accepted the recommendation with immediate effect and without further consultation. The MHRA were now tasked with working out the system for patients to register ADRs and raising awareness of the Yellow Card scheme. No greater sacrifice can a Minister make than to release a private secretary which I did in order to take forward this work in the MHRA.

It took until 17 January 2005 for me to be able to announce that the MHRA would publish anonymised data on ADRs on their website; and that researchers would be able to access more detailed data subject to approval by an independent committee accepting that the proposal was ethically and scientifically sound.[4] It took a long time to set up pilot schemes for patients to directly report ADRs to the regulator. Forms to report ADRs were eventually made available in 4,000 GP surgeries across the UK; and patients were also able to report on line. Subsequent progress was slow after my departure but the scheme for patient participation in notifying ADRs did progress. By early 2008 the MHRA had established a full scale patient reporting system as part of the Yellow Card scheme together with an online reporting system. By early 2009 the MHRA was reporting receiving about 25,000 ADRs a year under the scheme, with some 2,500 of these coming from patients and carers. There had been a 17% increase in ADRs notified in the previous year, with a 50% increase in those from patients. After 5 years the MHRA had come to terms with direct patient involvement and was even encouraging patients to notify ADRs.

The Seroxat story

While slow progress was being made on revamping the Yellow Card scheme I had my most difficult encounter with the MHRA over the anti-depressant Seroxat. There had been a Panorama programme in 2003 about Seroxat which was then being taken by about half a million people. The programme had revealed that many people taking higher doses were experiencing side effects of nervousness, aggression, irrational thoughts and in some cases feelings of suicide. There had been a number of cases of suicide among younger people that had attracted media attention. GSK, Seroxat's manufacturer, had sought to reassure the public ever since the drug was licensed around 1991. The MHRA was aware of the concerns and in January 2003 had launched their own review of Seroxat and similar drugs known as SSRIs (Selective Serotonin Reuptake Inhibitors).

This review included a small subset of patients for whom Seroxat was not licensed but was being prescribed by doctors. These were young people under the age of 18. An estimated 8,000 young people a year were being prescribed with Seroxat at the time. For some the results were disturbing. I received a report from the Committee on Safety of Medicines saying that children taking the antidepressant were more likely to self-harm or have suicidal thoughts. This report was based on information that was not current but had suddenly been provided by GSK. I had this published on 10 June 2003; and doctors were discouraged from prescribing Seroxat for young people under 18. The information was passed to regulators in Europe and the US.

The main review continued. MIND, the mental health charity, had demonstrated outside the MHRA's offices over Seroxat. As a result the MHRA, with a degree of shrewdness, had invited MIND's Chief Executive, Richard Brooks, to join the expert panel conducting the review. So far, so good. However in October 2003 the MHRA reviewed data from the earliest trials of Seroxat. In a number of the reviews of this data Richard Brooks claimed that the MHRA predecessor body had failed to pick up the salient fact that any dose of Seroxat above 20mg a day worked no better than a lower dosage but significantly increased adverse side effects. This caused, he said, serious problems for the 17,000 people a year taking the higher doses.

Matters worsened very rapidly in March 2004. Brook fell out with the MHRA and asked to see me. I was advised not to see him but did. He explained the situation to me and said that the MHRA panel wanted to kick the whole issue into the long grass by referring matters to the EMEA, the European regulator. What really incensed him was that the MHRA's Chief Executive had said he faced a criminal prosecution if he revealed anything that was commercially in confidence that he had learnt from his time on the panel. He felt seriously compromised as a patient representative and wanted to resign and tell the truth as he saw it. I had a good deal of sympathy with Brook and asked him to give me a few days while I talked to the MHRA.

I then had a number of robust discussions with MHRA staff in which I made it clear that threatening Brook was neither appropriate nor smart. I told the MHRA that I thought Brook would resign and tell his story but made it clear that I would not sanction a criminal prosecution. It was clear that the Expert Working Group had not completed their work but it was equally clear that there were very real concerns about excessively high dosages of Seroxat. The expert view was that the evidence was not clearly against Seroxat's use with adults. Even if the UK acted against it the EMEA might not, on the evidence available; and there could be a legal challenge by the drug company. As a compromise I settled for a reminder going out to prescribers from the Chairman of the CSM that the 20mg daily dosage of Seroxat was the recommended dosage for the treatment of adults with depression, social or generalised anxiety disorder and post traumatic-stress disorder. The 40mg dosage was only for adults with obsessive compulsive disorder and panic disorder. It was made clear that increasing dosages above the recommended levels would not increase the efficacy of treatment.

This letter was issued a few days after my meeting with Richard Brook. I talked to him again and tried to persuade him to stay on the Expert Working Group. He declined to do so and on 23 March 2004 wrote an article in the Daily Mail.[5] Unsurprisingly it was very critical of the MHRA but it did indicate that I had taken action. However this was not the end of the story. In November I received a final report from the MHRA along with some NICE guidelines on the treatment and care of people with depression and anxiety. I insisted on the report and the NICE guidelines being published together and they were on the 6 December 2004.[6] The report on SSRIs was hardly a ringing endorsement but nor was it particularly critical of most SSRIs. It came down strongly on the side of keeping dosages low as the evidence on greater efficacy from increasing dosage was poor. The advice was for careful and frequent monitoring, especially in the early stages of treatment and avoiding rapid withdrawal from SSRIs. It satisfied the drug companies by saying that SSRIs were effective medicines in the treatment of depression and anxiety conditions. But it left many lay people, including me, uneasy.

A further Panorama programme on Seroxat in October 2004 had given a roasting to GSK and the MHRA. It surfaced publicly the concerns I had about whether GSK had acted promptly enough in handing over to the MHRA crucial safety information from Seroxat's early days. This was the issue I had already been discussing with the MHRA because of my concerns over the evidence on Seroxat's effect on young people under 18 that GSK had mysteriously and suddenly handed over in June. A convoluted and unconvincing explanation had been provided to me for the delay in providing this evidence. The early clinical trials data on the use of Seroxat with under-18s had cast doubt on its efficacy and had revealed concerns over adverse reactions. However this data had been merged with adult data into a meta-analysis and the significance of the findings for young people under 18 was lost in the bigger adult numbers. Allegedly all this only became clear after the first Panorama programme on the 11 May 2003 and this caused GSK to disaggregate the data and provide it to the MHRA.

As far as I was concerned there was a respectable case for prosecuting GSK because they had failed to inform the MHRA in a timely fashion of information on adverse reactions in juveniles. However there would have to be a full investigation and the involvement of lawyers. This inevitably sank into a bureaucratic and legal morass and was far from completion when I changed Ministerial jobs in May 2005. To my astonishment I discovered that the issue limped on for another three years and was only concluded in March 2008. It turned into the largest investigation of its kind in the UK with over 1 million pages of evidence being scrutinised to try to establish whether GSK had failed to inform the MHRA of information it had on the safety of Seroxat in under-18s in a timely way. The company challenged matters all the way. The outcome was that government prosecutors finally took the decision not to prosecute GSK because they said there was no realistic prospect of a conviction, given the then state of enforcement legislation. All GSK received was a slap on the wrist, with the MHRA Chief Executive, Ken Woods, saying: "I remain concerned that GSK could and should have reported this information earlier than they did."[7]

Rebalancing the MHRA

What the Seroxat episode did was fuel the rumbling debate about the MHRA being in the pocket of the pharmaceutical industry and the Government being too weak to intervene. (The industry's counter view was that we did not do enough to support it as part of UK plc!) There were several strands to this argument: the industry funded the Regulator through fees; the MHRA staff came predominantly from industry and returned there; the MHRA did not publish the information to support its decisions; the industry did not disclose adverse reactions promptly; and patients did not play a big enough part in the decisions of the MHRA. I tried to tackle these systemic issues but at the same time bring the MHRA's committee structure more in line with the emerging legislative requirements of the EU on topics such as clinical trials and homeopathic and herbal medicines.

My main concern was to strengthen the position on declarations of industry interest and preventing Chairs of committees from having any current personal interest in the pharmaceutical industry; and to secure more lay membership on committees. We had a lot of internal debate and discussion, not all of it constructive, but the MHRA Chairman recognised that things had to change. In February 2004 the MHRA launched a consultation document that was clearly at the request of Ministers. This proposed an expansion of expert groups in line with EU changes, more involvement of lay people in committees and more rigorous arrangements over declarations of interest and avoiding conflicts. The consultation received around 100 responses from different bodies and was concluded in November 2004. I agreed a revised set of arrangements which came into full operation in October 2005.

There are now more lay people in the committee structure including two lay representatives on the Commission of Human Medicines, the new main body. Although I managed to improve what I inherited lay representation is still insufficient. Involving more lay people in pharmaceutical regulation is the best way to balance the inevitable involvement in these committees of people who have worked in the pharmaceutical industry. Removing these experts altogether would produce a technical deficit that would endanger public safety.

It was difficult to abandon the system of industry fees for funding the work of the regulator. This had been tried when the Medicines Commission had been established and had relied on a government grant. However successive governments failed to increase the grants sufficiently to keep pace with the growth of new drug applications. The result had been an enormous backlog of applications awaiting decision, with delays of up to 3 years before new drugs became available to patients. A change had been made by the Conservatives in 1989 so that the regulator charged applicants fees. I was challenged on this issue when I gave evidence in February 2005 to the Health Select Committee's Inquiry into the influence of the pharmaceutical industry. I explained that other countries such as Sweden and the Netherlands funded their pharmaceutical industries by fees and that government grants had not kept pace with the level of applications. This was not the answer that some members of the Select Committee wanted to hear but it sufficed.[8]

The Select Committee did not like the fact that I was the Minister regulating the industry, controlling NHS drug prices and the sponsor Minister for the pharmaceutical industry. I accepted that it could be argued that these were conflicts of interest but explained I had never found that in practice I felt conflicted. I was able to be tough with the industry on issues like Seroxat, lay representatives on the MHRA and patients registering adverse drug reactions but at the same time promote the interests of the UK-based industry in Europe and fight their corner on animal rights activists' illegal activities. I doubted whether the industry saw me as a soft touch in price negotiations. I did not convince all the Health Select Committee members on this so I had to let my record speak for itself.

One of the sub-texts to this issue of regulators being in the grip of 'Big Pharma' was marketing to the medical profession and the extent to which doctors were advocates for the industry. This was a difficult issue in that significant parts of post-graduate medical education were funded by the pharmaceutical industry through seminars and study days. If this was withdrawn then the public purse would have to fund more of this post-graduate medical education. My own sense was that most GPs were fairly sceptical about the pharmaceutical representatives that called on them and were happy to take samples without being particularly committed to individual products. Given the track record of GPs being overwhelming prescribers of generics – at levels of 80% or more of the prescriptions they wrote – it never seemed to me that the pharmaceutical industry had a compelling case to answer that they had brainwashed doctors into using their products.

Health Industry Task Force

One of the regular complaints from industry was that the NHS and the healthcare industries did not work well together in the best interests of UK plc. There was much disquiet in the medical devices industry about the NHS's low take-up of innovative devices - often invented by someone working in the NHS - together with the impenetrable nature of much NHS purchasing of the sector's products. In response to the growing criticism I set up the Healthcare Industries Task Force (HITF) which brought together government and industry leaders under the co-chairmanship of myself and Sir Christopher O'Donnell, the then Chief Executive of Smith and Nephew.

HITF brought together 200 experts from across industry and government, working in four groups. Chris O'Donnell and I chaired alternate meetings of the main taskforce. There was a lot of frustration within the industry representatives at the unwieldy structures and decision-making processes of the public sector. The DH/NHS purchasing machinery was thought to be too preoccupied with price rather than value for money. I had a good deal of sympathy with this view but equally had to tell industry representatives that they had to reduce their margins on their old staple products like mattresses if they wanted the NHS to have the money to pay for innovative products. My co-Chair and I managed to hold all the disparate interests together for nearly 18 months. We produced an agreed HITF report that we jointly launched in November 2005 at Imperial College London.[9]

Our report recognised that the global and domestic business environment was changing rapidly with huge technological advances transforming healthcare. NHS intelligence-gathering and purchasing had to change to reflect this. More focus on inventors and inventions within purchasing decisions was needed and the NHS needed to be more commercially-savvy about helping inventors coming from within its own ranks so that they could develop commercial products in the UK rather than moving across the Atlantic to do so. The HITF report had five main proposals:

- A new Devices Evaluation Service to make it easier to identify new devices and accelerate their take-up across the UK.

- A new Innovation Centre to be established to spread best practice in promoting and supporting the development of new healthcare technologies.
- Incorporating devices into the work of the new UK Clinical Research Collaboration with a focus on particular disease categories like diabetes so there would be more rapid take-up of innovative inventions.
- Maximising the UK's ability to influence international regulatory activity to prevent damage to the UK devices industry; and concentrating marketing efforts for these products on the USA, Germany, Japan, France and China markets.
- Improving training of NHS staff in the benefits of new technologies and strengthening industry involvement in NHS procurement processes.

Although the HITF report did not resolve all the problems it produced a better relationship between industry and government. Progress after publication was slower than I would have liked but the trade body, the Association of British Healthcare Industries still describes on its website the HITF work as "a substantial success". The pharmaceutical industry however was less pleased with the government over another area I was involved with, the attacks of animal rights activists on scientists and pharmaceutical industry staff.

Animal rights: activists or terrorists?

Animal rights activists had been taking direct action for some time against scientists, research laboratories and pharmaceutical companies. In the UK the focus of these activities was the Stop Huntingdon Animal Cruelty (SHAC) which campaigned to close down the company Huntingdon Life Sciences (HLS), Europe's largest contract animal-testing laboratory. HLS had been operating tests on about 75,000 animals a year from rats to primates. SHAC had been founded in 1999 and was bankrolled by wealthy anti-vivisectionists; and its founders had been involved in earlier campaigns against animal laboratories. The UK has a long history of animal experimentation as part of its strong tradition of biomedical research and discovery. SHAC would almost certainly have tried to close down Charles Darwin's experiments at his home at Down House, especially the somewhat gruesome experiments with pigeons that he conducted.

Research in laboratories using animals had been licensed by the Home Office for many years and since the mid-1980s there had been an annual audit of animal experiments. These experiments are now running at nearly 4 million a year, over a million more than when I was a Minister. The growth in experiments reflects an expansion in biomedical research in the UK which governments have encouraged. The advances in genetics and development of new drugs inevitably mean an increase in testing in animals and some use of monkeys before drugs are given to humans. The importance of this testing was demonstrated by the serious immune reaction in 6 students participating in trials at Northwick Park Hospital in 2006. SHAC and others want to stop all use of animal experiments, not just to reduce the numbers; and they have been prepared to take extreme measures in the support of their view.

In 2003 the animal rights activists were getting the better of the police. They would commit offences in one police force area then skip over the border to another. The police were slow to learn the lessons from tackling football hooliganism – as I regularly told them – and coordinate information, share it between forces and take concerted action. The pharmaceutical industry was up in arms and demanding that the Government became more active. None more so than the Japanese pharmaceutical industry on behalf of whom the Japanese ambassador wrote to me – in a very polite way – requesting more urgent action. A Ministerial Committee, chaired by the Attorney General, Peter Goldsmith, was established to improve the police and government response and I became a member of it.

Ministers were in no doubt that the police response was totally inadequate but it took time to appreciate how well organised and informed the SHAC activists were and the lengths to which they would go. In this country SHAC and their supporters were prepared to intimidate those who did business with HLS; and even write to the neighbours of businessmen making false allegations of rape in order to blacken their reputation. On one occasion they wrote to small investors in GSK telling them to sell their shares or else and smashed the windows of people who worked in companies that did business with HLS. Rape alarms were thrown in roof gutters to keep people awake at night; cars were wrecked; and houses daubed with paint. University and pharmaceutical company staff were intimidated and new buildings attacked. The body of a person whose company had provided guinea pigs for HLS was dug up from their grave. In the US some SHAC and Animal Liberation Front (ALF) activists had been more extreme and engaged in fire bombing and property destruction. They began to move in this direction in the UK when the ALF detonated a device at the home of a GSK executive in Buckingham when his wife and children were there.

Ministers realised that this was a war and that these activists had to be stopped. When I called them terrorists in a speech to the annual ABPI dinner in 2004, with over 1,000 people present, I captured the mood in the industry. More disturbing though was that a few people were so upset by my remarks that they walked out in mid-speech. It made me think that the activists may have penetrated the industry more than it realised. SHAC and their supporters were using encrypted messages to orchestrate actions across the country and appeared to have access to information from inside the industry. Under pressure from Ministers the police started to get their act together with improved information exchanges, a coordination unit and eventually penetration of SHAC with undercover officers. They discovered that there were clear links between SHAC and ALF despite SHAC claiming otherwise. The police asserted that there were a relatively small number of activists but I had the uneasy feeling that SHAC had wider public support than the police realised.

HLS secured injunctions under the Protection from Harassment Act but in 2004 failed to make these permanent. They tried suing for damages without success. The police said that they were hampered in their activities by the shortcomings of the existing legislation so we agreed to strengthen the law. This led to the passage of Sections 145–149 of the Serious Organised Crime and Police Act 2005 which was aimed at protecting animal research organisations. These new provisions prohibited criminal acts or threats designed to harm an animal research organisation "intended or likely" to cause someone "to terminate any contract", or "not to enter into a contract" or "not to perform any contractual obligations owed by it". The new Act also created an offence of intimidating any person connected to an animal research organisation (including employees and their families, research students, investors, suppliers and landlords). Sentences up to five years could be imposed for offences under the Act.[10] A doctor of molecular biology became the first person convicted under the Act in 2006 for attacking property owned by a company supplying equipment to HLS.

After I moved to other Ministerial duties the heat was turned up on SHAC on both sides of the Atlantic. In the US the so-called SHAC 7 were sentenced to a combined 24 years in prison and ordered to pay $1million in restitution. In Europe the police launched Operation Achilles against SHAC in 2007 with raids involving 700 police officers in England, Belgium and the Netherlands. Thirty two people were arrested, including Greg and Natasha Avery the co-founders of SHAC. They were found guilty of blackmail and eventually sentenced in 2008 to 9 years in prison, along with other SHAC activists who received long sentences. ASBOs were imposed also to restrict contact with the targeted companies.

The work started by Labour Ministers in late 2003 produced some significant results. The police have estimated that three-quarters of the most violent activists are now jailed. However if you visit the SHAC website currently there are a list of current protests against HLS, Novartis,

GSK and other drug companies both here and in the US. The worst of the terror tactics have passed for now but the mood also seems to be changing against using so many animals in experiments. When the Home Office published the latest increased figures of animal experiments in mid-2009[11] some scientists claimed that given the level of scientific expertise available now greater progress should be made with replacing animals with more advanced techniques. Although we have a longstanding ban on the use of great apes such as gorillas and chimpanzees in medical research we still use significant numbers of macaques and the numbers are rising. The animal rights issues around medical research may have calmed down since my time as a Minister but the story is not ended, however ethically justified the individual pieces of research may be. Ethical considerations were at the heart of another reform I pursued.

Medicines for children

When I arrived as the pharmaceuticals Minister in 2003 medicines for adults were subject to extensive clinical trials but this was not the case for paediatric medicines. So for a vulnerable 20% of the population there was an absence of extensive testing (including clinical trials) for the safety and efficacy of their medicines. Pharmaceutical companies were reluctant to invest in developing specific treatments for children because the market was small and of less commercial interest. Studies for paediatric medicines could be long, difficult and expensive. Formulating on an industrial scale a precise dosage of a medicine for a diverse child population group was technically difficult and costly. Drug companies could not easily make paediatric medicine pay so they had largely disengaged.

The result was that over 50% of the medicines used by children had not even been studied in the age group for which they were used. For doctors this often meant prescribing drugs for children for use "off label" or prescribing unauthorised products without evidence-based information to guide prescribing or without any risk-benefit assessment. The practical consequences of this were brought home to me on a visit to Great Ormond Street Hospital for Children. There I saw a child who had received pioneering, leading-edge surgery to save his life. On discharge his parents were taught how to cut up an adult tablet into four or six dosages, crush them with a mortar and pestle and then try to dissolve them in some liquid as a basis for getting the mixture into the child. I thought this situation was both ludicrous and scandalous and decided to do something about it. I found that the situation was worse than I realised. There was no British National Formulary for paediatric medicine. Some committed doctors led by Sir Alan Craft, President of the Royal College of Paediatricians were trying to rectify the situation but the DH civil servants claimed they could not find the money to complete the work, publish it and distribute it. £1-2million was involved. After much haggling I fixed on a DH budget-holder and instructed him to fund the project. The first British National Formulary for Paediatric Medicine was published in 2005.[12]

That was the easy bit. Harder was to engage with the drug companies, especially as this would have to be done on a Europe-wide basis for both licensing and commercial incentive purposes such as length of patent protection. I had a bit of luck because the UK was due to take over the EU Presidency in the first half of 2004. This meant that as President it could identify a few priority areas for progress during its Presidency. With some help from senior female doctors in the MHRA and support from John Reid I managed to infiltrate the Whitehall bidding process for UK priority areas and make the advancing of paediatric medicine a Presidency priority. This was facilitated by a changing mood in the industry where some industry leaders could see that resisting change in this area was indefensible and would not help improve their somewhat tarnished social responsibility reputation.

At EU Ministerial meetings I found a lot of support across Europe for progress on this issue. There was some tension with the industry over the length of patent protection, with the industry wanting 10 years and most countries' politicians not wishing to go beyond 6 years. In true EU fashion we secured the establishment of a Council Working Group in October 2004 to begin work on how to take forward paediatric medicine change on a Europe-wide basis. During the UK Presidency we progressed the drafting of an EU regulation on Paediatric Medicine and secured approval in principle to there being such a regulation.

Progressing this work required further meetings with European counterparts when Italy took over the EU Presidency so I was able to sample the Berlusconi approach to government. On one visit to Rome I was met at the airport and swept through immigration into a huge limousine and given a large motorcycle escort to my hotel. Furious Italian motorists were swept aside as we hurtled into Rome. This is the life I thought compared with my government car service Ford Mondeo with its iffy suspension and long periods in traffic jams. Berlusconi may have his faults but he knows how to look after visitors. Later when I described my experience to a colleague he said I was just lucky because I had been used as the rehearsal for Tony Blair's visit a week later – which sadly turned out to be true.

During the UK Presidency we established the 3 main objectives of increasing (a) the availability of medicines licensed for use with children; (b) the information to doctors, patients and parents (including clinical trials data) about these medicines; and (c) research into medicines for children. It took until December 2005 for political agreement to be reached by the Council of Ministers on the text of the Regulation and then agreement had to be reached between the Council, the Commission and the European Parliament which was finally achieved in 2006. Then the whole of Europe had a binding regulation on paediatric medicines. I was assured that achieving this in 2 years was remarkable by the normal timescales for EU legislation!

The new Regulation established a new body, the Paediatric Committee within the European Medicines Agency (EMEA); set out the rules for new products, the marketing and authorisation of existing products and for orphan drugs and off-label products; created a European database of paediatric clinical trials, some of which was available to the public; and created a symbol for packages of products authorised for use in children. There were many other detailed changes that took time in the various EU countries and some of these changes are still not complete in the UK. But from that decision to make paediatric medicines a UK Presidency priority in 2004 children across Europe became protected by a licensing system for their medicines.

Paying for NHS drugs

While these various changes were being progressed I had to renegotiate the prices the NHS paid for drugs. There were essentially two systems: how it paid for generic medicines; and a more elaborate scheme for paying for new branded drugs – the Pharmaceutical Price Regulation Scheme (PPRS). The PPRS had been around for nearly 40 years, since the 1960s. It had its critics but so far government and industry had been unable to agree on any alternative scheme. So every 5 years a reluctant set of combatants strapped on their armour for another round of jousting.

As the responsible Minister I had to pursue two conflicting objectives: protect a strong efficient and profitable UK research-based pharmaceutical industry and secure NHS access to new drugs at an affordable price. The UK industry was moving into a difficult period with clinical trials becoming cheaper to do in Asia with regulatory systems said to be less robust than in Europe. Across Europe governments, pushed by their Finance Ministers, were cutting drug prices and mainland Europe was losing its research-based pharmaceutical industry. The UK still had a lot of good science which attracted a research-based industry but the NHS was usually slower than many healthcare systems at taking up innovative medicines. Many of the existing patents would be running out in the next few years. More and more expensive new drugs were being found to have adverse effects when they were used in large populations so the cost of bringing them to market was also increasing. The pipeline of new drugs was getting smaller and potential new blockbusters were likely to be far fewer.

Alongside this the NHS had been one of the fastest replacers of branded drugs with cheaper generics. In the UK generic drugs were responsible for about two thirds of drug volume and the proportion would increase as many named branded drugs lost their patent protection. Over 80% of NHS prescriptions were written generically and we were moving towards letting pharmacists substitute generics for branded drugs unless the prescriber specified otherwise. I was also engaged in cutting the price of generics. In two exercises separate from the PPRS I had imposed a combined price cut of £400million a year on the generic sector – they barely seemed to blink which made me think I should have imposed heavier cuts! This was a useful signal to the research-based industry as was the move I authorised to prosecute a generics cartel organising price fixing (see Chapter 9).

In the UK new branded drugs were becoming increasingly expensive to produce and in volume terms were a shrinking proportion of the pharmaceutical market. To make matters worse for the industry the new National Institute for Clinical Excellence (NICE) – see below – was carrying out cost effectiveness assessments before a new drug became available in the NHS. Most but not all were approved by NICE but their processes meant new drugs came to market more slowly in the UK. As a result the pharmaceutical industry was feeling sorry for itself, with much talk of the UK losing its research-based industry. The industry came to the negotiating table with two main objectives – a price increase and protection of their right to fix the price of new drugs when these came to market. If they could push up the R and D tax allowance that would be even better. Their opening bid was a 3% price increase; and ours was a 10% price cut. In these opening stages the negotiations were conducted by DH officials and the ABPI negotiators on behalf of the industry led by a senior GSK executive. Ministers and the President of the ABPI – then Vincent Lawson of Merck, Sharp and Dohme – stayed in the background, although I was regularly consulted on various key points in the negotiations and I tracked progress regularly.

The first months were leisurely and technical with discussions about the allocation of costs and capital, returns on capital and sales, transfer prices from overseas affiliates, research and development allowances for incentivising innovation, and something dear to the industry's heart, marketing allowances. On these issues my job was to avoid the detail but ensure momentum without too many concessions. Growth of the marketing allowance needed to be restrained; return on capital needed to be contained to around 20%; and the R and D allowance could be increased only if this would produce a healthy price cut. My primary objective was achieving this substantial price cut and completing a new agreement before the old one expired at the end of 2004.

The ABPI negotiators had a difficult job because they had to keep well over 50 companies – with considerable diversity in size - engaged in the process. Many of these companies were overseas companies; and the two UK giants – Glaxo, Smith and Kline (GSK) and Astra Zeneca tended to dominate the negotiations. The PPRS agreement was theoretically a voluntary one for each company; but if they did not participate in the agreement they would be subject to a price control order under Section 34 of the 1999 Health Act. I made it clear that we would apply price control for those who did not agree changes. Periodically the top brass of the big pharmaceutical companies went to see the Prime Minister or the Chancellor to complain about the way the negotiations were going – i.e. no price increase. Fortunately neither Tony Blair nor Gordon Brown made any rash promises to them.

Negotiations had formally started in November 2003 and by Easter 2004 little progress had been made. I told the industry that we had to complete an agreement by November 2004 for introduction on 1 January 2005, otherwise we would make a price control order on expiry of the old agreement. This captured people's attention and moved the negotiations along a bit. As we approached the summer Parliamentary Recess the industry shifted from its no price cut position, subject to lots of safeguards around marketing spend, the R and D allowance and their right to fix the price of new products. I let it be known that we would move a little from our 10% price cut position.

There was then a further bout of serious lobbying of the Prime Minister, the Chancellor and the Department of Trade and Industry then under Patricia Hewitt (before her move to Health in 2005). The message was broadly that somebody needed to get a grip on these Health Ministers or there would be no UK research-based pharmaceutical industry, with foreign firms moving away and not selling into the UK market. Neither John Reid nor I were much moved by this sabre-rattling but the Ministerial letters flowed into DH seeking a substantial move away from a 10% cut. I wanted to go to an 8% cut, which John supported, and that was our first move. This served however only to encourage the big hitters in the industry to continue to lobby the Prime Minister, the Chancellor and the Secretary for Trade and Industry. Pressure to settle at a 6% price cut came from DTI; the Chancellor was less precise but wanted less than 8%; and Tony Blair was supportive of John Reid and me but wanted a deal struck.

I thought from my talks with the industry leaders that they would settle for a 7.5% price reduction but in the end John and I agreed on 7%. By this time we were into the summer holidays. I managed to track down the President of the ABPI, Vincent Lawton, to the South of France where he was on holiday. Somewhere in the French countryside through a dodgy mobile phone connection we agreed the 7% price cut at the heart of the 2005 PPRS agreement. There then followed an intensive two months of detailed negotiations before the final 2005 PPRS agreement was published in November, coming into effect on the 1 January 2005. The main features of this, apart from the 7% price cut, was an increased R and D allowance; and for the first time an allowance for developing paediatric medicines which I had kept alive in the negotiations.

I thought we had reached a reasonable deal with the industry. Some companies took a different view and continued moaning about the new agreement. They were not best pleased when the Office of Fair Trading (OFT) announced in September 2005 that they were launching a market study into the PPRS aimed at assessing whether the scheme was the most effective means of securing value for money for the NHS whilst offering appropriate incentives for pharmaceutical companies to invest in new medicines. Before then I had moved Ministerial jobs but not before I had gone on a "peace mission" to American pharmaceutical companies, with the Chairman of NICE. US companies did not like the 2005 PPRS settlement any more after our visit but it confirmed to me that they were not going to stop selling to the NHS and that they used NICE endorsements to help market their products in other countries – seemingly on the principle that if the mean NHS evaluator was prepared to endorse the products then everybody else ought to do so.

The 2005 PPRS settlement did not last its intended 5-year period. The OFT study produced a report in 2007 that suggested replacing the PPRS with what was called 'value-pricing'. This was aimed at stimulating innovative drugs that could be taken up quicker by patients, as opposed to the so-called "me too" drugs that were small refinements of existing drugs. There followed some further short-term price reductions in mid 2007 and a rather bad-tempered renegotiation of the PPRS leading to a new settlement that began in January 2009. This started with price cuts of 3.9% in February 2009 and a further 1.9% cut in January 2010, with small price increases amounting to about 0.5% overall during the final three years of the agreement. But before these changes took place the temporary price reductions were to be restored. Casting my eye over the five year period of the new agreement it looked to me to be likely to deliver a rather smaller set of savings to the NHS in real terms than the 7% John Reid and I delivered upfront in the 2005 PPRS negotiations. Although people continue exploring new ways of pricing research-based drugs we still have a PPRS in place in the absence of an agreed alternative.

NICE and its expanding role

Part of my 2003 Ministerial portfolio included NICE which had been established in April 1999 by Alan Milburn. Initially NICE had been a bête noir for the pharmaceutical industry who were concerned that it would lead to the rejection of drugs it had spent a lot of money developing and would slow down NHS market entry. By the time I arrived as a Minister the early tantrums and hostilities had largely passed and NICE had become part of the NHS landscape that pharmaceutical companies operated within. Some companies could even see benefits to NICE because a successful NICE appraisal could help with marketing their products outside the UK.

By 2003 NICE had established an international reputation and its findings on appraisals were freely available on an accessible website. Much of its success was down to its Chairman, Mike Rawlins and Andrew Dillon, the Chief Executive, both of whom are still in post now that NICE is over 10 years old. NICE had established acceptable procedures for their evidence-based decision-making that were free of political interference and secured effective public and professional involvement. All NICE recommendations were devised by independent committees that included industry and health experts as well as patients or members of the public. Just before my arrival NICE had set up a Citizens Council which was the UK's first advisory body made up entirely of members of the public.

NICE had started off with a single programme producing recommendations on the value for money of existing and new medicines and other treatments within the NHS with what were called 'technology appraisals'. There would be one or two waves of new technology appraisals starting each year so that there could be a proper pipeline for the evaluation process. My job as Minister was to approve what was included in each wave to ensure maximum likely benefit to the NHS but also to make sure that if all the drugs were approved the NHS budgets were likely to be able to accommodate them. Some were likely to lead to a cost increase but some might save money, so ensuring a measure of balance in each wave was important.

Some commentators have suggested that the Ministerial involvement caused delay but in my time the submissions on each wave were usually turned round by me within 48 hours. I thought the involvement of a lay Minister was sensible as it prevented wasting a lot of time on evaluating drugs that were too far away from obtaining a license from the MHRA. My approach was to ask intelligent layman's questions about the list submitted and occasionally shift the balance but not to include totally new drugs. I was never put under pressure from the pharmaceutical industry and I am not even sure they were aware of my involvement in the process.

This Ministerial involvement led me to ask some questions about the overall system which led to some useful changes. NICE had started to be asked about producing guidance on whole treatment pathways for particular conditions rather than just appraising specific drugs. This seemed to me likely to be of more value to the NHS so we began an expansion of clinical guidelines that has proved to be very useful and popular. We also began clustering the appraisal of groups of drugs for particular conditions so that there was more comparative information available about their respective merits for different types of patients with the same broad condition. All this meant splitting the technology appraisals of particular drugs into a separate programme from the clinical guidelines.

There were areas where I thought NICE could to do better. Two we made progress on but one we did not. There was a good deal of criticism that although NICE produced good appraisals and the NHS was supposed to implement them within 3 months once their recommendations were endorsed by Ministers (in effect as affordable), NHS implementation was not consistent. The postcode lottery that NICE was supposed to stop still existed. I asked NICE to give much more attention to implementation. This led in 2004 to them setting up an implementation team to help the NHS put their advice and recommendations into practice. They also produced "tools" aimed at managers and professionals to help them assess the cost implications locally of implementing NICE guidance. This meant that when Ministers signed off recommendations the NHS locally could no longer say they did not know how to implement guidance. This initiative did not solve all the implementation problems – particularly when drugs were expensive. There continued to be issues about some expensive cancer drugs. But a 2009 report by Professor Sir Mike Richards, the National Cancer Director, shows a year on year increase in 13 out of the 14 NICE approved drugs for treating cancer, with 7 of them increasing by 50% or more.[13]

Another complaint made to me by the drug companies was the slowness of the NICE processes, so I asked NICE to make improvements. In 2005 they introduced what was called a 'single technological appraisal' process to speed up appraisal of new drugs which resulted in decisions on some new drugs being made within 6 months of MHRA licensing. Later after I left this fast tracking approach was applied to clinical guidelines but there remain concerns about the speed at which NICE produces its verdicts.

The area I made no progress in at all was my attempts to get NICE to identify clinical practices or treatments that were out of date or poor value for money. I wanted to see some of these put forward in the waves of new technology appraisals but I made little progress, although I suspect my nagging on this issue had some impact over time. There remains an issue for NICE of how they root out costly, ineffective long-standing procedures and treatments in the NHS.

By the time I ceased to have responsibility for NICE the original single programme mainly focussed on technology appraisals had grown into three programmes: technology appraisals; clinical guidelines on treating and caring for people with specific diseases and conditions; and guidance on the safety of interventional procedures, tests and treatments that involve entering the body through the skin or a vein, artery, muscle or body cavity. All these activities were to grow apace in the rest of the decade. By the time NICE celebrated its tenth birthday in 2009 it had produced nearly 600 pieces of guidance ranging from cancer and coronary heart disease to the prevention of sexually transmitted diseases and the promotion of physical activity.[14]

These last two pieces of work arose from another decision that I took. When I conducted the Arm's Length Bodies Review described in Chapter 5 one of the bodies I had been under-whelmed by was the Health Development Agency (HDA) which was responsible for preventing ill-health and promoting good health. I decided that its processes would benefit from NICE's more structured and evidence-based approach. So I merged the HDA with NICE and this merger was completed in 2005. This led to NICE being slightly renamed as the National Institute for Health and Clinical Excellence, although the established acronym of NICE was retained. This merger led to nearly 20 pieces of new guidance being produced on public health in 4 years, an output the HDA was nowhere near achieving.[15]

Although NICE has grown in size, scope and reputation not everything has been smooth sailing. This is because there is an inherent conflict at the heart of what NICE does. There are few people who oppose in principle using NHS money efficiently and avoiding a postcode lottery on accessing treatments. The problems occur when particular treatments fall foul of NICE's assessments. Then their processes are challenged by those who dislike particular recommendations. This quickly becomes an issue involving patient interests and not one of simply fending off the drug industry. The issues are played out in the public arena and inevitably Ministers become embroiled because they have to sign off the recommendations and defend them.

I was involved in two of these uncomfortable episodes – the recommendations on IVF and Alzheimer treatments – and was a Ministerial observer of later disputes over cancer drugs. All these cases raised important public policy issues. One of the noisiest and longest battles was over drugs for Alzheimer's. In 2001 NICE had said that Aricept and drugs like it could be used for patients with mild to moderate disease but in 2005 it changed its mind. It then ruled that these drugs were not cost effective for people with all stages of Alzheimers and should only be prescribed by NHS doctors for those with moderate disease, not mild. More than 30 campaigning organisations came out against NICE's change of mind and the Daily Mail - ever ready to take a pop at the Government - supported the campaign.

Whilst I was responsible for NICE I was not responsible for the disease conditions involved in their appraisals. Some of my Ministerial colleagues wanted to overturn the NICE decision. My view was that if we rejected NICE advice in this case we could expect to see other campaigns against NICE recommendations, particularly where the drugs were life-saving but very expensive. (The Alzheimer drugs were relatively cheap which made it more difficult to support NICE.) With John Reid's agreement I asked NICE to look again at their model and calculations to see if they had made sufficient allowance for the benefits to carers. This produced little change but their model itself came under challenge and became the subject of judicial review. In August 2007 the High Court ruled in NICE's favour on 5 of the 6 counts in the judicial review of the process used to develop NICE technology appraisal guidance and NICE subsequently published an amended version of its guidance. However one of the pharmaceutical companies appealed over some details of the NICE model and NICE were required to reveal more details. In the end the whole issue limped on until 2009 when NICE finally issued a version of the guidance which despite all the noise was remarkably similar to their original guidance.

The IVF guidance in 2004 raised different issues. NICE recommended 3 cycles of IVF treatment on the NHS as this was more likely to produce a pregnancy for infertile couples – albeit multiple births might be involved. However this was a very costly recommendation overall even though some PCTs were already providing 3 cycles, as was Scotland. I raised the question of whether IVF should even be available on the NHS and favoured limiting our commitment to one cycle. That was the line that John Reid took despite some clamour - including from within the Ministerial team – but PCTs who wished could offer more cycles. The public noise level was considerably less than over Alzheimers drugs.

NICE had fewer doubts about Herceptin for breast cancer although lobbying started before they had reached their final decision. I was no longer responsible for NICE at this stage but breast cancer sufferers were lobbying all Ministers when we visited hospitals. Whilst I had great sympathy for the women I met facing death, sometimes with young families, I knew that their deaths were usually inevitable in a short space of time. The public policy question that was at issue was whether the NHS should be funding small postponements of death at great cost. When

NICE indicated in 2007 (after I had ceased to be a Minister) that it would turn down some kidney cancer drugs Ministers asked Mike Richards to investigate. This led to a rule change in which drugs to treat people at the end of life should have a higher cost effectiveness threshold (i.e. over £30,000 for a year of good quality life). Drugs could only be licensed for treating a patient population not normally exceeding 7,000 new patients each year; no other NHS treatment was available; and life expectancy of those receiving the treatment was unlikely to be more than 24 months. This meant that the NHS exposure to additional costs for relatively low value drugs was limited but the experience showed that lobbying on emotional grounds could get NICE recommendations overturned. Personally I thought it was a mistake to make these concessions. Tampering with the threshold for cost effectiveness is more damaging than phasing implementation. Once you have done it it is difficult to say you cannot tamper further again and again. This ruling will make it easier to challenge future decisions by NICE.

Overall however NICE has gone from strength to strength and has received relatively few challenges. The Health Select Committee has endorsed its work. Lord Darzi's Next Stage Review's final report in 2008 expanded NICE's role as part of increasing an evidence-based approach to improving quality in the NHS. Like me Darzi wanted NICE to speed up its appraisals process and for patients to be guaranteed access to NICE approved drugs and treatments. For the future NICE was to review and develop the indicators in the GP Quality and Outcomes Framework which governed about 25% of their pay; and would become responsible for setting independent quality standards and clinical priorities within the NHS.[16] This represented a major expansion of NICE's role and makes NICE the most powerful quality determiner in the NHS. It remains to be seen how it delivers this more ambitious role in a harsher financial climate, particularly as the Coalition Government seem to want to neuter its ability to reject new drugs on cost-efficiency grounds. This would be a major mistake after all the hard work put in by Labour to secure this challenge mechanism.

A changing world for Big Pharma

It is only 5 years since I had Ministerial responsibility in this area but in that time huge challenges have emerged for Big Pharma. Cost-conscious governments around the world have attacked expensive patented drugs and tried to boost the use of generics. There have been crackdowns on big pharmaceutical companies paying generics firms to delay launching generic versions of drugs coming off patent. Big Pharma has tried to sell branded versions of off-patent drugs at higher prices than generics; and in some cases bought generics-producing rivals. It is estimated that about half the nearly $400billion worth of patented drugs sold in the world each year will come off patent by 2015. Less than 10% of pharmaceutical sales are said to come from new drugs launched in the past 5 years.

Big Pharma have seen their highly successful business model of the blockbuster drug come under threat not only from the cost and high failure rate of producing new blockbusters, and the loss of existing patents but also from the advance of more personalised medicine through genomics. It is the rapid advance in scientific knowledge through completion of the human genome sequence that will force change both in the pharmaceutical industry and in healthcare systems. Rare single gene disorders accounted for a very small proportion of a nation's burden of disease; but recent studies have identified gene associations with large scale common diseases such as diabetes, coronary heart disease and several types of cancer. All this will make it possible in time to have more personalised treatments prescribed.

In the future we will still keep taking the tablets – because these are often the most cost-effective healthcare intervention, but they will be tablets more aligned with our own genetic make-up rather than 'blockbusters' trialled on large populations. Science will become an even bigger driver of change not only in the pharmaceutical industry but in their healthcare markets more generally as genomic medicine advances. The scientific driving of healthcare change often produces some of the most difficult political and public challenges. The implications of this 'March of Science' and associated problems of translation from bench to bedside are discussed further in Chapter 13.

11

Acute hospitals – cathedrals
of cures or expensive luxuries?

Hospital fantasia

Politicians and the British public are very attached to their hospitals. The 1960s District General Hospital (DGH) has become an established plank of the NHS. Governments like to brag about building hospitals, about expanding them and about the products of their buildings and services. The targets pursued by Labour were largely hospital-driven – inpatient and outpatient waiting periods, Accident and Emergency waiting times, cancer targets, hospital infection rates. These targets caused even more money to be poured into acute hospitals in terms of new buildings, new equipment and, most expensive of all, many more staff (as described in Chapter 6). It is acute hospitals that have done very well from the huge injection of extra money invested in the NHS over the last 10 years. The large Private Finance Initiative (PFI) programme of new and expanded hospitals has secured the future of many of them for years to come with 25-year contracts guaranteeing repayment for these medical Taj Mahals.

Yet this golden age of hospital building and renewal has not been without its problems. Mutating superbugs (as the media liked to call them) have damaged reputations and caused public anxiety and anger over dirty hospitals and sloppy infection control. Advances in medical knowledge and technologies and changes in disease profiles have called into question whether so much care and treatment should be provided in hospitals. The rise in medical specialisation and shorter working weeks for doctors drive the case for concentration of services in fewer hospitals. Increasing numbers of smaller acute hospitals have struggled to pay their way with a growing array of loss-making services and accumulating financial deficits. Still the idea of acute hospitals serving local communities with an impracticably wide range of services remains etched in the public and political psyche. The public expect their MPs to fight tooth and nail to keep the maximum number of services available in their local hospital. Too often politicians seem immune to legitimate concerns over the safety, quality and financial viability of particular hospitals, with clinicians reluctant to argue publicly for service reconfiguration and the movement of services elsewhere.

A classic example of how things can go wrong was the attempt in the 1990s to close the A & E Department at Kidderminster Hospital. A local consultant physician, Richard Taylor, led the medical staff in a campaign to save Kidderminster Hospital, a campaign he chaired from 1997 – 2001. In the 2001 Election Dr Taylor ousted the incumbent Labour MP who had supported closure of the A & E Department. In Westminster political circles a new verb – 'to be Kidderminstered' – entered the political lexicon, despite the fact that the Department was closed on safety grounds about a year or so after Dr Taylor's election. He was still re-elected in 2005.

Kidderminster and other dubious campaigns such as that to save the A & E Department at Chase Farm Hospital in North London – where three people were elected to the local Council to save the hospital – show the power of public campaigns to thwart medical logic and true public interest.

One of the most worrying aspects of these campaigns is the total public unwillingness to listen to arguments about the safety of services. 'Employ more doctors' ring out the voices even if these doctors cannot be employed sensibly or even at all. 'Our hospital deserves more money' even if achieving financial balance there means taking money from somewhere else in the NHS with greater needs. MPs' responses are predictable: they are reluctant to admit even in private that there is anything wrong with their local hospitals that a bit more money would not solve. They are reluctant to admit this in public or to support major change, even when they are a member of a government elected on a manifesto of NHS reform.

Too many MPs are in denial and too many Health Ministers want to ignore the clear warning signs of failure. Higher standard mortality rates, high rates of healthcare acquired infections, financial deficits and high use of locums and agency staff among doctors and nurses, all tell the story of a hospital in decline where major change is needed. £50million national steam cleaning programmes, sacking the Chair and Chief Executive or calling in the regulator for yet another report on failure are simply displacement activities rather than tackling the root problem – an acute hospital, often a DGH, that is not viable in its existing form.

It is unsurprising in this political climate that many NHS boards are reluctant to tackle service changes. They are faced with a process of public consultation that can continue for years with much bad blood locally: Chase Farm is a case in point. There is the prospect of determined local opposition campaigns with scope for legal challenges to their processes; doctors unwilling to stand up in public and say what they have said in private; nervous MPs; and the prospect of a changing cast of elected Ministers whose instincts are to take the line of least public resistance. History shows NHS boards that the process can go badly wrong and at the end of it Ministers or their officials will buy off trouble with some kind of financial fix – in football parlance 'a bung'.

There have been brave and competent souls who have re-engineered their local acute services successfully after a lengthy, skilful and determined process but too often these have been the exception rather than the rule. Too often the public has been encouraged to believe in fairies sprinkling gold dust over their local hospitals because that is what the NHS has usually done at the behest of their political masters. Many acute hospitals are given third or fourth chances to redeem themselves without carrying out the radical surgery needed. What this does is lock-up NHS resources – money, assets and people – in a failing or failed business model. It denies resources to innovative and more efficient ways of delivering health services.

This behaviour could be indulged during the years of financial plenty but is less likely to survive a period when the NHS moves from feast to famine. In 5 years' time the annual revenue available to the NHS in real terms is likely to be remarkably similar to that which it had before the huge Labour injection of money. The only differences will be that the NHS buildings and plant will be much better but also more expensive to run, public expectations will be greater, as will need. This means that politicians, doctors, managers and boards will need to tackle the examination question: 'Do we spend too much of our finite healthcare resources on acute hospitals and are they the good value for money that the public and politicians seem to think?' In considering this question there is now evidence and past experience to draw upon: the overall performance of acute hospitals; the issue of hospital cleanliness and infection; the deployment and use of NHS resources – revenue staff and fixed assets; and the barriers to change in the acute sector. The rest of this chapter examines these issues drawing on my experience as a Minister and in London where I tried to re-engineer change after Ministerial life but resigned in frustration in May 2009.

The performance of acute hospital trusts

At the end of 2008/9 there were 169 acute and specialist trusts in the Care Quality Commission's (CQC) NHS performance ratings. These trusts incorporated a mixture of specialist tertiary hospitals, district general hospitals (DGHs) and local hospitals. There were also a few community hospitals managed by PCTs - these are discussed further in the next chapter. DGHs tend to serve an average population of 200,000 – 300,000; but specialist hospitals derive their patients from much wider areas, sometimes nationally and even internationally. Local hospitals serve smaller communities of up to a 100,000 population and provide a much narrower range of services, often confined to little more than urgent care or minor injuries unit, outpatient clinics, rehabilitation and day care and possibly palliative care.

Much of the recent major arguments with local communities have focussed on DGHs and changes to their services. Since the 1960s the public have been used to DGHs providing a full range of clinical services, including an Accident & Emergency Department, emergency and elective surgery, maternity and paediatric services, as well as treatment for most diseases and rehabilitation services. Medical advances and specialisation, together with shorter working weeks for doctors as a result of the European Working Time Directive (see Chapter 6) have combined to cause many smaller DGHs to struggle to provide safe and cost-effective services across the full range of clinical specialties. Where these smaller DGHs are the only hospital in the trust relatively small shifts of patients and income can quickly threaten their financial viability and performance ratings by the regulator.

Some in the NHS will argue that the standards against which trusts are measured by the CQC are very demanding and that it is hardly surprising that some trusts seem to be failing. I would beg to differ. All trusts are measured against 24 core standards that have been in existence since 2003 when I helped to shape them and approved them. These standards are fairly basic, have 44 parts and you would expect the overwhelming majority of NHS trusts to be able to meet them. Indeed we set them in 2003 at a level that was designed to ensure maximum NHS compliance, with little prospect of trusts failing them. All trusts have to make a public declaration on whether they comply with these core or basic standards.

The CQC use 86 indicators across the different types of trust to assess performance, including meeting national priorities and targets. In 2008/9 the CQC assessed all trusts for overall quality and financial management. This was an assessment after 10 years of continuous investment that saw a threefold increase in the NHS budget in cash terms from £36billion in 1996/1997 to about £110billion ten years later. This was a doubling in real terms in revenue allocations apart from well over £20billion in capital investment in hospital buildings and equipment. The financial management of these trusts is discussed in more detail later.

In 2008/9 CQC assessed only 37 acute trusts as 'excellent' for quality of services - a reduction from 52 in the previous year. Only about half of this 37 – 19 – had managed to score 'excellent' in two successive years. Thirty trusts previously rated 'excellent' had declined to 'good'. In most of these cases the deterioration was due to failure on several – four, five or six – measures and could not therefore be dismissed as a 'near miss.' Although Trusts found national priorities challenging, it was in performance against core standards that CQC saw the most noticeable decline. Worryingly CQC found that in 2008/9 only 99 of the 169 acute and specialist trusts – 59% - fully met core standards by the end of the year; with only 41% of these trusts compliant throughout the whole year, i.e. from the 1 April 2008 to 31 March 2009.[1] In other words they could only meet the core standards for part of each year.

At the other end of the spectrum 43 acute trusts were rated 'fair' in 2008/9 compared with only 30 in the previous year. Eight were deemed 'weak' for quality, the same number (but not the same trusts) as in the previous year. One of these was Barts and the London Hospitals Trust – a prestigious body where a huge PFI building project is in progress that will make it even larger and even less financially sound. One, the Royal Cornwall Hospital Trust – scene of the birth of David Cameron's latest child - had been 'weak' on quality for four years in a row. One, Maidstone and Tunbridge Wells Trust, had been 'weak' for three years on the trot; and another one, Mid-Staffordshire Foundation Trust had been 'weak' on quality for two years in succession. Over 10 Trusts recorded continuing non-compliance in five standards: safe use of medical devices, decontamination, safeguarding of children, clean and well-designed environments and mandatory training. Amongst the areas considered consistently poor by CQC are stroke care, cancelled operations and maternity - all significant areas of activity for patients.

Two of these 'weak' trusts have managed to seriously hit the headlines in the last two years, searing their names into the public consciousness. In late 2007 a report into earlier outbreaks of Clostridium Difficile (which causes acute diarrhoea, especially among elderly patients) at Maidstone and Tunbridge Wells Trust in Kent found the infection had caused the deaths of 90 patients.[2] In 2009 CQC's predecessor the Healthcare Commission published a damning report into the emergency care deficiencies of Mid-Staffordshire Foundation Trust which had destroyed the local community's confidence in the services there.[3] Further later reviews commissioned by Alan Johnson confirmed how bad things were. There is now to be a further public inquiry into the wider lessons to be learned from this trust's failings even though I suspect we know them only too well but have failed to take effective remedial action.

A third name was added to the roll of dishonour when a CQC unannounced inspection found blood-spattered trays used to carry equipment and deeply-stained trolley mattresses in the A & E Department at Basildon and Thurrock Trust in Essex. That inspection had been prompted by concerns that the standardised mortality rates at the hospital had been unusually high. Adding fuel to the fire Dr Foster's analysis of healthcare data in its 2009 Guide to English Hospitals suggested that Basildon was not alone. It was one of twelve hospitals significantly underperforming on basic safety measures.[4]

These individual cases raised two concerns relating to inspection and regulation. First why are some trusts allowed to continue being 'weak' providers of healthcare; and second are the regulators using the right measures to assess quality. On the second issue, CQC's reliance on self-certification and spot checks when concerns are heightened could be said to give an unduly rosy picture of acute trust performance. Things could be a lot worse in the hospital world than the picture shown in the annual reports of CQC and their predecessor body. Bang on cue in March 2009, Professor Brian Jarman of Imperial College entered the fray to suggest they were. Examining deaths in 25 Trusts in 2007/8 Professor Jarman found there were 4,600 unexpected deaths – over 150 more than would have been expected at each of the trusts he examined. He acknowledged that these figures did not prove malpractice or inadequacy; and some of the trusts said their mortality rates had improved since 2007/8. CQC and the Department of Health have said rightly that mortality rates on their own do not measure the quality of care in the acute hospital sector. However it is worth noting that CQC imposed conditions on 10 trusts when the new system of licensing came into operation during 2010/11.

Taken in the round this data suggests that the picture on quality performance in the acute hospital sector is far from reassuring. After a decade of large and sustained increases in resources for acute hospitals most objective observers would have expected better. Given the poor performance on productivity cited in Chapter 6 one would have expected quality to have improved much more than it has across the sector as a whole. Shareholders of any business with this level of quality and productivity performance after a decade of massive investment would be a lot more dissatisfied with acute hospitals than NHS satisfaction surveys suggest that the public are. Or is it that the public has such low expectations in some parts of the country that they are simply resigned to acute hospitals underperforming? 'Hospital kills patients' is no longer a headline.

As Chapter 2 shows there have been some major NHS improvements in service access and deaths from killer diseases but there is still a long way to go on overall performance quality in the acute hospital sector. This was recognised in the final report of Lord Darzi's Next Stage Review, 'High Quality Care for All'. That report considered that progress had been made on the first dimension of quality which is ensuring we do no harm to patients by ensuring that the environment is safe and clean and we reduce avoidable harm such as excessive drug errors and HCAIs. Yet even on this basic level there is evidence of significant shortcoming as the report recognised on page 48. 'Nevertheless it is also true that progress has been patchy, particularly on patient experience. The local clinical visions found unacceptable and unexplained variations in the clinical quality of care in every NHS region. They identified important changes that need to be made to raise standards and ensure all services are high quality.'[5]

The Darzi report echoes the findings of the CQC and the Healthcare Commission. This patchiness is well illustrated in the area of stroke where CQC found only 37% of acute trusts met the required standard for stroke care, with only the South West and North East regions achieving 50% in 2008/9.[6] The National Confidential Enquiry into Patient Outcomes and Deaths, using 2006/7 data, found that in 25% of 1,635 deaths studied in detail there was 'a clinically important delay in the first review by a consultant'.[7] Poor communications between doctors, inadequate handovers at night and delays in contacting consultants are causing unnecessary deaths according to the report. It is this kind of evidence that have caused some to say that, unlike the university sector, the NHS may have renowned experts but unlike that sector it has no world-class acute hospitals.

On current evidence the jury is definitely out on whether all acute hospitals can be brought up to the levels that Lord Darzi rightly expected whilst maintaining anything like the current configuration of acute hospital services. In too many places too many hospitals are trying to provide too wide a range of services with the resources available or likely to be available in the future. Unless that changes we will continue with unacceptable numbers of underperforming and in some cases unsafe acute hospitals. All too often these underperforming hospitals are associated with another feature of acute hospitals over the past decade – the increase in healthcare acquired infections (HCAIs) and the associated deaths. It was during my time as a Minister that the public concerns about HCIAs and the related issue of hospital cleanliness rose rapidly up the political agenda. In the public mind acute hospitals all too often became associated with danger and even death rather than safety and recovery.

Healthcare acquired infections and clean hospitals

When I became a Health Minister in mid-2003 tucked away in my portfolio were the subjects of cross-infection and hospital cleaning. They did not look very significant and at that stage did not seem to attract much media attention. That changed dramatically in the autumn of 2003 when accounts of 'super-bugs' felling swathes of NHS patients began to appear with increasing frequency in the media. Newspapers became full of stories of MRSA (Methicillin-resistant Staphylococcus Aureus) and dirty hospitals. Vigilante visitors reported bloodstained and soiled linen, filthy toilets and unclean wards. Energetic but scientifically ill-informed reporters forged in the public mind a lasting link between dirty hospitals and HCAIs. The public spotlight then was on MRSA, although it was soon to be joined in the dock by other superbugs, especially Clostridium Difficile or – C.diff to the cognoscenti.

Getting to the bottom of causes and linkages in the infection pathways was to prove difficult, especially at a time of media hysteria. Few reporters understood that staphylococcus aureus is everywhere (and is usually harmless) and that it had been recognised as a very common cause of infections since late Victorian times. No-one bothered much all the while doctors could deal with the bacteria first with penicillin and then with methicillin. But between 1993 and 1997 5% to 30% of staphylococcus aureus became resistant to methicillin. MRSA became endemic in the NHS in these years when the number of reported cases rose most steeply from less than 1,000 a year to about 9,000. As I pointed out MRSA took up residence in NHS acute hospitals in the Conservative years. With drug resistance rising we had to change NHS behaviour on cross-infection and cleanliness.

Under Alan Milburn the collection of MRSA bacteraemia data from hospital trusts was made mandatory because the voluntary system in place since the 1970s had led to underreporting. This revealed that, despite some hospitals reducing MRSA, the total number of cases was increasing by nearly 4% a year. I began publishing data six-monthly rather than annually and later moved to quarterly publication. We started collecting data internally on a monthly basis to provide more up-to-date information; and local hospitals started analysing data by individual departments. It was clear that local practices in acute hospitals varied enormously and that more central involvement was required. By the end of 2003 the Chief Medical Officer had issued a report 'Winning Ways' to outline to hospital trusts the steps they should take to improve hygiene and infection control. All acute trusts were required to have a Director of Infection Prevention and Control to provide specialist advice, to require compliance with local guidelines and to start producing published reports on local progress.[8]

I decided that we should have a 'clean your hands' national campaign because the scientific evidence strongly suggested that better hand hygiene was vital to stopping the transmission of MRSA. The National Patient Safety Agency had been piloting this idea and I put them in charge of the campaign and making sure that alcohol-based hand sanitising equipment was available near every patient in acute hospital wards. A competition was held for firms to supply the NHS with these new alcohol rubs. We collected data on how many hospitals were pressing on with the hand hygiene campaign because the NHS response was mixed. The National Audit Office reported later in 2004 that 'there continues to be non-compliance with infection control practice'[9] and wanted to see all hospitals adopting the practices set out in 'Winning Ways'. It was to be the spring of 2005 before we could say with any confidence that all acute hospitals had implemented the 'clean your hands' campaign. Even then urinary catheter care which accounted for nearly 25% of HCAIs was still a great cause for concern

Improving infection control in NHS acute hospitals was seriously hard work with far too many doctors, nurses, managers and trust boards paying insufficient attention to the danger to patients. Only through unrelenting political and management pressure did we see cases of MRSA levelling off and slightly dropping in 2004. In the period April – September 2004 MRSA bacteraemia in NHS acute trusts were down over 6%, compared with the same period the previous year. But the variation between regions was considerable with London far worse than any other region; and the North East and East Midlands much better than any other region. It was clear from the visits I made and conferences that I spoke at that attitudes and attention to improvement varied enormously across the NHS. In most acute hospitals doctors and nurses were in charge of infection control but too often seemed unable to make their professional colleagues comply with good professional practice.

A new onslaught on MRSA was launched in 2004 with the announcement that we were reducing the number of targets to 20 but one of these would be reducing the number of MRSA bacteraemia in hospitals by 50% by March 2008. Each NHS acute trust was set an individual target and this was to be monitored by SHAs. But the media moved on from MRSA to other superbugs that the NHS was killing patients with. They had plenty to choose from because the Heath Protection Agency was now collecting data which showed virtually all these infections increasing during the 1990s. Cases of Escherichia Coli virtually doubled in that decade and it was one of the most rapidly increasing bugs emerging in resistant form. More significant were the hyper-virulent new strains of the bacteria Clostridium difficile (C.diff) which colonised sites left free by the effects of antibiotics and whose spoors lingered on indefinitely. It was causing unstoppable diarrhoea in elderly patients and leading to more death certificates blaming C.diff.

Public anxiety about superbugs was rising faster than NHS acute hospitals were able to respond. In too many hospitals there was a fatalistic acceptance of the inevitability of HCAIs and a reluctance to enforce better clinical practice. We extended mandatory surveillance to new HCAIs including C.diff in patients over 65 years which was later extended in 2008 to all patients over 2 years old. Unfortunately C.diff is spread by ingesting the bacterial spoors which then grow in the colon, so hand washing with alcohol does not work and alternative hygiene arrangements are required. Many acute hospitals have struggled to contain this widening range of HCAIs and have had to invest increasing amounts of money and effort to tackling them. Despite these efforts the number of people dying with HCAIs as a contributory or main cause of death on their death certificate increased. While MRSA received the lion's share of public attention the number of C.diff cases was far greater and more lethal: it was NHS-contracted C.diff that did for my 90 year old mother during my time as a Minister.

Despite the lack of scientific evidence most of the media and the public were convinced that cleaner hospitals would eliminate HCAIs. Trade unions like Unison claimed that the contracting out of hospital cleaning services was at the root of the problem. I was challenged to debate this with Unison in January 2005. I acknowledged that the number of NHS cleaning staff had reduced in the 1980s and 1990s but so had the size of the hospital estate – by 20%. Even if one disagreed in principle with contracting out cleaning to the private sector the evidence suggested that it mattered little whether cleaning was done in-house or by contractors: it was the quality of management at individual hospitals that counted. Independent inspections of hospital cleanliness by Patient Environment Action Teams (PEATs) revealed as many good - and bad - hospitals cleaned by contractors as those cleaned by the NHS in-house. Acute hospitals have shown the same variability in the way they tackle hospital cleaning as they have with controlling cross-infection.

The public needed reassurance that we were taking seriously the concerns over hospital cleaning because a clean hospital environment was probably the best platform for tackling HCAIs and increasing patient and visitor confidence in a hospital. To introduce some rational basis for choosing from the wide range of commercial products that began to be promoted for cleaning up the NHS I introduced a Rapid Review Panel in 2004 run by the Health Protection Agency to assess the scientific worth of these products. The HPA produced a rating scale to help the NHS decide what products to use and to deal with inflated claims. This mechanism had mixed success and did not live up to the 'Rapid' part of its title. I also raised hospital cleaning standards; let the Heathcare Commission toughen up the PEAT system; and produced a new NHS cleaning manual.

As the 2005 Election approached the public anxiety about HCAIs did not abate, as new superbugs surfaced. I became entangled in a debate with the NHS about whether infection was being imported into acute hospitals by elderly people admitted from residential care or nursing homes. There was evidence suggesting that about 5% of patients were bringing MRSA into hospital and passing it on to other sick people whose immune systems were weak. Five years ago testing for HCAIs was a lengthy business with NHS pathology laboratories; but I looked at some new tests producing results in two hours that were being used in the US. These were expensive but I arranged for pilots of two-hour swabbing tests for MRSA to take place in three hospital trusts (in London, Birmingham and Plymouth) to see if this could control imported infection. This led later to the Darzi

Report in 2007 proposing screening of all elective surgery patients for MRSA by March 2009 and for it to be extended to emergency admissions thereafter.[10] Where the swabbing has been done it seems to have reduced HCAIs.

I was told the NHS lacked sufficient single rooms to isolate patients and reduce cross-infection. At that time the average number of single rooms per acute hospital was about 15% but in some older hospitals it was much less. As I was responsible for hospital design I changed the recommended standard for new hospitals to be build with 50% of rooms becoming single rooms but this change would only help in the longer term.

Ideas poured in for the causes of infection: doctors' ties and shirt cuffs; nurses' uniforms and nurses taking their uniforms home to launder; hospital visitors, who needed to be stopped or restricted; face masks should be worn by visitors and staff. The cry went up to bring back matrons à la Hattie Jacques; and to put nurses more in charge of cleaning. We should sack contract cleaners and increase the pay of cleaners. New cleaning products were offered with the maximum of publicity to help their share prices. Where I ended up when I ceased to be the responsible Minister was that a few things were more important than others. Hand hygiene was critical and so was measuring performance on HCAIs, department by department. The culture and expectations on hygiene set by a trust board and their executive management team was critical. An authoritative doctor or nurse at Board level needed to drive the infection control agenda and enable clinical staff to improve cleaning and hygiene. Without these organisational and cultural changes patients will continue to die unnecessarily in NHS hospitals from HCAIs.

We had to do more to get hospitals to pay adequate attention to cross-infection. John Reid wanted to introduce fines but I had my doubts. We settled for a new hygiene code overseen by the Healthcare Commission who could issue 'improvement notices' to trusts requiring them to make improvements within a set period of time. This Code was eventually given a statutory basis in the 2006 Health Act which I piloted through the House of Lords.[11] new Code of Practice for the Prevention and Control of Healthcare Associated Infections outlined how organisations should work to ensure that patients were cared for in a clean and safe environment. It told trusts what their duties were in terms of systems and how they should assess and manage risks, implement clinical protocols and provide training to staff. Boards and Chief Executives were told clearly that they would be held accountable for cutting HCAIs and preventing cross-infection.

All this effort did eventually drive down MRSA infections in acute hospitals. The March 2008 target of halving MRSA cases from the 2003/4 level of 7,700 cases was achieved. The number of cases has continued to fall since then. The latest figures from the Health Protection Agency show that there was a 59% decrease in the number of MRSA episodes reported between the quarter October – December 2007 to the quarter October – December 2009 from 1,092 to 444. Currently the annual rate of cases is running at little more than 2000 cases a year – a dramatic improvement nationally from the position in 2003/4. But the numbers look as though improvement is flattening off and there remain major problems with HCAIs in some acute hospitals.

In mid-2008 the Healthcare Commission warned that a quarter of NHS trusts in England was still breaching the statutory hygiene code.[12] A similar picture showed in their 2007/8 assessment of trusts.[13] The problem had shifted in many hospitals from MRSA to containing the spread of C.diff which has a seasonal profile peaking in the winter quarter of January – March. In that winter quarter C.diff cases remained at about 15,000 cases a quarter in 2005, 2006 and 2007 but since then the numbers have fallen to around 13,000 cases in the 2008 winter quarter and then to under 9,000 in the 2009 winter quarter. The numbers appear to have continued falling and for the quarter ending December 2009 they were at about 6,000 cases in the quarter. However the improving trend looks to have flattened off and there is still major differences in performance between different acute hospitals.

C.diff is still a very dangerous issue in far too many acute hospitals as the 90 deaths in Maidstone and Tunbridge Wells Trust demonstrated. Some trusts are seriously struggling to contain HCAIs. Despite all the effort and improvements there are still about 25,000 cases of C.diff in NHS hospitals each year, a mixture of imported cases and those that are all a hospital's own handiwork. The UK death rates from HCAIs infections, especially C.diff, remain a continuing public concern and blot on the NHS's reputation. They still number in the thousands each year as main or contributory causes on death certificates. The NHS Litigation Authority pays out increasing sums of compensation for victims of HCAIs, including a record high one of about £5million to Lesley Ash, the actress.

The roll call of HCAIs continues to increase as do their name length: Norovirus, Escherichia Coli, Enterobactor, Glycopeptide-resistant Enterococcal Bacteraemia. Surgical sites, catheters and wards in NHS acute hospitals all present dangerous situations that can turn cure and care to danger and disaster unless there is constant vigilance and attention by hospital staff. The UK is short of microbiologists to tackle the epidemic and some of our doctors make matters worse by over-prescribing antibiotics compared to their German-Swedish, Danish and Dutch counterparts.[14] All these countries have far lower rates of MRSA bacteraemia than the UK; and have made more determined efforts to root out HCAIs in their acute hospitals – more 'search and destroy' than alleviation.

Despite the improvements in hospital infection rates for MRSA and C.diff under Labour, our acute hospitals face a very challenging future from HCAIs. Having more of these hospitals than we need and more of them underperforming and financially unviable will only make things worse in terms of infected patients and likely deaths. It is in these financially-challenged acute hospitals that corners are cut, good hygiene diminishes and cross-infection flourishes. It is these hospitals that are less likely to have the scope for separation of patients and barrier nursing to check the spread of infection. At the heart of the issue is how we spend taxpayers' money on the NHS and in this regard the financial performance of the acute hospital sector over the past decade is less than reassuring.

The acute hospital sector's use of resources

Whether in terms of fixed assets or control of revenue expenditure big question marks remain about the way the NHS acute hospital sector has used a decade of extra money. Investment decision-making, use of assets, financial management systems, changing business processes and labour productivity all leave much to be desired in too many NHS acute hospital trusts, including some household names. In too many of those trusts management has concentrated on delivering better access and clinical performance with insufficient regard to the most cost-effective way of achieving these improvements. Too many clinicians and politicians have blamed targets for the resulting financial failures that often occurred; but it is at least as reasonable to argue that it was possible – as some managers have demonstrated - to reconcile service improvements and better access with effective financial management.

These financial shortcomings have been exposed by the large number of acute hospital trusts – about 50% - lacking the financial management capability and business planning processes to convince Monitor that they can become FTs (see Chapter 3). To still have over 40 acute trusts carrying historic financial deficits at the end of 2009/2010 after the funding streams of the last 10 years is a serious indictment of those managing those trusts and those holding them to account.[15] Many of these deficits will continue well into the future.

The gulf in financial management between the FTs and non-FTs has been brought out well in the CQC's NHS performance ratings for 2008/9. 81 of 83 acute and specialist FTs were rated 'excellent' or 'good' for financial management. This is 98% of these trusts with such ratings; the same as in 2007/8. Among the non-FTs only 53 out of 86 – 62% - were rated 'excellent' or 'good'; only 6 of these non-FTs secured an 'excellent' rating compared with the 66 of the FTs. We go into a period of financial retrenchment after a decade of financial plenty with 20% of acute and specialist trusts rated as only 'fair' or 'weak' for financial management by the CQC.[16] This is a higher percentage than in ambulance trusts or mental health trusts. It does not bode well for achieving efficiency savings at a time of financial stringency without damaging services.

Some acute hospital trusts have only achieved a better financial position by overtrading and spending more than they should at the expense of their weak PCT paymasters. It is striking that in 2008/9 72 of the 152 PCTs were rated 'fair' or 'weak' for financial management by CQC.[17] This position has arisen largely because too many PCTs have allowed acute trusts to overspend. Too often SHAs switch money from financially well-managed providers and commissioners to bail out the under-performers. Then the whole cycle starts again the next year, rather than dealing with the problems of the weak financial management endemic in too many PCTs and acute hospital trusts. The best example of this is London SHA which I saw at first hand as Chairman of their Provider Agency for two years until my resignation. The CQC performance report for 2008/9 shows 14 of London's 31 acute and specialist trusts – 46% - as rated only 'fair' or ' weak' for financial management. This compares with 15% of such trusts in the rest of the country. The rate of improvement in London is glacial: between 2007/8 and 2008/9 one acute trust moved from 'fair' to 'good' and one from 'weak' to 'fair'.[18]

At the heart of this problem is a total failure – political, managerial and clinical – under successive governments to deal with the excess of acute sector capacity in London, especially in North London. Put simply in London (and some other places) money is pumped unnecessarily and unwisely into acute hospitals whose services should be delivered elsewhere and differently and provided to managements who are incapable of making the necessary changes. This approach is supported by MPs and local councillors across the political spectrum.

The position has been made worse in both London and elsewhere by the way the Private Finance Initiative (PFI) has been managed and used by the NHS. I described in Chapter 9 my attempts to curb the growth of the PFI hospital building programme and to reduce its scale from £12billion too nearer £7billion. By the end of the 1990s some new hospital building was undoubtedly required; and to secure new hospitals within a reasonable timescale the PFI approach had much to commend it: projects were built to time with few cost overruns. However the PFI programme required considerable rigour in assessing affordability and future income flows because the contracts for building these hospitals guaranteed real terms repayments over a quarter of a century. Locking themselves into inflexible contracts for such a long period was a very high risk strategy for some acute trusts especially with their hopelessly optimistic future income projections. We have ended up with too many PFI hospitals struggling to meet their repayment obligations.

A classic example of how PFI could go horribly wrong is the Queen Elizabeth Hospital (QEH) in Greenwich. In December 2005 QEH auditors issued a Public Interest Report noting that QEH was likely to fail to meet its statutory duty to break even and over a three year period would have a deficit of nearly £13million a year, about 10% of total income. QEH was a 'first wave' whole hospital PFI scheme with an initial contract of 30 years and a unitary charge fixed in real terms (linked to the RPI) for that period. The contract was signed in the late 1990s when the value for money test was that the proposed scheme should be cheaper than the public sector comparator – which at that time assumed that the cost of public capital was 6% in real terms. As the cost of public capital fell, this resulted in the new tariff for paying hospitals assuming a lower public dividend for capital. This meant that payments to QEH would not cover their unitary payments to the developer. An independent review suggested that QEH would incur excess capital costs of about £8.5million a year for 30 years.[19] Thus QEH was locked into a contract that would require it to generate a level of income from patient flows that were impossible to generate under the tariff system unless huge numbers of patients were diverted from other hospitals. The result has been a merger between QEH and two other South East London hospitals (one of which, Bromley, also has a PFI hospital which is struggling to generate the income to fund its unitary payments) so that patient flows can be moved to the PFI hospitals over time.

Whilst the QEH is an extreme example it illustrates, together with the Bromley example, how many acute hospitals are locked into inflexible long-term contracts based on over-optimistic assumptions about future patient income and with inflexible fixed assets that are difficult to change as models of patient care change. It means that future political and NHS management is going to struggle to meet many of the contractual obligations without a major (and difficult) renegotiation of the contracts or giving preference to these PFI hospitals in the location of services. This makes it highly likely that services will have to be moved away from some non-PFI older hospitals, even if they are better located for some patients, to bolster the income of the PFI hospitals.

An example of this, still unresolved, is the major PFI scheme costing well over £1billion at Barts and the London Trust mentioned in Chapter 9. When these new buildings open they will have far more capacity than the trust can use and this means attracting a sizeable flow of patients from other hospitals to meet the unitary payments for the PFI buildings. This in turn will make some other hospitals unviable unless they in turn reconfigure their services significantly. Much of this was known at the time that the PFI was given the go-ahead but in the face of a determined campaign led by the Evening Standard, Ministers and the hospital local management preferred to travel hopefully.

What the PFI building programme has done – especially in London, but also elsewhere – is to provide an even bigger challenge to the way the NHS uses its fixed assets and plant. While NHS hospitals have shown in their accounts a notional public dividend on capital there have been and remain few real incentives to use capital assets well. Expensive capital equipment can be installed with few requirements to see that it is used intensively: the contrast with the way I have seen imaging equipment and theatres used in Singapore and Hong Kong is striking. Buildings can be under-utilised or left unoccupied with few consequences for those responsible for their stewardship.

The land holdings of the NHS are considerable but vacant land and buildings are still held on to by local bodies, seemingly on the principle of 'saving for a rainy day'. As I was told by Lord Darzi in a 2009 Parliamentary Answer – "The Department [of Health] does not collect information centrally on what land and buildings have been declared surplus to requirements, neither does the Department audit for accuracy or completeness nor how long such property has been declared surplus by NHS bodies."[20] The DH has issued guidance but seems almost proud of its hands off approach and leaving hospital trusts unchallenged on the way fixed assets are used. Under prompting by the Treasury, as the fiscal screws tighten, Ministers also acknowledged to me in another 2009 Parliamentary Answer that they estimated that it would collect £200million in 2009/10 from disposal of surplus land and buildings from non-FT Trusts.[21] (For FTs assets have been handed over to the trust, without knowing what they will do with them.) But this estimate understates the scale of the problem.

From some work I did in London on the use of NHS land and buildings future governments may not wish to be so laissez-faire. This work revealed that the NHS in one part of London had something like 2000 different sites, excluding all the FT sites. This work related only to South West London which has about 20% of the non-FT sites in London. Scaling this work up to a pan-London picture showed that the building footprint on NHS owned land in London – where land is probably the most expensive in the UK – was only some 18%. Within that figure space underutilisation was another 18%; and about 25% of the buildings were functionally unsuitable. Alongside this the maintenance backlog was approaching £1billion.

As a picture of NHS stewardship and use of its facilities and fixed assets over the 60 years of its existence, this record is poor to say the least, especially given the extra money invested over the past decade. This London analysis does not suggest that NHS local bodies can be left alone, untutored and unsupervised, to manage their fixed assets if taxpayers' interests are to be properly protected. I asked the company who did this London work to estimate the opportunity cost of the underutilised non-FT fixed assets. On a market valuation of current use of the land (i.e. as a hospital, rather than as housing or commercial development use) the underutilisation was about 30% of the market valuation. For London as a whole this amounted to a figure in excess of £2billion, excluding the assets transferred to FTs. There is no reason to think that London is different from the rest of the NHS in the way fixed assets have been used and managed. Moreover it is clear that some of the surplus land could be used for non-hospital purposes where the market valuation is likely to be much higher.

The way money and assets are used in the acute hospital sector is indicative of a business leviathan that finds it difficult to adapt and change as medicine and public preferences change. In psychiatric care at least the asylums have largely given way to community services. In the acute sector too often the patients are sucked into the hospital rather than the specialist services adapting and going to the patients. This was highlighted by Lord Darzi in his work on the Next Stage Review. Transformation of hospital services is resisted for a variety of reasons but the way acute hospitals are paid and the way their fixed assets are used also fosters such resistance. The benefits of change in service configuration and delivery are rarely explained to a public whose learned behaviour seems to be that changing hospital services is a loss of amenity that should be opposed. The forces of change-resistance are indeed powerful in this sector.

Barriers to transforming the acute hospital sector

Re-engineering the acute hospital sector requires important changes of approach in several areas: the tariff system of payments; the consolidation of some hospital services in fewer locations; professionalising the use of fixed assets; and streamlining and depoliticising the process of change. Only by tackling these issues vigorously will we release resources from their wasteful deployment in the acute hospitals to deliver Lord Darzi's vision in the NHS Next Stage Review, 'High Quality Care for All' published in 2008. It is relocation of services in a consistent and timely way that will produce the necessary changes for patients, not just high flown and generalised speeches about quality and innovation. It is practical ways of releasing money, people and assets from the acute sector that will modernise and improve the cost-effectiveness of our NHS, not the pretence that change is avoidable and is bad for patients.

The death of the block grant as a way of reimbursing acute hospitals was an important step forward by the Labour Government, as described in Chapter 3. The construction of the new tariff system, payment by results (PbR) was a significant advance on what had gone before and mirrored similar developments in other countries such as Germany and Australia. The new tariff at least rewarded volume of defined activity even if it did not reward best treatment practice. However the change itself did not go far enough or fast enough. It has had the perverse effect of enabling savvy acute hospital managements to exploit the weakness of their commissioners by doing more work than agreed in order to generate extra tariff income – the so-called provider-induced demand. Because the tariff is an activity-related, average price system of payment it rewards doing as much work as possible in a year at an average price. Any payment over marginal cost is serious profit.

When the tariff was effectively launched in 2006 it was a job only partly done. Not all services were covered; it incentivised inpatient care; there were specialist services not covered; there was no provision for best practice to be recognised through the tariff; and community services were not provided for. These shortcomings were inevitable initially because in many of these areas the data was not available to make the tariff more refined. The effect however of this simplified partial tariff has been to tighten the grip of the acute hospital sector on finite resources. Although there has been a small fall in the proportion of PCT acute hospital expenditure covered by tariff payments – from 49% to 45% between 2006/7 and 2008/9 – this has been more than compensated for by local contracts with acute hospitals which have usually been highly favourable to those hospitals because of the lack of robustness among PCT commissioners. The need to bail out some PFI hospitals, as described above, has also not helped. Moreover most disputes between commissioners and acute providers have been resolved by SHAs in favour of the latter. Too often commissioners hold the deficits created by providers.

I attempted to secure faster DH work on disaggregating the acute tariff to incentivise elements of care deliverable in the community or to reward best practice for particular conditions. However this did not produce a very rapid response before I left as a Minister. The issue was pursued by Lord Darzi when he became a Minister with some success. He proposed in the Next Stage Review the idea of a Best Practice Tariff Programme.[22] This has just started with four high volume areas of work where there is significant unexplained variation in practice: cataracts, fractured neck or femur, cholecystectomy and stroke care. If this programme can be expanded it should see work being increasingly concentrated in the most efficient places and accelerate change in the underperforming hospitals but there is a long way to go before the tariff drives efficiency and quality in the acute sector.

Concentration of acute hospital work in the most efficient and highest quality facilities needs to be driven harder even if it involves extra travel for some patients. Stroke care is a good example of where it is in the best interest of patients to be taken to and treated at a specialist stroke centre as fast as possible rather than being taken to the nearest A & E Department. This is now starting to happen in London and elsewhere but it inevitably means a reduction in income for some A & E departments. There is a similar situation with trauma patients, for whom not all A & E departments can offer a full trauma service. Again in London this work will be concentrated at just four acute hospitals; with significant consequences for the income flows to other hospitals. In the area of cancer treatment the direction of travel may well be different with much more scope for work to be concentrated on specialist ambulatory care centres, as in the US. This would mean less use being made of inpatient treatment and so there would be fewer beds and probably lower costs and payments to many acute hospitals.

Changes of this kind inevitably alter the income flows to many hospitals and may well mean some DGHs becoming financially unsustainable in their present form. Such a trend will be continued by the growth of Academic Health Science Centres (AHSCs) which will bring together a small number of health and academic partners to focus on world-class research, teaching and patient care. Perhaps up to 10 AHSCs nationally will be established eventually, building on the 5 now established. The purpose of these new entities is to take new discoveries and promote them more widely, both here and abroad. The AHSCs will have the concentration of expertise and resources which enables them to compete internationally for research and clinical talent. These are the places where the big research breakthroughs will be pioneered and made available to NHS patients, but this can only happen in a limited number of acute hospitals.

In the field of diagnostics there is the same pattern of some increased dispersal to the community but also some greater concentration in more specialist facilities. On the one hand people want and can have more imaging and blood tests carried out in primary care rather than travelling to hospitals, with results more quickly available. On the other hand changing technology also means provision of interventional radiology and specialist pathology being concentrated in centres of excellence. Pathology is a key area where consolidation is essential, especially with the rapid growth of genomic medicine. But pathology has also shown how painfully slowly the DH and NHS make progress on consolidation when clinicians are in no hurry to change their practices and the system facilitates foot-dragging.

I commissioned in 2005 a review of pathology services by Lord Carter of Coles because of my concern over the waste in pathology services with too many underused laboratories and a failure to use cheaper and more efficient commercial laboratories for many of the high volume routine tests. The evidence suggested that there was scope for at least 20%-25% savings in a sector costing the NHS at least £2.5billion a year. The unwillingness of boards, clinicians (especially pathologists) and managers to group facilities, improve transport and IT and put work out to tender is deeply entrenched in the NHS. I received the first report by Lord Carter in August 2006.[23] Work on implementing it slowed after I left and continued at a snail's pace even with the production of a second report by Lord Carter in 2008 which went over much of the same ground as the first report.[24]

In a 2009 Parliamentary answer Lord Darzi told me that the DH was working with 5 of the 10 SHAs on 'developing approaches that responded to Lord Carter's recommendations'.[25] This was DH-speak for saying that they were making haste extremely slowly. In January 2010 I was sent a Pathology Programme Update showing how everybody was allegedly beavering away but with no indication of how much, if any, of the £500million of savings estimated by Lord Carter had actually been achieved or how much consolidation of services or contracting out had actually taken place. The review of pathology is a classic case of DH/NHS procrastination over securing greater efficiency and improved services to patients because the required changes to clinical practice cannot be enforced.

We have now a very strange situation in the acute hospital sector. A talented and innovative surgeon was brought in to review the way the NHS delivers services and he recommended major changes. His report, now over two years old, outlined a radical set of changes for the delivery of care and treatment with more work going out to the community and more work of a specialist nature being concentrated on fewer hospital sites. This inevitably means squeezing the income and reducing the viability of many of the smaller acute hospitals. The performance of some of these hospitals, as well as a few of their larger colleagues, has been shown to be inadequate by regulators but putting things right has eluded local management in many places for some considerable time. The big question now is whether there is the political and managerial will to push through the Darzi vision and deal with underperforming and unviable acute hospitals as we approach a period of straitened NHS budgets. The present political approach and system of public consultation looks ill-equipped to cope.

Even where change is in the best interests of patients and the NHS as a whole the public consultation processes represent a formidable barrier to change. Historically the critics of change have only had to run up the skull and crossbones flag of 'hospital cuts' and they can almost guarantee a protracted delay and probably a substantial reduction in the scale of change needed. Even where there is clinical agreement that the service reconfiguration is beneficial to patients, the clinical leadership to argue publicly for change is all too often lacking. Too many doctors and nurses prefer continuing as they have done for years rather than reshape services in ways that are personally inconvenient to them in terms of location, retraining and new ways of working. The consultation processes themselves are almost guaranteed to produce lengthy delay and the avoidance of change. Where unsustainable services can be preserved by taking money from elsewhere in the NHS, many NHS professionals prefer that to change.

The NHS now faces a paradox. It is possible with clinical advances to provide many more health services to people in their own homes and communities and at the same time provide more and better often life-saving treatments in fewer more specialist centres. Both these alternative service delivery systems produce benefits for patients but mean that the district general hospital in its historical form becomes less appropriate and less viable for such a wide range of service delivery. Yet patients can be mobilised by public outcry to keep services (and jobs) at a local hospital, often against their best collective interests. We have created public involvement mechanisms that encourage nervous politicians to respond to noise and to avoid contentious decisions on reconfiguration and relocation of services. In the name of local decision-making and autonomy, the naysayers to change in one area buy their victories at the expense of people in other areas because ultimately NHS expenditure is a zero-sum game.

After a lengthy public consultation on hospital service changes and appeals to the SHA, changes are passed to Ministers. They now refer all these cases to an Independent Review Panel (IRP) but invariably the cases end up on Ministerial desks before the IRP can finally decide. Throughout this process there is ample scope for procedural challenge, sometimes through the courts. This can mean the whole process starting again. Throughout the consultative and appellate processes MPs can raise the issues in Parliament and lobby ministers. As general elections approach, nervousness sets in amongst Ministers and MPs and it becomes a political badge of honour to retain the status quo.

The time taken to achieve services changes can stretch into years in many cases. The management effort to achieve change is enormous. The status quo in the acute hospital sector has almost become the default position for much of the NHS. In some cases a merger – even if inappropriate – becomes easier to achieve because it can be done often without immediate service changes which are left until later, in the hope that people's memories are short. What we have now in the NHS is a backlog of acute hospitals requiring significant service reconfiguration – many of them in London. Instead of making these changes during a time of NHS resource plenty, they will need to happen at a time of resource shortage, when the scope for taking the sharp corners off change is reduced. The lack of financial consequences for poor and unprofessional use of NHS fixed assets makes it much easier to avoid painful change.

A new way of delaying significant change has now appeared called 'vertical integration'. What is being proposed is that acute trusts merge with the community services provider arms of PCTs. This would create bigger organisations with larger turnovers and some savings on overheads. It also enables PCT providers to avoid competition from the private or voluntary sectors. Many of these PCT providers are serious underperformers, as are some of the acute trusts that they will be joining. Merging two relatively unsuccessful organisations may do little more than create a larger unsuccessful organisation, as well as reduce competition locally. More than a third of the PCTs in London have been seeking this option of vertical integration. I return to this issue in a later chapter. Suffice it to say here this approach does little to solve the problem of underperforming and unviable acute hospitals.

Concluding remarks

There are major problems with some of our acute hospitals; and a major reconfiguration of services in many of them is both essential and inevitable. If the NHS is to deliver the vision set out in Lord Darzi's report 'High Quality Care for All' this change is needed quickly. At the heart of those changes is the requirement to use resources – money, fixed assets and staff – very differently from the way they are used today. It requires a redirection of resources to different services and different places and many hospital staff working differently. Changes of this kind cannot be done painlessly and they require stronger political, clinical and managerial will than we have seen so far in the NHS, together with leadership that is much better at explaining the need for change to the public. As we move to a period when NHS resources are scarcer there has to be redeployment of resources to new services from the existing configuration of acute hospitals.

It is said that the best predictor of future behaviour is past behaviour. In which case, we have no reason to believe that a new generation of elected politicians will behave much differently to a past one. The reconfiguration of services needs to be handled by a more streamlined system that does not have Ministers at its apex. I discuss this further later, but in the meantime I turn to examining whether the NHS services outside hospitals are ready to take on an expanded role.

12

Getting closer to home

The state of the nation

After the 2005 Election it was clear that simply pumping money into improving hospitals would not deal with the health challenges the country faced. The nation was getting older and more obese, especially our children. About a quarter of the population – over 15 million people – had long-term health needs such as diabetes, stroke, high blood pressure or cardiovascular conditions. These conditions needed better prevention and earlier care rather than waiting for emergencies that required hospital treatment. As the population ages, dementia has been growing faster than the care system across the health/social care divide could respond to adequately: 750,000 people and their families are struggling to cope, with the prospect of this number growing to a million in 10-15 years. At the end of life most people want to die in their own homes, not in hospital but we have managed to achieve the opposite for most people. End of life care has not received the attention given to acute care and too often is unable to respond to people's preferences.

Tackling these problems has not been helped by investing more resources disproportionately into acute hospitals, particularly underperforming ones. These hospitals have received a huge investment but continuing along the same path will not resolve the health problems facing the country. Nor will it secure improvements in health inequalities. Despite having a National Health Service for 60 years with a founding principle of equity of care it remains the case that where you live has a huge impact on an individual's health and wellbeing and the care they receive. A graphic illustration of this in London: Westminster and Canning Town are separated by eight stops on the Jubilee Line but also by a 7 year difference in life expectancy.[1] Health inequalities remain stark between the different parts of the country and communities and across class and income groups.

Both when I was a Health Minister and today the contradictions in health policy and strategy remain striking. The variations in GP distribution are considerable with many fewer GPs per head of population in some of the areas in greatest need. Nowhere is this more apparent than in London. Dissatisfied with the availability (and sometimes the quality) of GP services at night and weekends many Londoners flock to the improved A & E Departments for their urgent care. The more we improve those A

& E Departments, the more many people take the perfectly rational decision to choose those them for their care rather than inadequate or inconvenient GP services. We have poured resources and management time into driving down the maximum waiting times for treatment in all acute hospitals from GP referrals to 18 weeks – a major task for me as a Minister - but not the same effort into preventative services. In London – and I suspect elsewhere – some of these hospitals have population catchment areas far too small to meet the specialised care needs of their populations effectively, yet we continue to divert staff, money and effort to them instead of improving the community services that are badly needed. This was brought out very effectively by Lord Darzi in his 2006 review of services in London before he became a Health Minister.[2]

We have known for a long time that we have the wrong balance of effort between hospitals and community health and social care services. About 90% of people's contacts with the NHS take place outside hospitals; at any one time adult social care services are providing support to over 1.7million people, most of whom also receive health services. As medicine, technology and disease profiles have changed we have singularly failed to re-engineer services so that people receive more treatment, care, support and advice without going to a hospital. Patients still go backwards and forwards to hospitals for tests and consultations under arrangements more concerned with the convenience of professionals than that of patients – again well brought out by Lord Darzi in his report on London's NHS.

Talented NHS clinicians and managers have done a remarkably good job of enhancing and protecting the budgets of their acute hospital citadels and convincing the public and politicians that resources need to continue to flow in ample quantities into these institutions with their costly and often underused fixed assets. The professional structures supporting hospitals – clinical and management elites, professional bodies, unions and career structures – all reinforce hospital-based health services at the expense of community-based services. In my time as a Minister it was clear to me that the power structures of hospital services out-punched those of community and social care services in the political contests for finite resources. Many of the senior people advising me and other Ministers have built their careers in the acute hospital sector where their networks are powerful. Social care remains the poor relation within DH.

Rebalancing the focus of services away from hospitals remains difficult but was something that Patricia Hewitt, Liam Byrne and I tried to do in 2005. As I was responsible for GPs and community health services I took the lead in producing a new White Paper on developing services outside hospitals. Tony Blair, impatient for reform as his time as Prime Minister ebbed away, wanted a new strategy by the autumn of 2005.

We persuaded him that he would get a better product if he gave us until the turn of the year.

We did not start work on this White Paper with a blank sheet of paper. Prior to the Election, a consultation paper on social care had been published setting out a 10-15 year vision for adult social care but making clear this would have to be met from existing resources.[3] It promised more control and choice for service users, wider use of direct payments and piloting individual budgets. Stronger emphasis on preventative services, better partnership between local authorities, health and other agencies and greater acceptance of risk among service users were important themes. There was recognition of the need to improve the skill and status of the social care workforce, many of whom were low paid and lacked qualifications. To sceptical Whitehall watchers like myself, this consultation paper looked like a low-cost holding operation when there was no political appetite for diverting more resources to long-term care of the elderly but the responses to this consultation published in October 2005 were useful in producing the White Paper.

There had been several earlier attempts to produce a stronger focus on wider public health issues and better health outcomes. When Virginia Bottomley was Health Secretary the Conservatives had produced a respectable public health White Paper but at the time public expenditure was tight and little change had resulted. In 1999 Labour had produced a rival product suggesting, a bit unfairly, that their predecessor's effort was a scatter-gun approach to improving public health. This document focussed on what the Government then regarded as the main killers: 'cancer, coronary heart disease, stroke, accidents, mental illness'.[4] It was very much a document of its time with an emphasis on what were called 'tough but attainable targets'. Cancer death rates for the under 75s were to be reduced by at least a fifth; CHD and stroke targeted the same population group but the target reduction in death rates was 40%; for accidents the target was to reduce the death rate by a fifth and serious injury by at least 10%; and for mental illness the death rate from suicide and undetermined injury by at least a fifth. These reductions were to be achieved by 2010 and would, it was claimed, prevent 'up to 300,000 untimely and unnecessary deaths.'

In October 2009 the DH released some encouraging figures showing progress on achieving these targets from a baseline of 1995 – 1997 and using the latest data from 2006 – 2008.[5] The mortality rates for cancer amongst those aged under 75 had fallen by 19.3%. If the trend line continued the 20% reduction target by 2010 would be achieved but this masked the fact that for more deprived areas progress was much less good. The 3-year average mortality rate for circulatory diseases in the under 75s had fallen by 47% against the baseline, so the 40% reduction target for

2010 had been met ahead of schedule and was going well in the deprived areas. For suicide and undetermined injury the 3-year average had dropped by 15.2% since the baseline and was theoretically on track to meet the 2010 target; but between 2007 and 2008 the rate had gone up which was a setback. The rate of accidents had not decreased, with a small increase in the latest figures, so the target was not going to be met.

The targets were well intentioned and they did help to reduce many unnecessary deaths. What, however, they demonstrated was that it was more difficult to reduce killer disease mortality rates in more deprived groups and that the targets had no impact on accident reductions. Where behavioural change by individuals was more important than clinical interventions, the NHS was much less successful. Much of the extra money made available for this programme went into the hospital sector. I have never seen a cost-benefit analysis of the 1999 initiative; and there was little by way of results data available to us when work on the 2005 White Paper began.

The 'Saving Lives' publication had been followed 5 years later in 2004 by a document 'Choosing Health'.[6] This went from the narrowness of the 1999 targets approach to the other extreme of a Government-wide set of initiatives to improve the public's health. Although the Government wanted to build health regulatory impact assessments into all future legislation most of the initiatives to improve health were made the responsibility of the Health Secretary. There was to be new funding for stimulating demand for health through campaigns, more school nurses, the introduction of health trainers and better obesity and sexual health services. Funding priority was to be given to areas of greatest health inequality; and the emphasis was to be on partnership working between different agencies at the local level. There was to be action to improve the nation's diet and to increase physical activity, especially amongst young people.

The Healthcare Commission was to work with other inspectorates into looking for how health improvement was being secured rather than just examining the treatment of ill-health. The Prime Minister's Delivery Unit was to be involved pursuing issues like effective performance management, better data and clearer pursuit of priorities. This 2004 document was a broader and clearer statement about a health rather than an ill-health agenda for the NHS but somewhat silent on how this change of emphasis was to be delivered.

The idea of delivering health services closer to people's homes with more emphasis on prevention was an attractive idea in principle but history and circumstances did not appear to be on our side. Many of the lifestyle changes going on in early 21st Century Britain were working against better health. After 60 years of existence the NHS had build up a particular configuration of services, staff deployment and buildings and plant, together with a set of expenditure patterns that supported them. In this configuration there was a strong emphasis on treating ill-health through specialist services located in hospitals where the latest advances in expensive life-saving medical technologies and treatments were located and consumed much growth money. Only with pharmaceutical advances were we seeing more innovative treatments that did not rely so much on a trip to the hospital.

This wider public health agenda required the DH and NHS to work in a more negotiative way with other agencies such as local government, social services, voluntary and private sector providers, housing interests and others. This partnership approach has never seemed to me a strong feature of DH or the NHS. There is a self-absorbed introspection among many senior NHS and DH managers and clinicians. Too much attention is given to protecting NHS interests and budgets rather than looking to see how those interests might be better pursued by working more cooperatively with others. The longstanding failure of DH top management – political and official – to see how boosting adult social care budgets for long-term care of the elderly - especially dementia - might reduce pressure on NHS hospital beds and budgets was and is a classic example of this failure to look outwards for solutions to NHS problems. Similarly with wider public health programmes that required behavioural change by individuals rather than treatment responses.

The history of health centres and public health illustrates how the wider health agenda can, almost absentmindedly, be forgotten by the NHS in its preoccupation with the work of treating people in hospital. At the beginning of the NHS in 1948, health centres were seen as an important part of the new service's future. They had started in the 1930's and continued to be developed in post-war Britain by local authority medical officers of health who had a statutory duty to report annually on the state of the public health locally. There was a health centre building programme for local government. When I worked as a Private Secretary to Dick Crossman, when he was responsible for both health and social security at the end of the 1960s, he had on the wall behind his desk a map of the country showing all the health centres built and to be built. The emphasis on public health in these centres was strong.

In the cause of greater integration NHS local authority responsibility for health centres, health visitors and district nurses was swept away in 1971, along with medical officers of health. The health centre building programme lapsed as more money was poured into funding improvements in GP premises – again almost absent-mindedly - enabling independent contractors to build up private capital assets at public expense as part of their pension kitty. A platform for preventative health was lost and the new

Directors of Public Health became less powerful influences locally; and at the regional level they became cut off from the NHS by being despatched to Government Offices. It has been left to the Chief Medical Officer and his annual report to carry the banner for public health instead of a flotilla of flag-wavers spread around the country who are able to influence local government about the health and wellbeing of their populations. However the disease and demographic profile of the country has changed greatly since the days of medical officers of health.

The disease and demographic profile

The disease and demographic challenges to which the 2006 White Paper needed to respond were considerable. The bulk of the work of the NHS related to the over 15million people in England with longer-term health needs. Every decade the estimates suggest that the number of people with these conditions will increase by over a million from the ageing of the population alone. By 2025 the number of people aged 85 and over was projected to rise by three-quarters. The number of people with severe disability will also increase as the prevalence rises among children, partly as a result of the increased survival of premature babies. Over two-thirds of NHS activity relates to the one-third of the population with the highest needs and they account for an estimated 80% of what we spend on health and social care. Carrying on the way we have been has massive resource implications for the NHS and social care as the ageing of the population continues. The burden on the taxpaying working population can only increase with a tax-funded NHS and at a time when that working population is likely to shrink in proportion to the non-working population.

At the other end of the age spectrum the picture was equally alarming. Obesity in childhood was increasing and was forecast to continue doing so. Physical exercise was declining as car and bus replaced walking to school and as school PE and sport declined. All types of diabetes were increasing among children and young people and were not being well-managed in terms of blood sugar control targets. As an increasingly obese younger population grows into adulthood, the result would be an increased prevalence of circulatory diseases, cancer and diabetes. As we pushed up NHS performance in dealing with killer diseases for one generation, we were doing a remarkably good job of ensuring a continuing flow of customers for the healthcare system with our children. As a country we face the possibility that unless our children's lifestyles change many of them will not live as long as their parents. A minority of children are also copying adults by drinking more, the equivalent of about five pints of beer a week. In 2005 there was more than a 25% increase in under-16s admitted to hospital with conditions related to alcohol compared with a decade previously.

The working age population had their own sets of problems and in some cases could hardly be said to be setting a great example to their children. In 2005 22% of men and 24% of women were regarded as obese and the obesity rates were rising steadily. The rates had nearly doubled for men and increased by about 50% for women since the early 1990s. Higher obesity rates predict a rise in strokes, angina, heart attacks, hypertension and Type 2 diabetes. In the 2004 Health Survey for England only 37% of men and 25% of women were achieving the recommended physical activity levels of 30 minutes or more of moderate-intensity activity for five days a week.[7] Alcohol-related deaths (chronic liver disease and cirrhosis) in the UK almost doubled between 1991 and 2005 from 6.9% to 12.9% per 100,000 population. We found that between 15,000 and 22,000 deaths and 150,000 hospital admissions each year were associated with alcohol misuse. In ten years those hospital admission rates had increased by about 80%. Binge drinking was on the rise and a significant proportion of the population was drinking more than the maximum recommended weekly amount (21 units for men and 14 units for women). Excessive drinking was rising fastest amongst women.

Much had been done by successive Governments to deter people from smoking: higher taxes on cigarettes; transport bans on smoking; stark warnings on cigarette packets that smoking kills; and NHS smoking-quitter programmes. Yet smoking was still the single biggest cause of illness and premature death in England. In 2005 smoking was estimated to be killing over 85,000 people a year and accounted for a third of all cancers. About 22% - 23% of the population still smoked but this was higher among manual workers where it was over 30%.

Sexually-transmitted infections (STIs) were continuing to rise. Much of the public concern related to HIV/AIDS but it was other STIs like gonorrhoea and chlamydia that were on the march as a result of unsafe sex. Up to 10% of young people aged under 25 were thought to be infected with chlamydia. This could lead to pelvic inflammatory disease, ectopic pregnancy and infertility. Sex education programmes had a rather mixed record on changing individual behaviour.

Among those off sick from work, mental illness and stress-related conditions were now the most common cause of sickness absence. One in four consultations with GPs concerned mental health problems. Being 'stressed out' was now a common topic of conversation in public places and soap operas, as more people went to their doctor complaining of anxiety and depression. Forms of mental illness are now a common cause of social isolation and exclusion amongst older people. Dementia has been on the rise, especially among the over 80s and has caused major care problems within families. People out of work for longer periods are known to be at greater risk of losing their sense of wellbeing and confidence, sometimes leading to longer-term mental health problems. It was this term 'wellbeing' that was now entering the lexicon for Health Ministers and that was to feature very strongly in the public consultation discussed in the next section.

In the profile of disease and demography for the White Paper two things stood out. First, that the misery of disease was not spread evenly through the society; and secondly that the health of carers posed particular problems. There have been some dramatic improvements in people's health in the UK since the mid 1980s. Average life expectancy had increased for men by about 5 years and for women by more than 3 years. The number of infant deaths fell from around 9 per 1000 live births in 1986 to around 5 per 1000 live births in 2003-2005. However the gap in life expectancy between those living in the most deprived areas and the population as a whole had continued to widen. There was a difference of 10 years between the life expectancy of men living in the least and most deprived local authority areas in England. Income, education and housing have all been shown to have a profound influence on health outcomes but so has access to health services.[8]

It is these deprived areas that have the lowest density of healthcare professionals, especially GPs. Since the beginning of the NHS the distribution of GPs has been uneven. Research has shown that those areas with the poorest health outcomes are also those with the fewest GPs. The variation in GPs is large. We found in 2005 that those PCTs that had the most GPs per 100,000 weighted population had more than double that of the most deprived areas. If we were to combat the inequalities of income and education there was a need to compensate by better access to health services, especially primary care, in deprived areas.

There was a similar problem among the 6million people in the country who care for family or friends. Over a million of these provide care for over 50 hours a week; and some 400,000 combine full-time work with caring more than 20 hours a week. About three-quarters of carers are financially worse off because of their caring responsibilities.[9] Caring for someone has life-changing consequences. If you are a carer caring for more than 50 hours a week you are twice as likely to be in bad health as those who are not carers. This had been brought home to me well before I was a Minister when I had been a trustee of the Carers National Association and had undertaken research on carers. Leaving aside the humane arguments there was and remains a strong public interest argument for supporting carers more – as Labour has done – because public expenditure would be higher by many billions of pounds if it had to fund the care that carers provide free.

As Ministers we found daunting this profile of disease and demography that we needed to respond to in our White Paper. The profile remains much the same today, only worse in some areas: ageing continues, dementia has increased, as have obesity, diabetes and chlamydia rates. Although overall life expectancy and infant mortality continue to improve, the gap between rich and poor areas continues to widen. Labour has done a good job in reducing mortality rates in targeted killers – cancer, all circulatory diseases and suicides; and in these areas we are now much closer to the average for the 15 countries who were members of the European Union before 2004. But the prevalence of obesity in England is the highest in the EU-15 countries. We are the fat men (and women) of Europe. And we have risen above the EU-15 average for death rates for alcohol-related diseases.[10] Many of these diseases are avoidable if lifestyles change and we could persuade people to make those changes. In 2005 the next step was to find out what people thought were their priorities.

The 'Our Health, Our Care, Our Say' consultation

We had 6 months as Ministers to come up with a fundamentally different strategy for the NHS which would place more emphasis on improving health rather than providing healthcare. We also had to ensure that adult social care was given proper attention. Many senior DH personnel did not have a good understanding of the needs of social care, how it could help the NHS and why integration of health and social care was important to many people with long term conditions. Also DH policy capability on social care was weak with the transfer of the Social Services Inspectorate to the Department of Children, Schools and Families. Liam Byrne who was responsible for social care wisely reached outside DH for help in this area. We needed also a process for discussion with the main NHS professional interests to keep them engaged in the debate; so I set up and chaired a group of senior people which secured their involvement in the exercise and led to later support for the White Paper. Most important of all we had to find out the public's preferences and priorities.

Patricia Hewitt wanted the White Paper to be informed by a comprehensive engagement process with the public: something that went beyond the usual surveys and putting out ideas for consultation. She took personal responsibility for hiring Opinion Leader Research (OLR). Throughout the processes devised by OLR's Deborah Mattinson and her team we wanted to demonstrate that as Ministers we were genuinely listening to what the public were telling us. Too often public consultation is tokenistic but on this occasion we did our best to engage directly with people, to find out what they thought about services and how they wanted them changed and to feed back our thinking to a group of fellow citizens.

We called this exercise 'Your Health, Your Care, Your Say.' The scale of the exercise was large for the time available. I suspect that some civil servants thought these Ministers were mad to adopt this process, not least because we might be told uncomfortable things that would be difficult to respond to. It was also clear that Patricia was putting Deborah Mattinson, not the civil service, in charge of the processes. The scope of the programme was considerable and the views of over 40,000 people were heard. There were four regional deliberative events accompanied by a range of local events and activities which involved about 10,000 people. Special efforts were made to ensure that seldom-heard groups were included in the consultation. A questionnaire was available to people who wanted to have their say but were not involved in a deliberative event: this attracted a response of about 30,000 people. This material was supplemented by magazine surveys which attracted several thousand responses. The whole process was to culminate in a national event in Birmingham on a Saturday which about a 1000 people would attend from across the country. The Ministerial team would participate in this event and hear what people had to say and observe the voting process in which people would determine their priorities.

I was unaware of any similar public engagement process leading to a government White Paper. We established a 'citizen panel' to ensure that the consultation was genuinely citizen-led. It had ten members of the public recruited to match the demographic profile of the delegates at the deliberative events. The youngest was 23 years and the oldest 82 years. One member was unemployed and other members included a retired machine operator, a fashion designer, a gardener and an underwriter. The panel vetted material to make sure that language and format were easy to understand and free of NHS jargon. The panel also met the Ministerial team before the White Paper was written to act as a sounding board for the policy themes to be included in it. This was deliberative democracy in action and was a process that the NHS should use more frequently when difficult choices have to be made.

The consultation on social care launched in March 2005 was brought to a conclusion while we were working on the White Paper. Around 100,000 people were involved in this consultation. The results were published in October 2005;[11] and these were brought together with the results of the wider health consultation in the preparation of the White Paper. Broadly speaking the vision in the March 2005 consultation document was strongly supported but this was hardly surprising given that most of the ideas were what people had wanted the government to do for some time. The difficult bit was delivering this vision in a future where there was little, if any, growth money proposed for adult social care and there was a political reluctance to ask people and their families to pay more out of their own pockets as the population aged and personal wealth increased.

Some clear themes and views came out of both these public consultation exercises and they almost certainly hold true today. The public have a strong desire for more help to support people to maintain their independence and to feel included in society, with more emphasis on tackling loneliness and isolation, especially among older people and those caring for others. People knew that prevention was better than cure and believed that it would reduce the risks and costs of long-term illnesses and their treatment. They recognised their own responsibility for their health but wanted more support to stay healthy. They wanted the NHS to become a service with a focus on prevention rather than concentrating predominantly on treating illness. 86% of the nearly 1,000 people who attended the Birmingham Citizen's Summit thought that professionals in local GP practice should provide people with more support to manage their own health and well-being. They wanted to see a wider range of professionals – particularly practice and community nurses and pharmacists – involved in health improvement, disease prevention and the promotion of independence. Some 61% said that being given more information about their health and the services available to them locally would make a big difference. They particularly wanted to know more about the availability of social care services. The public believe health checks could be cost effective if done in the right way and they strongly support the idea of regular check ups.[12]

This consultation made clear that the public want services to fit the way they live their lives and do not want to be made to fit around the way public services choose to organise themselves for their own convenience. They see as a priority a wider range of times when services are available and there was a clear desire for GP services to be open at more convenient times. People wanted to be able to get rapid access to advice and care and to be able to book appointments in advance. They did not expect 24/7 services from GPs but they did expect more flexibility around evenings and early morning opening times during the week and on Saturday mornings. My conversations with people at these events confirm my view that we had gone too far in the 2003 GP contract in letting GPs off the hook on their opening times and that we were right to claw back the access agenda (as described in Chapter 7). The public are in a different position on service access to many health and social care professionals and they want to be treated more as customers – an idea many health professionals simple do not accept. People have had to show more flexibility in their own working lives and do not see why public sector professionals should not do the same.

There was a lot more altruism among participants at these events than I had expected. Most people thought that priority should be given to those with the greatest needs and most at risk, especially older people so they could remain independent and thereby reduce their need for expensive residential and nursing care. To do this they wanted to see better joining up of public services, especially health and social care. A common complaint throughout this engagement process and the separate social care consultation was the way different agencies assess people separately and make them repeat the same information to every professional they meet. The public simply do not understand or accept that the public services cannot integrate their assessment processes better; and they are much more relaxed about agencies sharing information about them if it improves assessment processes than many campaigners against data-sharing would have us believe.

Public support for greater personalisation for services is very strong. People often think that they are treated too impersonally and this is reflected in the strong support for individual budgets and direct payments. People know their own priorities for keeping themselves active, with a reasonable quality of daily life; and they believe they are more likely to achieve this if they have more control about the way money is spent on them. Time and time again the point was made to Ministers that the public want advice and support from professionals, not excessive direction and control.

The culmination of the 'Your Health, Your Care, Your Say' public engagement was the voting on people's top priorities at the Citizen's Summit in Birmingham in the autumn. Much of the day was spent in groups discussing the findings from the regional deliberative events and the 36,000 questionnaires; and then testing arguments with each other. This led to the production of a list of specific changes that people wanted Ministers to deliver through the White Paper. The Ministerial team wandered around the groups listening to the arguments, responding to any questions people asked but we deliberately declined to influence people's thinking. Nearly 1,000 people (986 to be precise) were then asked to vote 'yes' or 'no' for 13 items that they had chosen as the most important.

Four priorities dominated the voting by securing support of 40% or more.[13] The top priority by some way was a regular health check for everyone, with 75% support. Second was more focus on mental well-being with 62%. For me, and I think other Ministers, the big surprise of the whole process was the public's concern about what they saw as an increasing mental health problem across society with more and more people feeling unhappy about their lives, anxious, depressed and generally miserable. The term 'well-being' was something that was put on the political agenda by this engagement process and became much more commonly used in Departmental discussions. The political class has been slow to realise that even as national wealth and prosperity was increasing, more people seemed to be made miserable by the lives they lived. Now political leaders want to measure happiness as well GDP but in 2005 that was still a novel idea for many politicians.

The third and fourth priorities, with just over 40% each were more help for carers and a trained nurse as a first point of contact for patients. In fifth place there was a lot of support – about 30% - for incentives for healthy behaviour. A significant proportion of the public believe that more incentives would drive a change of behaviour on health if only we could find the right incentives. Others however wanted to take a punitive approach: the ninth priority, penalties for inappropriate use of services and the tenth, penalties for unhealthy choices, both attracted support from just over 10% of participants. I had expected the punitive approach to prevail but it was clearly outvoted by people supporting incentives. More discouraging however is that about half the public think neither incentives nor penalties will drive an agenda for healthier living. There is much more thinking and research to be done about how to persuade people to change behaviour that adversely affects their health and what role the State should play in this. The research evidence on how to do this still leaves a lot to be desired.

One slightly surprising feature of the consultation was the level of concern over transport. Better transport to health and social care services (at number 8) attracted over 15% support; and public transport being better integrated with services (number 11) was supported by nearly 10%. So about a quarter of the public consider transport is a problem for accessing health and social care services. This supports the idea that we need to work harder at bringing more services closer to home.

Nearly 20% of participants supported patients holding their own medical records on smart cards. There was considerable understanding among some participants about the potential of IT to empower patients to keep their own medical data and produce it when necessary. It showed a public awareness of the need for patient information to flow between services much better than it does currently. Two stragglers at number 12 (improved services for drug users) and number 13 (allowing other organisations to set up local health centres) attracted little support, with only about 5% of participants voting for either of these. Perhaps more surprising was the over 20% support for the sixth top priority which was offering more treatment options including complementary therapies on the NHS. It is clear that some of the public are not convinced by the lack of scientific evidence to support many alternative medicines and treatments.

The overall messages from these consultations were clear and consistent. People had a lot to say that was good about the services and the expertise of many of the professionals they encountered. They praised many of the recent reforms and innovations such as social care direct payments, NHS Direct, walk-in centres, on-line booking of appointments and text message appointments. However they thought service quality was often uneven and that they had been lucky personally to get good service. They wanted more personalisation, more preventative work and more say in how services are designed and delivered whilst recognising that finance was limited and staff can be hard pressed. People thought more emphasis should be placed on assistive technologies to support people and carers in their own homes and to monitor some long-term conditions such as diabetes.

People were interested in providing more hospital services such as diagnostic tests and routine surgery in community settings but there was some nervousness about whether this would adversely affect convenient access to emergency or more complex care at local hospitals. Nevertheless over half the people at the Birmingham Summit supported in principle moving some hospital services to community settings, whilst recognising that this would have implications for general hospitals and that local people would need to be engaged in decisions about shifting services. These were the challenges we faced when producing the White Paper and that we still face today.

The 2006 White Paper

In preparing the White Paper we concentrated on strengthening the NHS approach to securing health and well-being; improving access to both general practice and community services; increasing support for people with longer term needs; finding ways of delivering care closer to home; more public empowerment; improvement in commissioning; and greater integration of health and social care. The agenda was driven by Ministers with little involvement by the DH top management who never seemed engaged with the process and were more preoccupied with acute hospitals, current targets and NHS finances. The only time top management became involved was when we started discussing the idea of ring-fenced budgets for health promotion and preventative services. Mandarin cold water was poured on the idea with much talk about how difficult this would be to do. Suddenly people who had let the NHS finances get totally out of control became very concerned that we might be thinking of transferring relatively small sums of money from traditional NHS conduits. As the NHS financial crisis described in Chapter 9 worsened at the end of 2005, there was suddenly a lot of official concern that all proposals in the draft White Paper should be backed by detailed costings. Without a trace of irony we were advised that there would be virtually no new money in 2006/7 despite the fact that this was the same that had mismanaged the huge extra resources poured into the NHS and DH central budgets.

In November 2005 we had a Ministerial away day with officials to discuss and settle the structure and content of the White Paper which Nigel Crisp attended. Ministers made it clear that the White Paper was intended to set a new strategic direction for the NHS and the DH that would help people to live more independently in their own homes and focus much more on their own well-being. This strategic shift was to support choice and give people more say over decisions affecting their daily lives; and we wanted the White Paper to realign the way the health and social care systems worked. More services were to be delivered safely and effectively in settings closer to home and they would be integrated and built more around the needs of individuals rather than the convenience of service providers. I was under no illusions about the obstacles we would face in delivering this change of direction and the associated expenditure flows. That is why I told officials that we needed a timetabled implementation plan as part of the White Paper.

Under pressure from No. 10 we produced a White Paper called "Our Health, Our Care, Our Say - a new direction for community services" by the end of January 2006 setting out key recommendations to help people to improve their health and well-being. A new NHS 'Life Check' service would be developed and evaluated in 2007 to help people to assess their own risk of ill health, based on a range of risk factors and awareness of family history. There was a renewed commitment to expand access to psychological (or "talking") therapies by planning two demonstration sites that focussed on people of working age with mild to moderate mental health problems; and taking forward computerised cognitive behaviour therapy (CBT). The Quality and Outcomes Framework (QOF) in the new GP contract would be refocused on wider health and well-being outcomes. A range of activity was promised to realign planning, budget-setting, commissioning and regulation of health and social care to improve service integration.[14] These changes were modest relative to need but a more ambitious programme of early action was thwarted by two things: the financial crisis in the NHS and the absence of proven new models of care that would deliver better health and well-being.

What was clear was if this agenda was to be pursued general practice would need to be strengthened and access improved. In some ways the new contract had curtailed access to family doctors outside the Monday to Friday, 8am to 6pm period, with access shifted to out of hours services in evenings and weekends. We had also identified a problem with GPs in some areas showing their lists as 'open but full' which had the same effect as making the list 'closed'. We had four key recommendations in the White Paper which promised tough negotiations with the BMA. Patients would be guaranteed acceptance onto a list shown as 'open'. Successful practices would be encouraged to expand through contractual incentives. There would be a national procurement of additional practices in under-doctored deprived areas. And we would push hard to secure GP opening hours that reflected patients' preferences. All these changes required a considerable change of attitude by many PCTs, GPs and the BMA, with few financial sweeteners available.

A large number of changes in community services were proposed.[14] Urgent and emergency care was becoming complicated and overlapping. Apart from A & E Departments and GP services, there was NHS Direct, some new walk-in centres, minor injuries units, pharmacists, local out-of-hours services and for mental health, crisis resolution teams. So a review of urgent care was promised. A new screening programme for bowel cancer would be provided; piloting self-referral to physiotherapy would be undertaken; more choice for women over the place of their babies' birth would be provided; and easier access to immunisation services. Coordination of end of life care would be improved through establishing networks of services. In social care use of direct payments would be expanded, with the prospect of individual budgets spanning health, social care and possibly other services. The Expert Patients Programme would expand to train more people in self care. Integrated care plans covering health and social care for those with long-term conditions would be developed, together with increased support for carers.

Much of the White Paper was more a 'to-do list' than a carefully calibrated scheme of reform. Because we were in the middle of restructuring PCTs and had to avoid a further political row over separating PCT service provider arms from their commissioning role, little was said unfortunately about much needed reform of PCT community services. A wider role for the voluntary sector and social entrepreneurs was promised which did lead to the setting up of a Social Enterprise Unit in the DH before I left as a Minister. But what the White Paper lacked was a major commitment to wholesale reform of community health services to ensure they concentrated more on health promotion, undertook more work outside hospitals and were integrated with social care more effectively.

As Ministers we recognised the need to do more to demonstrate on a wider scale the scope for shifting care safely from hospitals to the community. I had chaired a group of professional leaders while the White Paper was in preparation to look at which specialties had the best prospects for transferring work out of hospitals. This work had identified six specialties where there was some work going on that looked promising and where we needed to collect evidence on how to take matters further. These specialties were ENT, trauma and orthopaedics, dermatology, urology, gynaecology and general surgery. I set up six groups under expert leadership to identify sites where promising work was in progress or in prospect with the scope for assessing their potential for wider application. These groups reported back positively in time for including in the White Paper a proposal that over the next year the DH would work with specialty associations and Royal Colleges in 20-30 demonstration sites to define clinically safe patient pathways and appropriate models of care for doing work outside hospitals in the six specialties. At that time there were nearly 45 million outpatient appointments in England every year. For some specialties there were reliable estimates that up to half these could eventually be provided in a community setting. I agreed that Manchester University should be appointed to carry out an independent evaluation of these projects.

The purpose of these demonstration sites was to convince sceptics that community settings for services would work and save money. Investment in intermediate care and related community services since 2001 had already resulted in a reduction in delayed discharge from acute hospitals of 64% by September 2005. This released about 1.5million bed days per year with more than 360,000 people benefiting annually.[15] There was also evidence that community hospitals provided better (and cheaper) recuperative care than DGHs.

The White Paper committed the Government to a new generation of community hospitals providing diagnostics, day surgery, rehabilitation and outpatient facilities where specialists could work with community-based staff. Community hospitals would be one of the places where we expected to see more co-location of services – health, social care and other public services. We wanted to expand the 350 or so existing community hospitals and also stop the inappropriate closures that were going on. The White Paper said that any PCTs threatening to close community hospitals would be required to demonstrate to their SHA that not only had they consulted locally but they had tested their proposals against the principles in the White Paper. A further document inviting proposals for new community hospitals was promised for mid-2006.

The White Paper made clear that "we intend to shift resources and activity from acute hospitals to local settings, in direct response to patient feedback". PCTs, SHAs and acute hospitals were required to review their capital plans accordingly. Unfortunately we too readily accepted civil service advice and backed away from a firm commitment to start shifting resources from secondary care to primary and community care, as I had argued for. Instead the White Paper said that from 2008 we would look at PCT annual plans to see if this was happening and would "examine the case for setting a target for the percentage shift from current secondary care to primary care and community services" if health reform drivers would not do the job. This was the most I could achieve but I still regard it as a major mistake that we did not, as Ministers, insist on a required shift of revenue resources of a given percentage. I come back to this issue in the final chapter.

The White Paper also showed how the UK lagged behind the US, Germany, Netherlands and France in the proportion of its health expenditure that went on prevention and public health. It promised to establish an expert group to develop robust definitions and measures of preventative spending and to look at establishing a 10-year ambition for preventative spending based on comparisons with other OECD countries. In six months Ministers with some supportive officials and external professional leaders had produced a game-changing NHS White Paper despite DH top management indifference. The question was would DH and the NHS implement it?

The White Paper's aftermath and the Darzi review

It was clear that if Ministers were to get the NHS to change direction we had to come up with an implementation plan that set timetabled and enforceable requirements. Our message to the NHS in the White Paper was clear: acute hospitals were places where people went when it was really necessary, not as a matter of routine. We needed to get the NHS to make primary and community services more centre stage in a more integrated health and social care system. Implementing the White Paper was supposed to involve a fundamental shift to care being provided closer to home and a shift of expenditure away from acute hospitals to preventative and community work. Unfortunately at the very time that we published the White Paper the NHS finances were in meltdown as a result primarily of the acute hospital sector spending more than they should but also because of the weak demand and financial management of many PCTs.

Much of 2006 was spent trying to construct a road map for local change in line with the White Paper vision. This was "management stuff" that rarely excites politicians, the commentariat or the public, but without different management activity little change would take place in the NHS. A picture was needed of what successful implementation would look like – something all too rarely done in changing public services where people often do not know where the winning post is. For the White Paper to be seen to be working there would need to be better prevention and earlier intervention for improved health, independence and well-being. There would need to be more choice and a stronger say being exercised by individuals and communities. Inequalities would need to start reducing, with access to services, especially primary care, in poor areas improving. There would need to be demonstrably more support for people with long-term conditions and needs. For all this to happen, the NHS had to become more pro-active over health and well-being rather than reacting to the ill health presented to it. Community services and social care had to advance in terms of resources and people with a compensating slowdown in the growth of acute hospital care. Capturing evidence that these things were happening was essential but difficult particularly if the way money was spent was not clearly changed.

We wanted service users to become partners in the design and delivery of services; and this would require more public engagement, developing self-care through the Expert Patient Programme, and improving patient access to meaningful information through initiatives like the NHS Choices website. The expanded use of direct payments and individual budgets were key. Better leadership locally was required with partnership development between the new Directors of Adult Social Services, Directors of Children's Services and PCT Chief Executives committing to the White Paper goals. Regular survey evidence from users about their experiences was required even though the idea was often resisted by professionals. The range of services commissioned needed to change with better use of practice-based commissioning and the PbR tariff; and Local Area Agreements (LAAs) and development plans shifting resources into community services. There were significant organisational and cultural barriers to these changes but only if they were overcome would the White Paper vision become a reality.

We set out the required changes in a document published in October 2006 called "Our Health, Our Care, Our Say: Making it Happen", which explained what people needed to do over the next three years. It also indicated what the Department would deliver in areas like the GP contract and improving the QOF; starting health checks; improving carers support; aligning health and social care budget cycles; expanding primary care; establishing a social enterprise to run the Expert Patient Programme; developing an urgent care strategy; and legislation on direct payments. There was a timetable for various actions to the end of the 2008/9.[16]

My greatest difficulty in this period was battling with DH and the Treasury over money to start this work in 2006/7 and continuing it in 2007/8. The NHS and DH had so mismanaged their budgets (see Chapter 9) that there was little money that could be found to kick-start this new agenda that would use NHS resources more effectively. It was a classic public sector Catch 22; the financial situation was so bad you could not finance the changes that would improve it. Accessing start up money caused the 'Making it happen' document to be delayed until the autumn of 2006 while we put the DH management and NHS finances in better order. However we used the time to start a wide-ranging programme of pilots, early implementers and demonstration sites so that practical applications

of the White Paper's ideas were planted around the NHS and social care.[17]
   This programme included:

- Pilot schemes to test self-referral to physiotherapy;
- 3 pilot sites covering a population of a million people to test whether a comprehensive integrated approach to care supported by assistive technologies like telecare could show a significant shift from hospital care – the so-called ICAT demonstrations;
- Testing and evaluating of individual budgets on 13 sites over 2 years;
- 30 demonstration sites covering 6 specialties to define and test new care pathways for national use to shift care closer to home for dermatology, ENT, general surgery, gynaecology, orthopaedics and urology;
- Scoping and designing the online health and well-being assessment tool for NHS 'Life Checks' and an associated website, along with 4 pilots for teenage health demonstration sites that would start by the end of 2006;
- 18 month pilots to run at two sites to establish the evidence base for psychological therapies to support people in and to return to work, including the use of computerised cognitive behavioural therapy;
- Partnerships for Older People Projects – about 30 in all in two phases – to provide examples of how innovative partnership arrangements could lead to improved outcomes for older people, thereby reducing hospital admissions and residential care stay;
- Testing the idea of information prescriptions that would signpost people with long-term health and social care needs and their carers to the information and advice that would enable them to self-care better.[17]

All these pilots were to be spread around the country. Most were to start in 2006/7, would last up to 2 years and would be independently evaluated. They were the White Paper legacies that Patricia Hewitt and her Ministerial team left behind.

Alongside this work I tried to re-energise the community hospital building programme that had been promised in Labour's 2005 Election Manifesto and again in the 2006 White Paper. This turned out to be something of an uphill struggle with little enthusiasm for it among officials. I discovered that DH never spent their full capital allocations so there was capital money in the current year which could be earmarked for expenditure in future years. Defining what we meant by "a community hospital" proved more difficult. I ended up with a broad definition that covered a wide range of services and encouraged co-location but excluded complex medical procedures. It was left to local people to come together to agree and configure the services they wanted in particular buildings.

I launched in July 2006, with a personal foreword, an invitation to the NHS to come forward with bids for new or refurbished community hospitals and services.[18] PCTs and local communities could bid for money from a £750million fund created for a 5-year building programme. We envisaged 3 different funding models: straightforward public capital through the NHS; Local Improvement Finance Trusts (LIFTs) which was an existing model for bringing together public capital and private sector expertise; and community ventures, which was a new approach for capital investment using a joint venture between PCTs and a partner such as a private or voluntary organisation. We wanted PCTs with advanced plans to put them forward by the end of September 2006 and those with schemes ready for 2007/8 to come forward with those schemes by the end of December. At the same time we stopped further closures of community hospitals without full scale reviews by SHAs. I personally intervened in proposals in Gloucestershire to stop the proposed closure of nine community facilities that would have taken service configuration back into larger hospitals – the completely opposite direction of travel from that set out in the January White Paper. This was a classic example of local NHS managers totally ignoring an elected government's community-based policy favoured by local people in order to protect larger acute hospitals in financial difficulty.

Despite having little money to take forward the 2006 White Paper I believed that this programme of pilots and demonstrations projects and the community hospital initiative, together with the 'Making it Happen' road map did start to embed in the NHS psyche the ideas of bringing care closer to home and placing more emphasis on prevention and health promotion. These projects kept alive the White Paper's ideas for when the NHS moved to financial balance and then into surplus; but not much had changed on the ground when Lord Darzi's Next Stage Review was launched by Gordon Brown when he became Prime Minister in July 2007. Brown wanted to put his own imprimatur on the NHS; and there was little political interest in promoting the ideas in the 2006 White Paper. The new review was to be medically-led and to produce a new vision for the NHS in time for its 60th Anniversary in July 2008. The Darzi Review was part of Brown's political strategy of looking different from Blair and reassuring the NHS workforce and the public sector unions after the turbulence of the Blair health reforms. Competition and care closer to home posed threats to hospitals and their staff and were less popular with the new Prime Minister. The 2006 White Paper disappeared into the new review although Ara Darzi kept some of the White Paper ideas alive and was personally supportive of many Blair reforms.

The Next Stage Review

It must have seemed a political masterstroke to put a doctor in charge of an NHS Review but Brown was then stuck to some extent with what Darzi proposed. For a while it looked as though the person setting the NHS agenda was the surgeon from Imperial College and St Mary's Hospital – who still carried on operating on Fridays and Saturdays. He was said to have the Prime Minister's mobile number and the new Health Secretary, Alan Johnson, seemed almost invisible. Ara Darzi quickly established his own agenda in October 2007 in an interim report, with his picture in surgeon's scrubs on the cover in case anyone had missed the point that a doctor was now in charge of shaping the NHS. This Report began by Darzi saying that he had detected little enthusiasm in the NHS for doing something completely different from the NHS reforms and that they should be seen through to their conclusion. He went on to say that "No-one should see this Review as a way of slowing down or diluting what we need to do. If anything we should …be more ambitious".[19] his may not have been what Gordon Brown had in mind.

The immediate steps proposed for primary care were very much in line with the 2006 White Paper's approach. New GP practices – 'whether they are organised on the traditional independent contractor model or by new private providers' – should be brought into those areas where they were most needed starting with the 25% of PCTs with the poorest provision. Darzi wanted to see newly procured health centres in easily accessible locations; and PCTs introducing more choice over when patients could see their GP by expanding opening hours into the evenings or weekends. The emphasis was to be on a safer more innovative NHS, with a new combined health and social care regulator – as I had proposed – with tough powers backed by fines to inspect and intervene where hospitals had poor hygiene and infection control.

The next step in the review was to be groups of health and social care staff – over 1,000 in total – established in every region to discuss how best to achieve a fairer, more personal NHS delivering more effective and safer care in a locally accountable manner. This was to be a much more staff-led review than the 2006 White Paper's public-led approach. From the outset the Darzi Review rather boxed itself in over changes in hospital services by indicating that changes could only be initiated when there was a clear and strong local clinical basis for doing so and resources could be made available to open new facilities alongside old ones closing. These requirements may seem sensible but they make it easy for local opponents to delay necessary change, particularly as the NHS moved from feast to famine. As it progressed the Darzi Review started to look more like an exercise designed not to upset the acute sector too much or take NHS professionals out of their comfort zone.

The interim report lacked the emphasis in Ara Darzi's pre-Ministerial review of healthcare for London on developing alternatives to hospital and grouping more hospital services in major specialist centres. In his London review published in early 2007 Darzi had described a radical change in the models of healthcare for London.[20] The most significant of these was "a new kind of community based care at a level that falls between the current GP practice and the traditional district general hospital". He called these polyclinics although I had tried to persuade him to call them "community hospitals" which I thought would be more publicly and politically acceptable. In London Darzi called for more healthcare to be provided at home and polyclinics, with local hospitals providing the majority of inpatient care and elective surgery centres where most high-throughput surgery should be provided. Major acute hospitals should be handling only the most complex treatments with existing specialist hospitals being valued and increased; and with Academic Health Science Centres being developed as centres of clinical and research excellence. All this would have involved major upheavals for London's hospitals and GPs. True to form the BMA immediately protested about polyclinics which were quickly redefined so that groups of GP practices could be regarded as a polyclinic if a diagnostic hub was provided. Most of the hospital changes never happened because as I discovered later there was little appetite – political, clinical or managerial – for the reconfigurations required.

The NHS as a whole did not get the radicalism of Darzi's London Review. Instead each SHA conducted its own change agenda through clinical leads. When the Next Steps Review Final Report, 'High Quality Care for All' was published in June 2008 – ready for the NHS's 60th birthday party in July – it produced 10 regional reports covering maternity and newborn care; children's health; planned care, mental health; staying healthy; long-term conditions; acute care; and end of life care. These were heavily influenced by staff views, although ideas from the 2006 White Paper survived in both the regional reviews and the final national report.[21] The latter had a preface by Gordon Brown, a foreword by the Health Secretary and a letter to them and the Chancellor from Ara Darzi. It looked as though the "system" – Ministerial, official and NHS – had neutered radicalism. Terminology had changed with no more talk about 'reform' but describing the NHS as on a journey, without too much clarity about the destination. Apparently Ara Darzi had been joined on this journey by 2,000 clinicians and other professionals but not apparently by any managers because the word 'manager' is completely absent from his Final report.

Although the 2006 White paper was little acknowledged much of its thinking was incorporated in the immediate steps identified by the final report:

- Every PCT was to commission comprehensive well-being and prevention services in partnership with local authorities to tackle obesity, reduce alcohol harm, treat drug addiction, reduce smoking rates and improve sexual and mental health.
- There was to be a Coalition for Better Health between the Government, private sector and voluntary organisations to improve health outcomes, focusing initially on obesity.
- A new programme of vascular risk assessment was to be provided for people ages between 40 and 74.
- GPs were to help individuals stay healthy by improving the QOF to provide better incentives and indicators.
- Choice of GP practice for patients was to be extended by providing more information on the NHS Choices website about primary and community care services.
- A personalised care plan was to be provided for everyone with a long-term condition and individual health budgets were to be piloted.
- Practice-based commissioning was to be reinvigorated and more freedoms were to be given to high-performing GPs.
- New integrated care organisations covering health and social care were to be piloted; and the NHS would be encouraged to set up social enterprise organisations and other enhancements of community services.

These were however not much more than a rehash of the 2006 'Making it happen' document described above.

What was new in Darzi's Final Report was the emphasis on quality issues: stronger enforcement powers for the CQC; independent quality standards and clinical priority-setting through NICE and a new National Quality Board; new quality accounts; best practice tariffs for paying hospitals. There was also more emphasis on supporting innovation; improving NHS staff education and training; enhancing clinical and Board leadership. The major proposal in the Final Report was the proposed NHS Constitution that it was claimed would secure the NHS for the future in terms of its 'enduring principles and values'. Although this was espoused in the Darzi Review it sprang really from Labour's political leadership who wished to put the Conservatives in a political straightjacket on the NHS, especially if they created an independent NHS Board as they threatened to do. Although the Next Stage Review reprised many of the ideas in 'Our Health, Our Care, Our Say' it did not really tackle the implications of bringing care closer to home. Those implications for acute hospitals were nowhere mentioned in the final report. One senses that the political handcuffs had been placed on Ara Darzi on this issue as all the political parties vied with each other to promise the public that their hospitals would be saved if people voted for them in the 2010 Election.

The ideas in Darzi's final report on issues like quality, innovation, health outcomes, inequalities and personalisation are all perfectly sensible. However by promising no further structural change and leaving everything to local decision what the Next Stage Review ended up doing was to duck the hard choices that have to be made. The NHS cannot improve health outcomes, bring care closer to home and concentrate specialist services to improve quality but at the same time go on pumping money into the existing range of acute hospitals and their service configurations. Leaving an unnecessarily large number of weak PCTs in place – many of them uncomfortable with replacing NHS service providers with people from outside the NHS – was never likely to deliver Ara Darzi's vision anytime soon. Moreover the world of adult social care – the NHS's poor relation - which had been brought into the fold in the 2006 White Paper had been largely cast adrift again and received virtually no attention in the Next Stage Review.

As we approach a lengthy period of public expenditure austerity we still face the need to tackle the agenda of bringing care closer to home and its implications for acute hospitals. The NHS still needs to shift faster from an ill-health service to a more balanced health service, with a stronger emphasis on health promotion and wellbeing as part of the closer to home agenda. We have frittered away much of the momentum that was building in early 2006 with the 'Our Health, Our Care, Our Say' White Paper. As the money gets scarcer the NHS needs even more radical changes, as I discuss later and the Coalition Government seems to be planning.

13

Lost in translation – science, healthcare and politics

A week into my first Ministerial job I found myself sitting with Tony Blair and John Reid launching the first government White Paper on genetics to an audience of distinguished scientists.[1] (My only consolation was that Tony's and John's grasp of the human genome was probably as sketchy as mine!) Not long after, I opened the new £40million Biobank laying down genetic lines for future research before an even more distinguished scientific audience. Soon I found myself answering Parliamentary Questions, speaking in debates, piloting legislation and talking to the media on a range of controversial scientific topics: stem cells, genetics, use of human tissue, human fertilisation, contaminated food, variant CJD, animal experiments, alternative therapies, MMR immunisation among others. As a result I was forced to grapple with the complicated relationship between science, politics, faith and public expectations in an age of rapid scientific discovery surrounded by much uncertainty.

Science and politics in an age of uncertainty

We live in a world of phenomenal scientific advance and rapid change and in which the established economic order is under challenge from Asia, Latin America and Eastern Europe. Climate change, major population migrations, religious fundamentalism and fuel and food insecurity all create uncertainty and often pessimism in the minds of electorates. At the level of the nation state – even one as large as the US – it is often impossible for individual governments to achieve the level of security and stability their electorates want. Scientists, politicians and the public are caught in a vortex of information overload, with time for validation and assimilation often a major casualty. It is not easy to absorb rapid scientific change, particularly when increasingly specialised scientists are in their own language bubble which makes little sense to outsiders. As a result scientists and politicians can find it difficult to communicate with each other and with the general public on many issues which require public assent.

In this fast-changing and complex world it is hardly surprising that some people reach for the certainty that religious faith seems to provide. In a democracy elected politicians have to deal with the voting public they face and cannot simply ignore religious beliefs, however misguided they may believe them to be. In handling legislation on scientific issues I had to resist the temptation to quote the message on the Humanist Bus – "There probably is no God so stop worrying and enjoy life". But some scientists, especially the evolutionary fundamentalists, seem not to accept that in this complex and fast-changing world scientists do have to reach some accommodations with organised religion. Politicians cannot simply ride rough-shod over religious beliefs that are held with varying degrees of conviction and fervour by significant proportions of their electorates. None of this means bending the knee to religious fundamentalism which is not only hostile to science but also to human rights and civil society as well. As the journal New Scientist said in an editorial in November 2007 "...the idea that science can simply replace religion in the public consciousness is not only fanciful but also bad for science. Trying to tell people how they should think is likely to alienate them."[2] Most experienced politicians have discovered that truth, sometimes painfully.

Recent UK governments have seen science and innovation as critical to making the UK economy knowledge and high-value based and thereby able to compete with lower cost emerging countries. The title of a 2008 review of the UK's science and innovation policies by Lord Sainsbury, a former Labour Science Minister, says it all – "The Race to the Top".[3] Ministers find themselves, as I did, working hand-in-hand with scientists, universities and business trying to protect the national economy, high value jobs and prosperity. At the same time on an issue by issue basis, life can be more complicated. This is because public perception of risk on a particular issue is often different from science's assessment of risk. Two very good examples of this in recent UK history would be genetically modified food and nuclear power. In both cases government found it difficult to follow the advice of its own Chief Scientist. The Chief Scientist recommended regulation of GM products on a case-by-case basis but then public unease about GM crops and food meant there was little support for early commercialisation of GM crops. There has been a similar position with nuclear power as an alternative to fossil fuel, despite the UK having been world leaders in nuclear power after the war. Until recently most UK politicians have been more influenced by public anxiety about safety than advice from scientists. It is only with greater concern over climate change that nuclear power as a fuel source has made a political comeback in the UK.

These two issues illustrate how science and politics can have a difficult relationship, without any religious intervention, sometimes depending on where the media positions itself on an issue. When GM foods were introduced into UK shops in the mid-1990s the media almost immediately expressed scepticism about them on health and environmental grounds. The BBC replaced Professor Peter Raven as a

Reith lecturer when they discovered his botanic garden had received a large donation from Monsanto. The Daily Mail waged a masterly campaign against "Frankenstein foods" – a label that stuck with the public. Media coverage of the combined MMR vaccine created similar public anxiety, starting with an ill-judged article in a medical journal on a possible connection between the vaccine and autism. This resulted in a massive reduction in vaccination which in turn reduced public resistance to measles, leading to a rise in child deaths. This was despite the scientific evidence clearly showing that MMR does not cause autism. Science was overwhelmed by media hysteria and a lack of authoritative scientists able to argue publicly the pro-MMR case.

However the public attitude to science has been changing compared with a decade ago. The latest survey of public attitudes to science in 2008 showed a positive shift in attitudes to science and the generation of new ideas and knowledge.[4] 62% of people agreed that it is important to know about science in their daily lives. More people felt better informed about science than previously – 56% of adults compared with 39% in 2005. The public wants to hear directly from scientists themselves; but a quarter of people still say the more they learn about science the more worried they are - although this is down from 35% in 2005. There is still considerable public suspicion of science and an expectation that science and scientists should be regulated. This is the public and political context within which I and other Ministers were and are operating. Most of the scientific issues I handled related to 4 main themes which remain of current concern: meddling with nature; the search for cures; safeguarding personal information; and the translation of research into practical healthcare, particularly in areas like genetics.

Meddling with nature

GM foods were a good example of scientists presented as meddling with nature – the so-called "Frankenstein foods" – and losing the public argument because they were unable to provide the guarantees that the public were seeking, particularly after the history of chemical spraying of crops and contaminated animal feedstuffs. The food industry's apparent lack of transparency over nanotechnology and its possible long-term effects on the human brain shows how history could repeat itself in the food area. There has been a similar range of arguments over the issues of stem cell research and assisting human fertilisation where not only were scientists meddling with nature but were getting involved in matters of life and death.

As a Minister I was a strong supporter of stem cell research and the benefits it could bring but there were powerful opponents. In 2004 I found myself confronted with a US-backed UN motion seeking to restrict the world-wide use of embryonic stem cells in medical research. Despite an overtly Christian Prime Minister and a Health Secretary with a large Catholic population in his constituency I was allowed to pursue the best interests of scientific research and patients. Working with DH officials and a good link-up with the FCO and our man in New York at the UN I was able to ensure that the UK vote was cast with the opposition to the US-backed motion – even though this meant voting with Iran! No.10 and John Reid were kept in the picture throughout but this was a good example of how the UK was not rolled over by George Bush and how the best interests of UK science and patients were protected by defeating the US-backed motion.

I was helped in this action by a 2003 survey showing that 70% of the UK public supported the use of embryos for health research.[5] Nevertheless it can still be difficult sometimes to counter those with a strong religious belief that human life begins when an egg is fertilised, so it is morally wrong to use cells from human embryos, particularly if there are stem cells available that can be represented as just as good as embryonic stem cells, even if they are not. When debating these issues with people holding firm religious beliefs on the start of human life you struggle to persuade them to accept embryonic stem cell research because there is a regulatory system that destroys embryos at 14 days. Embryo disposal at 14 days just makes matters worse for the devout. As I discovered this minority religious viewpoint has had a disproportionate influence on the public debate on stem cells in the UK and on some politicians, including members of the UK Cabinet.

For some people, their religious views on the start of life overlap with the other main objection often voiced to stem cell research – that it interferes excessively and dangerously with nature. Scientific fantasies, as well as hardline religious views, especially within the Catholic Church, have influenced much of the public and political debate on two related issues – cloning and hybrid embryos. Concerns started before my time as a Minister with Dolly the sheep, the first cloned mammal, in 1996. They were given impetus nearly a decade later by the scientists in Newcastle who became the first group in the UK to generate a human embryo by nuclear replacement. It was the wish of researchers to generate stem cells by cell nuclear transfer using cow eggs with human nuclei that pushed hybrid embryos into the political limelight. Somewhat reluctantly the Government was forced to look again at the regulatory legislation in this area – the 1990 Human Fertilisation and Embryology Act, itself a world first.

As I resigned as a Minister a White Paper was published in December 2006 reviewing the 1990 Act which came down against science by proposing that the creation of hybrid embryos in vitro should not be allowed on ethical grounds.[6] There had been considerable opposition to their creation in the public consultation leading up to the publication of the White Paper and much of this had surfaced in the House of Lords. Fortunately the scientists regrouped and got at another group of politicians, the House of Commons Science and Technology Select Committee. In early 2007 that Committee produced a report saying the Government had got it wrong. They said that outlawing the creation of embryos which are part-human, part-animal was unacceptable and threatened to undermine Britain's leading position in stem cell science. They called for permissive legislation which would regulate research using animal-human hybrid and chimaera embryos through licensing.[7] ll such embryos would continue to be destroyed after 14 days and it would be illegal for them to be implanted.

The Government climbed down in the face of an onslaught from scientists, patient groups and fellow politicians. In September 2007 the regulatory body indicated that it would license hybrid and chimaera embryos. New legislation was introduced at the end of 2007 to do this but was fiercely debated in both Houses of Parliament, with further attacks from the Catholic Church hierarchy which I observed from the backbenches.[8] Around Easter 2007 Catholic sermons across the country condemned the proposed revising legislation and scary language like "creating monsters" was used to try to bring Catholics and others into line. The Head of the Catholic Church in England and Wales and other church leaders lobbied the Prime Minister to change tack. Catholic government Ministers said they could not support the Government's own legislation and were given personal dispensations not to vote. The Prime Minister to his credit put his personal reputation behind the legislation and backed science against organised religion. Even so the final stages of passing the legislation were deferred until later in the year for fear of upsetting Catholic electors in a by-election that the Government needed to win. On stem cells the majority of the public have supported the scientists and politicians against organised religion because at its heart was clearly the issue of the search for cures.

The search for cures

We are all living longer. Human beings seem to prefer this to the alternative. Medical technologies and pharmaceutical products have built on public health improvements to increase life expectancy, even though some people make poor lifestyle choices around diet and exercise. Finding a cure for health problems seems increasingly to be part of mainstream public belief. It was this search for cures that won the public argument on stem cell research and hybrid embryos. The shortage of human eggs was going to slow down stem cell research into many unpleasant diseases and using animal eggs was the only way of allowing researchers to push ahead unhindered. It wasn't only the scientists who persuaded the Government to change its mind on hybrid embryos but the letter to the Prime Minister signed by 223 medical charities and patient groups. These groups were not going to let a few bishops and cardinals prevent scientists getting on with finding cures. They were quite happy to have nature meddled with because they didn't much like what nature was producing in people near and dear to them.

However other aspects of the search for cures can cause problems for science, notably experiments on animals and alternative therapies, both of which I have been involved with as a Minister. As I indicated in Chapter 10 experiments on animals have had a regulatory system that affords the greatest protection for animals genetically closest to humans, like the great apes. Scientists have been on the receiving end of the campaigns against animal experiments and it took real courage for scientists to speak out against these campaigns as the former Director of the Medical Research Council, Colin Blakemore, did. However it was government Ministers who pushed the police hard to improve their intelligence gathering, who legislated to deal with animal rights terrorists and who carried the fight to the opponents of science.

On alternative therapies, Ministers have been more cautious, not least I suspect because members of the Royal Family use these therapies. The heir to the throne is a staunch advocate for many alternative therapies and homeopathic medicine has been available under the NHS since its beginning in 1948. As many modern drugs have become even more toxic in order to tackle the conditions they are trying to cure, so the appeal of less toxic natural cures seems to have increased for many members of the public, even if supporting scientific evidence is scanty or non-existent. The conspicuous absence of randomised clinical trials for alternative therapies infuriates the scientific community. Periodically as a Health Minister in the House of Lords I participated in debates on these issues as both sides berate each other and try to persuade you to come down on their side of the argument.

Slowly a European-wide system of licensing is developing together with some degree of minimal registration of practitioners but even this is a source of dispute. This new regulatory approach convinces few scientists, some of whom would like the NHS to ban the use of homeopathic remedies and stop using public money on unproven therapies - a view I have a good deal of sympathy with. At the same time the supporters of the therapies continue to lobby for preventing any regulation that will result in the disappearance of their favourite remedies in what is now a sizeable industry. My approach as a Minister was to act on any evidence of real harm caused by particular products – as happened with some Chinese products; shelter behind the EU; and try to soothe the fevered brows of the more strident advocates of alternative therapies – some of whom were in positions of influence. I suspect this will continue to be the approach of most Health Ministers of whatever political complexion for some time to come.

A much more contested area has been the research use of human tissue which raises several issues – ownership, storage and consent for usage: these were all the subject of new UK and European legislation which I had to handle. The political focus on this issue in the UK arose from the way parts of dead children had been kept rather unceremoniously in Alder Hey, a Liverpool children's hospital, instead of being returned to their parents for burial. Following an inquiry the Government decided to legislate to introduce more public safeguards; and it used this legislation to incorporate into UK law new EU legislation. As I watched representatives of the bereaved Alder Hey parents keeping a beady eye on me while I took this legislation through the House of Lords I was constantly reminded that some scientists need to behave with a lot more sensitivity than they have done in the past.

The 2004 Human Tissue Act required consent for the research use of tissue consisting of or including human cells from living people (apart from embryos, hair and nails). A tissue sample must be anonymised and the research must have the approval of a Research Ethics Committee. Patients had the right to give their consent and to be sure their identity was not revealed; the material had to be stored correctly; and the research required ethical approval. As Ministers we were on the side of the individual's right to control access by scientists to their human tissue, much to the annoyance of some senior scientists. Throughout the passage of the legislation members of the scientific community continued to moan about what they regarded as bureaucratic barriers to scientific research that would damage the UK's science-based industries. I had a number of meetings with medical scientific leaders with my Ministerial colleague Rosie Winterton who had policy responsibility for the legislation. We were told that research and scientists would leave the UK for countries where controls were less onerous. Pressure built up in the Lords but there was not much room for manoeuvre within the EU Directive. Apart from tea and sympathy and a few modest amendments little of substance was conceded. Scientists have continued to complain about the European Clinical Trials Directive incorporated in the Human Tissue Act. The UK does not have much room for change unless the EU accepts a loosening of patient safeguards, although some of the coverage of the Directive could be reduced and it could be a little less energetically policed.

Similar issues of human rights in relation to scientific research cropped up with embryos during the passage of the Human Fertilisation and Embryology Act 2008, already discussed. The Government had taken the legal view that the use of a person's genetic material without their express consent to create embryos and their subsequent use and storage would interfere with a person's rights under Article 8 of the European Convention of Human Rights. As someone who had written the Labour Party policy paper on incorporation of the Convention into UK Law leading to the Human Rights Act, I had considerable sympathy with this view. This interpretation meant that new legislation had to ensure that informed consent was given to create or alter an embryo or hybrid embryo but this posed problems for existing banks or cell lines for which no individual consent had been obtained in the past. Effective political lobbying by scientists led to the Government discussing with those working in stem cell research whether existing stores of cells were vital to the progress of stem cell research. As a result exceptions to consent requirements were made for existing collections.

In the search for cures scientists claim that they have the public on their side – and they usually do – but people do like to be asked for their permission to use bits of themselves and to know what the scientists are going to do with those bits. On detailed issues the scientists have sometimes been effective lobbyists but usually they have lost attempts to be given carte blanche on use of human tissue for research. The majority of the public seem keen to control access to their personal information, including their genetic information – whether scientists or Ministers like it or not. So the safeguarding of personal information has become a political issue that has to be taken into account in the onward march of science. Access to that information is not something that scientists can take for granted, whatever human benefits they claim for their research.

Safeguarding personal information

The growing use of large public (and private) databases with massive amounts of personal information has focussed public attention on the security of that information. Personal identity theft through financial institutions has undermined confidence in those institutions and created a major new crime category across countries. In the UK the failure of public bodies to protect the confidentiality of personal data has reduced significantly the credibility of Ministerial reassurances on this issue. Research scientists cannot escape from this public anxiety about institutional holding of personal information, much as many would like to.

In the UK we have now three pillars of reassurance on holding personal data for medical research: individual consent, anonymity and independent ethical approval of the proposed research. The debate on individual consent has to a great extent been settled as a result of the recent legislation on human tissue and embryos operating within the umbrella of the Human Rights Act. There are a few exceptions for existing collections where individuals cannot be traced and for mental incapacity. Otherwise the informed consent of the individual has to be given for the use of data or material relating to them. I will turn to the issue of anonymity later but first let me deal with independent ethics committees which continue to be a source of irritation to scientists despite my efforts to improve matters.

For some time local ethics committees have been in place to safeguard those participating in medical research. Like many regulatory bodies, these committees have engaged in "mission creep", particularly by questioning the methodology of the science rather than sticking to the ethical basis of the research proposal. By the time I became a Minister in 2003 these committees had become a source of continuing complaints about their bureaucratic procedures by scientific researchers and drug companies. These procedures were said to be leading to the UK losing research work to Asia where the rules were fewer. To respond to these concerns I set up an independent review led by Michael O'Higgins (now Chair of the Audit Commission) with a remit to streamline the ethics committees' processes and speed up decision-making. Ethics committees were directed to safeguard participants in research rather than checking research methodology; their processes were streamlined and time limits were introduced; and a central bureau exercised stronger oversight of their activities. Although improvements have been made, complaints rumble on and I suspect that a more robust statutory framework with enforceable time limits will be needed if autonomous local ethics committees are to cease being unnecessary barriers to UK medical research.

So far individual consent, anonymity and ethics committees have been regarded as adequate public safeguards for medical research. Whether this scientific/political settlement is robust enough to cope with the growth of genetic data remains to be seen, particularly in the area of anonymity. This has been brought home to me by my involvement in the 2009 House of Lords inquiry into genomic medicine.[9] The increased access to genetic information continues at a phenomenal pace, and the potential for patient benefits is huge in terms of more personalised and targeted medicine for common diseases. Given what has gone before on medical research and human tissue use, it is hard to argue that individual genetic information should not be under the same control of the person to whom it relates, particularly if in the future it is linked to an individual's electronic patient record. However, matters are not straightforward. Unreasonable withholding of individual consent to access genetic information could jeopardise genetics-based research which requires large population-based databases and DNA collections in which inevitably individuals will be identifiable to some extent.

There is a wider public interest in the benefits of this research that transcends individual rights so governance of these databases poses difficult political questions not just scientific ones. Moreover genetic data can have relevance for people other than those from whom it derives because it could reveal unexpected information on paternity, or provide information about a disease risk to a relative that may manifest itself in the future. Giving the individual from whom the genetic information derives an absolute veto on access and use is unlikely to be in the best interests of wider public policy. Throughout my time as a Minister the tensions were considerable and growing between individual rights to confidentiality and the march of science and the potential benefits offered by accumulating personal (including genetic) data. These new databases and how they are accessed present both huge opportunities for good and considerable scope for misuse. They will present a major challenge for politicians and scientists in terms of new systems of governance and controlled access, together with the need for serious sanctions for misuse or negligence. We are only in the foothills of understanding the problems to be faced, let alone identifying solutions to handling the governance of this mass of genetic-rich individual information combined with inevitable IT advances.

The problems that can arise were illustrated by a rumpus that occurred at the end of 2008 when the DH consulted on a proposal to allow researchers for the first time to write to patients who shared a particular set of medical conditions to seek their participation in trials.[10] Nothing wrong with seeking consent you might think but to write these letters medical researchers had to trawl through personal medical records to select the people they needed to ask to participate. This caused uproar, with Harry Cayton the Chairman of the National Information Governance Board for Health and Social Care that I had initiated (see Chapter 8) criticising the proposal publicly. Here we had a straight conflict between the understandable wish of government to boost the UK's research-based pharmaceutical industry for the good of some patients and UK plc and the rights of patients to control access to their personal data whatever the consequences for other patients. When the then Information Commissioner, Richard Thomas and Mark Walport, Director of the Wellcome Trust produced their report on data sharing in 2009 they described this situation as a "Catch 22 dilemma".[11] It posed the problem of how do researchers gain the consent to identify the people needed for their research in the first place in order to gain consent to use their individual information. By definition "Catch 22s" are rarely easy to resolve and some legislative arbitration is likely to be needed eventually.

Alongside these ethical issues involved with science and its regulation, I spent much time on how to translate medical discoveries into healthcare practice – the so-called 'bench to bedside' issue arising under the DH system for managing NHS research and development.

The problem of translation

The UK has a formidable international reputation for basic scientific research as measured by things like Nobel prizes, citations in published research and the flow of overseas students for PhD places in UK universities. Eminent UK scientists proudly claim that we punch well above our weight, given our population size and our level of investment in basic scientific research. On most of the measures scientists use in these international comparisons we look to be second only to the US, although we may be losing ground to other countries as well. Our biomedical and genomic research is up there with the international best. It offers huge potential benefit for the UK and this ought to be easier to deliver with a National Health Service which provides universal health coverage to its population. Sadly this translation of discovery to NHS care is something the NHS continues to struggle with.

There are two stages to the translation process. The first is moving the basic scientific knowledge through processes such as clinical trials to the creation of a particular clinical product such as a drug, a medical device or a new procedure that is fit for general use with patients. The second is the adoption and widespread use of these new products with patients across the NHS. Both stages present potential barriers and bottlenecks but as the Minister responsible for NHS R and D and the pharmaceutical and devices industries I concentrated initially on trying to improve the first stage.

In 2003 we did not know accurately what the NHS spent on R and D because historically the NHS had used money labelled as "research" for other things, including balancing the books. Even when the money was spent on R and D it was often more to do with the interests of particular researchers and their ability to secure money than with any national priorities. The UK lacked any system similar to the US where there were identified centres of excellence funded through federal national institutes who concentrated their research resources and effort on these centres of excellence. I supported the head of NHS R and D in the Department of Health, Sally Davies, a doctor who then still saw patients, to begin the process of bringing some order into this chaos. The first step – which was not concluded until I moved on in 2005 – was to stop the random distribution of money to the NHS; and to refocus the research effort on a smaller number of places, pursuing clearer national priorities on the basis of competitive tendering for grants. This produced unrest in the NHS because some prestigious institutions saw their budgets cut and did not want to compete for funds by demonstrating the quality of their research work. It took 2-3 years to work through this reform process and required support to Sally Davies and her team to carry out this long overdue change.

The second element of reform was to attempt greater coordination of research funding between the different funding streams for medical research. These were DH's NHS R and D which was re-branded as the National Institute for Health Research (NIHR); the Medical Research Council (MRC) – which received its money from another government department; industry – mainly the pharmaceutical industry; and the large medical charities, particularly the Wellcome Foundation and Cancer UK, who fund a major part of UK medical research. I asked Sir John Pattison, the former DH head of R and D to see if he could find a way of bringing these various interests together in some kind of forum. His diplomatic skills were impeccable and he recommended the establishment of a UK Clinical Research Collaboration. I accepted his recommendation which was a step forward within DH but did not go far enough, as I agreed later with Lord Sainsbury, then the Minister for Science. Just before I left this Ministerial post in 2005 Sir David Cooksey, a former Chairman of the Audit Commission and a venture capitalist was asked to review the whole system of UK health research funding.

In 2006 Cooksey's "Review of UK Health Research Funding" identified a number of cultural, institutional and financial barriers to the translation of publicly-funded research into clinical practice.[12] Unless these were tackled the UK was at risk of failing to reap the full economic, health and social benefits that should flow from its investment in health research. The two stages of translation described above were still too weak. Cooksey wanted to see better coordination of health research and improved funding arrangements to support translation. He recommended a new Office for the Strategic Coordination of Health Research (OSCHR) to coordinate research between NIHR and the MRC and to monitor progress; the inclusion of additional but ring-fenced funding streams for DH research; and additional funding, including for Health Technology Assessments, to support the take up of new ideas and technologies. In 2007 after I had left government OSCHR was finally established.

OSCHR was the logical completion of the reforms that Sally Davies and I had started in 2003 but it had taken 4 years to achieve. It now coordinates a public sector health research budget which grew under Labour to about £1.7billion a year. Much of the overlap that existed between DH and the MRC has now been eliminated. The MRC is responsible for the early development of new opportunities from discovery to early-stage clinical trials. NIHR is responsible for large scale clinical trials and health technology assessments. The Wellcome Foundation as a large funder of medical research and other charities have supported these changes and there have been real improvements in coordination and funding for translation research. But serious continuing challenges on translation have been highlighted both by OSCHR in its first progress report and by others. In January 2009 a report by the Bioscience Innovation and Growth Team said that despite all the work done to improve translation of health research into clinical application "the adoption of new therapies, drugs and procedures in the NHS remains painfully slow... and the translation of these improvements into patient benefit has not materialised".[13] One of the witnesses to the House of Lords Inquiry into Genomic Medicine - the PHG Foundation - said that although genomic science was in a "robust state", "progress is dramatically slower in evaluating the clinical and public health relevance of these scientific advances and in developing systems for effective translation of validated tests and interventions into clinical practice". It went on to say "insufficient attention has been paid to the final stage of translation, which bridges the gap between assessment /evaluation and implementation".[14]

The pace of change in genetic knowledge, as demonstrated in the House of Lords report, will bring a whole new range of translation problems for the NHS.[15] We have known for some time about the many single gene disorders like cystic fibrosis and Huntington's disease but, terrible though they can be, they affect relatively few people. In the last 5 years or so the completion of the human genome sequence and other knowledge has led to the identification of more than 500 new susceptibility genes for common diseases affecting very large numbers of people – for example coronary heart disease, diabetes, and rheumatoid arthritis. Although cures and treatments may not be imminent these discoveries will change NHS clinical practice significantly and highlight NHS weaknesses in translating discoveries into clinical practice.

Strengthening NHS approaches to translation

Industry has long complained about slow NHS take up of innovative treatments, drugs, devices and procedures; and I discussed some of this in the previous chapter, including the work done on the HITF Report. There have been many complaints about UK health discoveries and inventions not being taken up here but being commercially developed and used overseas. When you visit abroad as a Minister people cannot understand why, with the NHS, we cannot ensure better take up of our own inventions. In 2009, the Medical Technology Group – a large UK coalition of patient groups, research charities and medical device manufacturers produced "An Action Plan for Medical Technology" in the NHS. In this document they noted that "the UK lags behind many of our European neighbours in utilisation rates as well as total spending, with overall expenditure on medical technologies almost 2.7billion euros, less than the EU average each year".[16] They gave many examples of where we are slower to take up these technologies; and Lord Darzi's Next Stage Review recognised the inadequate NHS take up of innovation.

The nub of the problem is what fails to happen at the end of the second stage of the translation process so that there is widespread use by patients of proven new products and procedures. The procedures and funding for translation research have now been strengthened considerably following the Cooksey Report, although genomic medicines will require further strengthening. What is lacking are effective policy and operational systems and processes within DH and the NHS to ensure that clinical practice changes faster and speeds up patient access to new technologies. This requires a cultural change and investment in knowledge transfer on a different scale from the past. It is not sufficient to rely on bodies like OSCHR and NIHR – who are responsible for funding and overseeing research and its translation - to bring about the necessary operational changes with the NHS for the use of new technologies.

Action needs to move much more now to the NHS/DH policy, practice and operational arenas from which NIHR and OSCHR are too removed at present. It is striking that in a 52-page NHS operating framework for 2010/11 sent out by the NHS Chief Executive in December 2009 there is no reference to R and D and little relating to new clinical practices.[17] Although the NHS is expected to improve its efficiency and quality over the next 3-4 years in a tough financial climate the role of R and D and its application in making these changes is not mentioned. Improving the translation of these new discoveries to widespread patient use and benefit requires new approaches that involve the people who can make this happen across the NHS on a day-by-day basis. The research world's work needs to be linked more closely with the wider clinical community (and not just those involved with research), patients' representatives, service managers, commissioners, Trust non-executives and regulators. Whatever the QUIPP system, established after the Darzi Review, will achieve this is a matter on which the jury is still out.

Changes of this kind are likely to require new forums and ways of transferring knowledge to those in day-to-day clinical practice and operationalising that knowledge to those who buy services and products. When a new operational framework for the NHS is being prepared the world of NIHR and OSCHR should become more involved.

Commissioners, Trust Boards and Executive Management teams and the wider clinical community, especially GPs, need to be more aware of how the proven new products can be used for their patients in the here and now. It is not sufficient to leave it to the scientific and research community to spread the word. NICE has an important role to play in this area because of its assessment of new clinical products and practices, although many of the new genetic and diagnostic tests are still in an evaluation no-man's land. The NHS tends to respond to priority-setting if there are incentives. Bringing an R and D implementation element into the annual NHS operating framework seems to me crucial if we are to improve the knowledge brokering and transfer required for effective translation of discoveries into the NHS.

14

Who's in charge? – accountability and regulation

The issues of accountability and performance

Two good questions to ask about any organisation is "Who's in charge?" and "Who controls how the money is spent?" Leadership, looking ahead, reading the environment, motivating people, communication skills and many other attributes are important contributors to organisational success. But it is the way resources are distributed and used that ultimately shapes organisational achievement over time. Accounting for the use of resources and relating performance to expenditure should be a key part of running public services like the NHS to ensure that they are run in a businesslike manner and achieve their public service objectives within the resources made available politically in an efficient and effective way. To do this involves keeping up with technological advances and customer or service users' needs, preferences, and expectations. It does not mean allowing particular service providers dominating the decisions about how things are run. This more managerial approach also means not treating public services in an opportunistic way simply because your stewardship of them is likely to be short and you want to make impact for reasons of personal or Party advantage or both. In my case it turned out to be an approach somewhat at odds with the way much of the NHS operated and many elected politicians related to the NHS. Good management turned out too often not to equate with political advantage and success, both of which can run counter to taking difficult decisions and allocating resources wisely.

The conventional wisdom about the NHS is that the Health Secretary is accountable to Parliament for the way he/she and their governing Party have used the taxpayer's money. Parliament through its scrutiny can hold the government of the day to account. If the electorate doesn't like the way things have been done they can throw the governing party out at the next election. In practice Parliamentary scrutiny has limited effectiveness. No matter how good and embarrassing are the reports by the all-Party Public Account Committee or the Health Select Committee – and some are very good critiques indeed – they rarely secure a significant change of personnel, spending priorities or service direction. These reports become another bit of turbulence to be dealt with by

Ministerial incumbents. Although Parliamentary scrutiny and political accountability are important and necessary they are not sufficient in themselves to ensure that the NHS is well run and delivering value for the large amount of taxpayer's money invested in it.

It was the need to show the public what they were getting for the extra money being pumped into the NHS that led to the Labour Government's increasing use of targets, as described in Chapter 3. Targets, whatever their critics say, imposed some conditionality on the NHS in that Ministers could indicate the service access and performance that the public had the right to expect from the NHS in return for the extra money provided. Targets made it possible to shift the political dialogue away from bragging about inputs – more nurses, more doctors, and more hospitals – and start to talk instead about outputs and occasionally even outcomes. As has been shown targets did measure some aspects of NHS performance and help to improve them significantly but they were a far from perfect system for holding the NHS or Ministers to account. Used to excess, targets alienated many of the clinicians who make the individual patient decisions that ultimately determine the use of NHS resources.

Some argue that it is doctors who make most decisions that determine NHS expenditure and patient outcomes so they should be put more in charge of budgets. Doctors regularly moan about targets, managers and political decision-making/interference but there has hardly been a long queue of doctors fighting to get into clinical management or to be held accountable for the use of resources. Many doctors prefer not to be put into a position where they have to require other clinicians to behave in a particular way or to make choices between the priority given to particular service areas. Published comparisons of individual doctor performance has not been a feature of NHS accountability; and relatively few doctors are willing to stand up in public and explain the conduct of their peers in the way local services operate. It is much more congenial to look after their own patients, call for more money and more clinical independence and to blame managers and politicians for any service shortcomings. Of course some doctors do take very well to management and are competent and responsible budget-handlers; and we need to encourage more take on these roles with good data underpinning. However politicians who want to hand the lion's share of the NHS budget to doctors will still have put in place adequate systems of performance measurement and public accountability as the Coalition Government will find. Those who want to hand more budgeting control to doctors should beware of getting what they wish for at a time of constrained resources and patient empowerment unless the performance measurement and accountability is robust.

Moreover many of the NHS resource decisions are not clinical. Buildings and plant and their use, IT and information systems, staffing levels and deployment, supplies and back office services are just some of the areas where the NHS spends large sums of money but doctors simply do not have the expertise to be responsible or accountable. Currently it is managers and boards who are held accountable collectively for the way money is spent and services delivered in a particular geographical area or facility but many would question the rigor of that accountability. Boards are not democratically accountable although like managers they can be sacked; and many NHS chief executives have a dual accountability, both to local trust boards and to the NHS Chief Executive, if they are not FTs.

With the exception of targets, most of the current accountability arrangements have changed little since the beginning of the NHS, although early on local authorities played a larger part by running services like health centres, district nursing and public health. Until the 1980s local authorities had representatives on hospital management committees but this more formal engagement in the NHS has lapsed. There is, in my view, a strong case for increasing local authority involvement with the NHS, particularly if securing health and wellbeing is to play a much larger part in its work. More recently the Mayor of London has been given powers to become more involved in Londoners' health; and some have suggested that Primary Care Trusts should have a democratic element in their membership or be wholly elected. I believe the time has come to involve local government much more formally in the running of the NHS, especially on local commissioning priorities and integrating health, housing and social care. This would reduce the democratic deficit in the way the NHS is run currently at the local level.

Periodically the cry goes up that the NHS should be taken out of politics and run by an independent board. The advocates of this model often seem to have in mind something that looks rather like the 1940s and 1950s nationalised industries model for running utilities like electricity, coal, water and railways. A major problem for these nationalised bodies was their inability to raise investment capital for investment thereby making them reliant on a Treasury reluctant to part with the capital these sectors required. It was these capital needs that drove much privatisation of utilities, as well as the fact that whenever a major problem – or strike – arose it was the responsible minister who was held accountable and expected to sort it out. The NHS has partly overcome the capital problem but the highly emotional and often controversial nature of the NHS and the large sums of public money involved have made it difficult for Ministers to hand over NHS operational accountability. As Nye Bevan said, if a nurse dropped a bedpan in Tredegar the noise echoed round Whitehall and Ministers got involved. The Coalition Government will face this problem with their reform proposals.

Although handing over complete responsibility for the NHS to an independent board may pose political problems, there are some aspects of running the NHS where it looks increasingly necessary to distance Ministers from decision-making. Setting the tariff for payments to hospitals is one such area. In Germany there is an independent body collecting the data and using it to set the tariffs on an annual basis; and, as I indicated earlier, this is an area where we should shift responsibility in the way we operate our own PbR tariff. The endlessly debated system for resource allocation for local areas is another area where there is a strong case for taking the methodology for resource allocation and its application locally out of Ministerial hands. Ministers would settle the total sum to be made available for publicly-funded healthcare and the broad priorities within that between hospitals, community services, adult social care, and public health/health promotion but not be involved in geographical allocation. Perhaps more controversially hospital reconfigurations and dealing with failing and unsustainable trusts would benefit in terms of effective decision-making if so much responsibility did not rest in Ministerial hands.

Under Labour there has been considerable interest in trying new approaches to accountability and pepping up performance but always within the conventional framework of a Health Secretary being accountable publicly and to Parliament for the NHS, its finances and performance. These new approaches have included developing markets with more competition and user choice; stronger patient empowerment through better access to information, direct payments and individual budgets; improving commissioning of services; and more latterly the ideas of an NHS constitution and quality accounts. All these initiatives have required action by government because relying on the local NHS to generate the necessary change was likely to mean a very long wait. This has led to the development of a much-needed performance framework with measurement, monitoring, comparison and publication of data - effectively public naming and shaming. What this has revealed is that although NHS overall performance has improved as a result of the extra investment, the rate of improvement has varied considerably between institutions, areas and bodies in terms of quality of services and financial management.

Much of what is now known about this variability in performance comes from the performance assessment work of a new generation of inspectors and regulators who have done much to keep the public, Parliament and the media informed of the NHS's progress, or lack of it. Some within the NHS do not like this extra light being shone on some of the darker corners and have been quick to criticise these newcomers. We already have professional bodies, traditional audit and SHAs and DH crawling all over us, so why do we need the added bureaucracy of these new inspectorates and regulators? The data is unreliable so the comparisons are unfair. Regulation has gone too far and should be reduced. But has it?

The growth of inspection, performance management and regulation

The huge increase in public expenditure on the NHS has required a closer look at where the money has gone, what it has delivered and whether the improved performance has been as good as it should have been. People want to be reassured about the safety of their treatment and care, particularly when things go so badly wrong in particular places. It is no longer Nye Bevan's Tredegar bedpan that echoes round Whitehall but major scandals like handling dead children's remains at Alder Hey, child deaths at Bristol Children's Hospital, HCAIs deaths at Maidstone and Tunbridge Wells Trust and Accident and Emergency failures at Mid-Staffordshire Trust to name a few of the more celebrated examples. If Ministers are accountable for the NHS and the extra money they have committed to it, how do they find out what is going on and try to prevent the disasters occurring? However 'hands-off' Ministers want to be in managing the NHS they cannot absolve themselves totally from gross failure in a tax-funded NHS, particularly if consequences for serious failure do not automatically follow.

Until the last decade or so, central government had a very traditional approach to monitoring and regulating the NHS. All authorities were audited through accredited auditors - since the 1980s overseen by the Audit Commission who were also responsible for auditing local government and the police. The National Audit Office audited DH and together with the Audit Commission would periodically examine in depth particular NHS and social care topics to assess value for money. Large amounts of statistics on NHS inputs and outputs – mainly in relation to hospitals – were collected annually by DH but were little used for any critical examination of performance. It took the arrival of Tim Kelsey and his company, Dr. Foster, to start turning this mass of material into useful management information which was then sold back to the NHS as described earlier. Little of this information was made available to the public so that they could make their own judgements about NHS performance.

Medical Royal Colleges inspected hospitals doing teaching to see that they were up to snuff for training doctors. Because the private sector had a profit motive and was outside the NHS, private hospitals and nursing homes and independent sector residential care homes were inspected and regulated. However equivalent NHS establishments were not regulated in the same way even though some NHS hospitals for the mentally handicapped and the mentally ill had been shown to be highly unsatisfactory. Regional Hospital Boards, later to become Regional Health Authorities, were used to oversee local hospital bodies, usually with some form of annual accountability review; but Alan Milburn lost patience with these regional bodies in 2000 and abolished the remaining four (see Chapter 5). The publication of the NHS Plan in 2000 set a new direction for regulation when Alan Milburn established the Commission for Health Improvement following the 1999 Health Act.

This new Commission was the first organisation to assess the clinical performance of NHS hospitals in a systematic and regular way; and had doctors as its first Chair and Chief Executive. Its aim was to improve the quality of patient care by assessing NHS organisations and publishing its findings; investigating serious failure; advising on best practice; and checking that the NHS was following national guidelines. When I arrived as a Minister in June 2003 I took over responsibility for CHI and the star rating system it had introduced for hospitals, giving them one, two or three stars on an annual basis. CHI had delivered one set of star-ratings and I had to oversee the publication of its second (and what turned out to be its final) version in July 2003. I had to wind up CHI as the decision had been made to merge it with the private hospital functions of the National Care Standards Commission (NCSC) and some of the NHS performance review functions of the Audit Commission. A new enlarged Commission for Healthcare Audit and Inspection (CHAI), later to be called the Healthcare Commission, was to be established to take over these functions, together with reviewing unresolved complaints about the NHS and handling complaints about non-NHS hospitals. CHI had done a workmanlike job but there were tensions within it and between it and the DH.

The Healthcare Commission came into operation in April 2004 through the 2003 Health and Social (Community Health and Standards) Act which I had to pilot through the House of Lords in time. The 2003 Act also brought into being Foundation Trusts, (FTs) as described in Chapter 3 along with their own regulator, Monitor – legally just called the 'Independent Regulator'. Suddenly the NHS had two new and powerful regulators – one a quality regulator (the Healthcare Commission), the other more akin to an economic regulator (Monitor) who relied on the Healthcare Commission for quality information but lacked powers to ensure competition. Monitor had to assess the financial strength and business acumen of hospital trusts along with the Healthcare Commission's quality information, to see if trusts were capable of becoming FTs and coping with the independence (including borrowing) that went with FT status. Having licensed FTs, Monitor had to go on overseeing their financial and clinical performance and could suspend or withdraw licences. Monitor could also agree mergers of FTs and the takeover of other trusts by FTs.

The 2003 Act also created a new social care regulator, a Commission for Social Care Inspection (CSCI) which assumed the responsibilities of the DH Social Services Inspectorate for adult social care together with the inspection work of the National Care Standards Commission and the Audit Commission's social care value for money activities. During the passage of the legislation I was criticised – quite fairly – for reorganising health and social care inspectorates so quickly. Defending these decisions was not amongst my finest hours as a Minister and was only excelled when I proposed later the merger of the Healthcare Commission and CSCI as part of the review of Arm's Length Bodies in 2004/5 (described in Chapter 5). This was a period when Tony Blair and Gordon Brown competed with each other to reduce the number and cost of public sector regulators that Labour had largely created. Although we needed these regulators – and still do - to improve the NHS, the way we went about creating them was ill-considered and messy.

Alongside these new regulators the 28 new Strategic Health Authorities established in 2002 had been used for performance managing hospital trusts, largely focussed on delivery of national targets. This operated through the chief executive line – trust chief executive to SHA chief executive and onto the NHS chief executive. It led to a by-passing and disempowerment of many clinicians and trust boards, as already discussed. There was a strong incentive to escape from the clutches of SHAs and the DH by becoming FTs with a regulator who might be demanding but was fair, consistent and transparent and did not raid your financial surpluses. When I reorganised the NHS in 2005/6 to correct the mistakes of the 2002 reorganisation the SHAs were reduced to 10, with performance management of PCTs and non-FT hospital trusts as one of their functions.

How has all this worked? Monitor has been a robust and effective regulator of FTs and has not lowered the bar for becoming an FT. Some FTs have failed to maintain standards – clinical and financial - but usually remedial action has been taken promptly. The exceptions were Mid-Staffordshire and Basildon and Thurrock FTs which inexcusably slipped under the net; but these exceptions do not negate the achievements of Monitor. I considered that Monitor's systems for scrutinising FT financial performance were better than the DH system used to let Ministers know what was going on within the NHS. I tried to get the Monitor system introduced in DH but had not succeeded by the time I left. Monitor has defended robustly its independence and that of FTs despite occasional attempts by the top echelons of DH to challenge its independence.

I always saw Monitor as having a limited set of functions if, as was our policy, all trusts were to become FTs but I regarded it as the likely basis for conversion to a fully-fledged economic regulator embracing competition.

The Healthcare Commission was a considerable success also. During its time – April 2004 to March 2009 – NHS performance improved and public satisfaction with the NHS increased. The proportion of the NHS that met national standards and targets increased, with evidence to show this. The Commission carried out over 30 national reviews of services and when they followed these up they found that generally their recommendations had been acted upon. Its surveys of NHS organisations showed that the NHS found their reports to have been an important driver of improvement. The Commission expanded enormously the volume and quality of information about NHS performance; and its information has been seen as independent and credible by MPs, journalists, DH, patients, clinicians and the NHS generally. The Commission began the process of moving more of this information to an outcome basis by monitoring death rates, length of stay and re-admission rates. It initially struggled with the high volume of complaints it received for review but redesigned its processes and reduced the time it took to close complaints by nearly two-thirds. It had become respected and trusted both by the NHS and those outside when it closed its doors in April 2009. My only regret was that I could not achieve my merger with CSCI through the Healthcare Commission simply absorbing CSCI and retaining its existing Chair and Chief Executive who had made such a success of the Commission.

This is not to diminish CSCI's achievements in improving the quality and cost-effectiveness of regulating adult social care. CSCI had inherited a disparate system of local authority inspections with highly varied customs and practices and a rigid system of annual inspections that failed to target inspections where most needed. CSCI had done much to create an effective and modern inspection and regulatory system covering a wide range of social care services.

Both Commissions, unsurprisingly, disliked the idea of a further merger and a budget reduction and were slow to recognise that the political and public mood was turning against the continuing growth of public service regulation. The budgets of inspectorates and regulators were growing at an unsustainable rate, as were the demands they made on services in terms of inspection time and for information. CSCI and the Healthcare Commission disliked the pressure I exerted on them in 2004/5 for reduced budgets; and there was a degree of shroud-waving about the risks to elderly people if CSCI budgetary cuts reduced the frequency of care home inspections. I had to take my regulatory proposals to a Cabinet Committee chaired by John Prescott where I received short shrift from my

Ministerial colleagues for my attempts to secure some moderating of the proposed budget reductions for health and social care regulators who now had to cut their regulatory coat accordingly. The merger of CSCI and the Healthcare Commission was incorporated into a broader cross-government strategy to reduce the number of public sector inspectorates. In the 2005 Budget the Chancellor announced there would be a single health and social care regulator that would incorporate the work of the Mental Health Commission. The new body was to be established during 2008 subject to legislation: in practice it came into operation as the Care Quality Commission in April 2009.

Further regulatory reform and the 2006 consultation paper

In mid-2005 it was apparent that even with the creation of a single quality regulator we needed to examine some wider issues. What was the relationship between inspection/regulation and the performance management role of SHAs? If choice and competition were to advance in a more marketised NHS how were we to ensure fair competition and market entry? If there was a market how did government deal with service failure whilst safeguarding public access to essential NHS services? In a commissioning-led NHS, how could the competence of commissioners be guaranteed? And what should happen to unregulated services like GPs and primary care that accounted for 90% of the population's access to the NHS? Did we need a separate regulator for the growing number of FTs or should Monitor be merged with the Healthcare Commission? What were the distinctive roles of economic and quality regulation in healthcare and should they be separate or combined? As we battled with financial meltdown of the NHS it became apparent that we needed answers to these questions and to some extent still do.

By 2006 the Government was saying that it wanted to shift from top-down, target-driven performance management of the NHS to a more bottom-up self-improving system based on individual patient needs. The trouble was that it lacked the mechanisms to make this happen without unacceptable financial and other risks. Choice and competition were still weak; quality improvement was still in its infancy; NHS providers retained considerable monopoly power; patient access to information about service providers was still inadequate; and commissioning remained weak, especially in respect of powerful acute hospitals. National targets and standards were the only sure way of guaranteeing some consistency of performance across the NHS. We lacked other mechanisms that could guarantee the informing of the public (and Ministers) on what was going on in an NHS gobbling up an increasing share of national wealth. It was all very well saying we wanted to cut bureaucracy and reduce the cost and burden of regulation but how were we going to safeguard the public and its investment and discharge our Ministerial accountability responsibilities? A coherent system of performance management, inspection and regulation still required more work than simply merging existing regulators.

In Spring 2006 Patricia Hewitt chaired a meeting with me and another Health Minister, Jane Kennedy, together with officials and a few regulatory experts from outside the NHS. Its purpose was to work our way through the regulatory intellectual landscape. It was clear from this discussion that there was no simple regulatory model from other industries like rail, telecoms, the Royal Mail and water that could be applied to the NHS. However there were lessons to be learned from the regulatory experience of other industries which had previously been state-owned monopolies as well as ideas from economic theory. The NHS reforms themselves had produced incentives to improve quality, fairness, responsiveness and efficiency through choice, competition, commissioning and requirements placed on trust boards. It was important that we did not crowd these out by a fixation with nationally-determined standards and targets. We commissioned further research on the lessons from regulation of other industries and other healthcare systems; we published it in November 2006.[1]

When one looked at other state monopoly industries the underpinning assumption was that regulation should support competition. Quality and price regulation were both important but were handled differently in different industries: they were in the same body in, for example, post, telecoms and rail but separated in others like water where quality was thought to be especially sensitive. Regulators used a number of tools to drive efficiency. Several regulators had concurrent powers with the Office of Fair Trading (OFT) to ensure effective competition but with the sector regulator able to develop deeper industry knowledge. Government and regulators had also restructured industries to separate monopoly segments (e.g. gas pipes, electricity transmission, telecoms local loops) from competitive segments (e.g. gas and electricity supply, retail telecoms) so that there could be full de-regulation of the competitive segments.[2] Many of these lessons had considerable appeal to those of us who thought the NHS needed a healthy dose of competition but caused great anxiety amongst NHS stalwarts and those worried about how the Labour Party (and its trade union supporters) would respond.

The other healthcare systems we looked at were the US, Australia, Germany, the Netherlands, Norway and Singapore. Most countries adopted either direct public provision (e.g. Norway) or had created distinct commissioning/payer institutions, whether public (e.g. Germany) or private (e.g. Netherlands). A number of countries were seeking to create a contestable provider market (e.g. Australia, US, The Netherlands, Germany). Apart from

The Netherlands with its private payer/commissioners, none of the countries appeared to use an economic regulator, including the US which had a public-funded contestable market for Medicare and Medicaid. All countries had some mechanism for checking quality but only The Netherlands and Norway had quality regulators with a degree of independence. Patient choice of payer and provider, accreditation, licensing and professional regulation were all used to varying degrees; but in all countries primary care was self-regulated by professional associations. There was no equivalent of Monitor acting as a guardian of public assets when public providers acted in an autonomous way. Most countries used independent experts in setting payment tariffs (usually for hospitals) but with the national Health Ministry retaining ultimate control over tariff rates. Systems for regulating hospital failure were relatively scarce because in Western Europe hospitals are very rarely closed; and financial or quality distress were dealt with by each hospital or owner.[3]

Over the months following the initial Ministerial meeting our research, analysis and thinking enabled us to identify key functional elements for effective healthcare regulation in England, much coming from economic theory and experience. Monopoly providers – which abound in the NHS – do not have the same incentive to drive up quality or efficiency as a provider whose customers can choose to go elsewhere. NHS hospitals have effectively created a natural local monopoly because of their high fixed costs and the high barriers to NHS market entry. Vertical service integration between hospital and community services – which as a Minister I was reluctant to support – merely creates new local monopolies. Providers have more information about their services than commissioners and a lot more information than service users. In a tax-funded, free at the point of use, NHS patients have little incentive to choose the most efficient delivery of treatment and care. They will choose on the basis of quality and convenience – potentially driving up costs – despite the overall budget constraints of a cash limit. There is no direct connection to the ultimate payer for these services – the taxpayer.

Although competitive markets create incentives to improve quality they do not necessarily achieve equity of provision across geography or population groups – a critical requirement for UK health and social care. We had to disentangle the elements of functionality to be provided for in a future regulatory system for health and social care where competition and individual choice were supposed to play an important role and where much depended on effective commissioning. Our analysis showed that there were five key risks of market failure in the NHS: monopoly power; asymmetric information between provider and user/commissioner; unintended consequences of service decisions; lack of a price mechanism for service users; and equity needs. If a service like the NHS was to have some market disciplines that would improve quality and efficiency a clearer description of functions and who exercised them would need to be put in place.

It is worth summarising these features of an effective NHS regulatory system because they still remain to be put fully in place:

- Safety and quality assurance – covering national standards, registering providers as safe, monitoring providers against standards, investigating and dealing with failure.
- Promoting choice and competition – including assuring sufficient level of service and continuity, minimising barriers to entry and ensuring level playing field for providers.
- Commissioner assurance – performance managing and assessing commissioners and replacing them where necessary.
- Information availability – including performance information for commissioners and users that compares providers, using robust cost and performance data.
- Price-setting and allocations – fair and equitable allocation of funds to commissioners and defining and updating tariff prices consistent with overall budget constraints.
- Stewardship of public assets – safeguarding public assets and ensuring their effective and efficient use.
- Financial distress and failure regimes – including intervening on financial grounds, loans, overseeing insolvency and provider replacement and ensuring continuity of essential services.[4]

We recognised that there were important differences between the NHS and adult social care; the latter had a mature pluralist provider market but the NHS needed more choice and competition. In healthcare staff were highly qualified and largely employed in the NHS but in social care there were far more unqualified staff and most staff were employed outside the statutory sector. The NHS was far more complex than adult social care and was currently experiencing far more reform and investment. Perhaps most significantly of all was the means-testing of social care, with a third of users funding their care directly, so providing market discipline. Although the architecture for system management and regulation for health and social care needed to be adapted accordingly, there was no reason to abandon combining their regulation in a single regulator.

The more contentious issue, then and now, was the extent and organisation of economic regulation. My view was that the distinctive function of economic regulation meant we should separate it from quality regulation. To avoid a further expansion of regulators this would almost certainly mean converting Monitor into a fully-fledged economic regulator with the power to ensure competition and market entry to the NHS of new providers on a level playing field basis. At the end of 2006 there was little DH appetite for strengthening the role of Monitor and its robust and independent-minded Executive Chairman Bill Moyes. I was in a very small minority in favour of a strong, separate economic regulator and I was running out of Ministerial road as I knew privately that I would be resigning at the end of 2006.

On 27 November 2006 we published a 70-page consultation document – "The Future Regulation of Health and Adult Social Care in England" – which set out our analysis and conclusions. The proposed future regulatory structure gave the bulk of the regulatory power to the new integrated regulator. Safety and quality assurance regulation across the NHS, private healthcare providers and adult social care would go to what was to become the Care Quality Commission (CQC). For the NHS CQC would share promoting choice and competition, commissioner assurance and information/performance assessment with the SHAs: this turned out to be a serious mistake. Stewardship of public assets and financial distress and failure would be shared with SHAs (for non-FTs) and Monitor (for FTs) – again we were not bold enough. DH would remain responsible for price-setting and allocations which was unlikely to be sustainable in the future. The Office of Fair Trading would be responsible for competition in the private healthcare sector and adult social care (shared with local authorities). This document was put out for public consultation due to end in February 2007.[5] As it turned out a final set of proposals would not be promulgated before Gordon Brown took over as Prime Minister and a new Health Secretary, Alan Johnson, was in place by which time the Ministerial appetite for competition in the NHS had diminished considerably.

A changing approach to regulation

The response to the consultation document was not published by Alan Johnson until 24 October 2007.[6] This revealed that the responses to the consultation showed broad support for a single health and adult social care regulator but a lot of concern over a common registration system for all care providers. There was considerable NHS and professional concern about extending the new registration system to primary care, community services and public health/health promotion, so a separate consultation was launched on these aspects. There was no change to the proposed timetable for bringing the CQC into operation from April 2009 but full implementation of a new registration system was delayed to April 2010. The one significant change from the 2006 consultation that exerted a profound effect on the NHS was the decision to remove from the integrated regulator any responsibility for promoting choice and competition.

The argument then in the October 2007 document was that people supported SHAs and PCTs having responsibility for choice and competition but "there was less support for the Care Quality Commission having a national role".[7] In other words it would be left to NHS organisations to determine whether there should be any competition from outside the NHS in providing a competitive challenge to NHS providers. This was all of a piece with the post-Blair regime's lack of enthusiasm for competition in NHS service provision. Without an independent regulator to keep PCTs and SHAs honest on competition issues, they would conform to the prevailing Ministerial climate which had moved on from NHS reform and more competition to the more emollient Darzi Next Stage Review of the NHS. So the problem of NHS monopoly that we had identified and laboured over in our analytical work leading to the November 2006 regulatory consultation document was quietly abandoned by new Ministers anxious to avoid conflict with NHS unions and staff over competition. The Coalition Government has now decided that this is not good enough and has committed itself to converting Monitor into an economic regulator which is where we should have been in 2006/7. They should learn from Labour's mistakes and ensure that NHS service providers are subjected to a robust competition regime under the watchful eye of an independent regulator.

The Next Stage Review absorbed a lot of NHS time and effort during late 2007 and the first half of 2008. When Darzi's final report was produced in June 2009 with the upbeat title of 'High Quality Care for All' the emphasis was on quality and how it needed to be improved. It proposed a new NHS Constitution to secure the NHS for the future, provide public guarantees and improve accountability. Rights for patients and staff were to be the order of the day. Quality was to be at the heart of everything the NHS did with new 'quality accounts' to be published by NHS providers from April 2010 alongside their financial accounts. Change would not be driven from the centre but NHS staff would be supported to deliver high quality care.[8] The language of the report was about values, principles, empowerment, leadership, and partnership – all splendidly warm words that gave people an inner glow as the NHS celebrated its 60th birthday. Quite how change was to be secured remained something of a mystery to some of us, as did how failing organisations would be dealt with.

The robustness of Darzi's earlier review of London's NHS was lacking in the final Next Stage Review report, with little about the importance of regulation in driving change and improvement. 'Choice' was sprinkled liberally through the report but 'competition' was completely absent. The CQC received two modest mentions in over 80 pages: to provide assurance for the public that information about the quality of care was reliable; and it was to use its new enforcement powers to tackle healthcare acquired infections.[9] It was almost as though at the top of government the idea of using challenge mechanisms to improve the NHS had been removed from the political and managerial lexicons. Despite this 2008 atmosphere of an NHS love-in the issues of competition and proper failure regimes did not go away.

Underperformance and failure

A year into his premiership Gordon Brown and those around him realised that failing public services after years of hefty public investment was a political problem. In September 2008 the DH launched a low-key consultation document on a regime for unsustainable NHS providers. This acknowledged that a minority of organisations would under-perform and that these had to be tackled, particularly if they were not only 'challenged' but 'seriously under-performing' – subtle semantic distinctions probably only fully understood in DH offices.[10]

A new performance regime would go live in 2009/10, with an acknowledgement that a failing organisation might need to be replaced and that CQC could suspend or de-register a provider in its entirety on clinical quality grounds. 60 years after the birth of the NHS the DH finally acknowledged that "there is currently no clarity about the process by which the Secretary of State will use these powers (to transfer services or dissolve NHS Trusts) in relation to unsustainable providers". The document acknowledged that boards might not be able to turn round trusts because there were "clinically unviable service configurations" or there was "over capacity" in the area. To the credit of some officials, what had been staring many NHS observers in the face for some time - namely the existence of failing and unsustainable hospitals and the lack of process to deal with them - was now clearly articulated in a public document.[11]

However rather than placing responsibility for identifying these failing institutions on an independent body it was all to be kept in-house. It would be for SHAs to decide what to do about failing trusts and to make a recommendation on those identified as failing to the NHS Chief Executive to decide whether to advise the Secretary of State to designate a trust as unsustainable. If this happened then Ministers would have to lay a statutory instrument before Parliament and appoint a 'Trust Special Administrator' who would report to somebody called a 'Receiver-General' – who on closer inspection turned out to be the Health Secretary. There was then to be a long process of reports and consultation stretching over the best part of a year before the Health Secretary made a final decision on a trust's future. Winding up a failing trust would not be for the politically faint-hearted and new legislation would be required to both appoint Trust Special Administrators and to de-authorise FTs after applying the TSA regime to an FT.[12]

Before the failure regime document another one was produced in May 2008 called 'Framework for Managing Choice, Cooperation and Competition'.[13] This was supposed to help SHAs get the balance right in terms of choice, cooperation and competition or, as sceptics suggested, to ensure that SHAs did not behave in too red-blooded a way over competition. A new entity was to be established – with the contradictory title of a Cooperation and Competition Panel - under the Chairmanship of Lord Carter of Coles, a Labour peer. The new Panel was to go live at the end of January 2009. An introductory letter about the new Panel was sent to the NHS by the NHS Chief Executive which stated that the Panel would help what was called the 'rule-based approach' and would support SHAs and provide advice as to compliance with the overarching rules in individual cases.[14] The Panel was advisory to SHAs, the DH and, in relation to FTs, Monitor; and could not decide anything itself. It was another hurdle to be cleared before any drastic action could be taken with an individual NHS trust that was seriously failing. To complete these new failure, merger and takeover processes legislative changes were introduced in the 2009 Health Act to give legal force to the new regime of Trust Special Administrators for failing Trusts and to enable the de-authorisation of failing FTs.

When the new CQC came into operation in April 2009 and began the process of registering NHS independent hospital and social care organisations it found the regulatory landscape somewhat changed since I had proposed merging its two predecessor bodies 4 years previously. On the quality front there were new quality accounts; and a new NHS Constitution. SHAs were to have first shot at dealing with failing hospital trusts and separating the provider arms of PCTs. A Cooperation and Competition Panel would advise on any mergers of Trusts and PCT provider arms. There was a new lengthy and bureaucratic statutory process for handling unsustainable trusts; and for enabling Monitor to de-authorise FTs. Reconfiguration of hospital services between trusts were still subject to the same lengthy public consultation process, ending up in contested cases with the Independent Review Panel advising the Health Secretary. The NHS was blanketed in processes and obstacles before any significant action could be taken to replace failing or unsustainable trusts; and local populations with these failing services just had to put up with them until these processes had been worked through. When it came to reconfiguring unsatisfactory services or replacing failing and unsustainable hospital trusts all roads led to the Health Secretary. With an election in the offing rapid changes were not going to happen and the new, bureaucratic process web would thwart speedy introduction of any new providers to take over failing services.

To add insult to injury Brown's second Health Secretary, Andy Burnham, made a speech to the King's Fund in September 2009 announcing that in his view the NHS was to be regarded as the 'preferred provider' of services. This turned out to mean that underperforming NHS providers should be given two formal chances to put things right before they faced contract termination. It effectively drove a coach and horses through what Lord Darzi had assured me two months previously in a Parliamentary Answer was still the government's policy, namely that PCTs should commission services from whichever public, private or voluntary provider best met their population's health needs.[15] The Burnham doctrine of NHS preferred provider was questionable in terms of competition law and caused confusion among those SHAs and PCTs who were still pursuing what they thought was the government's provider policy.

The East of England SHA was looking to market-test the provider arms of their PCTs but before the Cooperation and Competition Panel could act on a reference to them the DH had told the SHA to withhold action so that new PCT procurement guidance could be issued. Following protracted negotiations over the meaning of the term 'preferred provider' a new guide to PCT procurement was issued at the end of March 2010 just before an election was called. Currently EU rules did not require clinical services like PCT provider arms to be formally tendered but did not prohibit market-testing either. The new guidance said that contracts must comply 'with the overarching principles of transparency, equality of treatment and non-discrimination, as well as an objective evaluation process for assessing expressions of interest'.[16] This seemed to suggest that the 'preferred provider' policy was dead in the water but it was hardly a ringing endorsement of competition either.

Where we are now

Early in 2010 the new Chair of CQC resigned and Steve Bundred took over as Chair of Monitor. The new Coalition Government announced that it would strengthen the role of the CQC so that it 'becomes an effective quality inspectorate' and would develop Monitor into an economic regulator that would oversee competition and price-setting in the NHS.[17] The separation of quality and economic regulation that I was hoping for in 2006 looks as though it will take place, alongside independent tariff-setting that some of us thought would eventually come (as in Germany) when Payment by Results was introduced. The activities of the Cooperation and Competition Panel will be folded into Monitor but it remains to be seen how much streamlining of dealing with failing trusts takes place. Establishing an independent NHS Commissioning Board should remove from DH the allocation of resources for commissioning to the local level and make that Board accountable to the Health Secretary for managing the overall commissioning revenue limit. The Board will hold local commissioners to account, commission some services themselves and be required to deliver improvements against certain health outcomes.[18]

The proposed reshaping of regulation, resource allocation and commissioning supervision will mean major changes in the NHS system of accountability, involving the abolition of SHAs and PCTs. There is also the prospect of the kind of fair competition and more open access to the NHS market by a wider range of providers that some of us were trying to achieve at the end of Tony Blair's premiership. Market-testing of PCT provider arms will be a test of the Coalition Government's resolve to introduce more competition into the NHS. Ministers are still likely to have the last word on some things but there is now the possibility of more sharing of power outside the traditional DH/SHA closed bureaucracies. It looks as though more power is to be placed in clinical hands and that local government will be allowed a bigger say on how the NHS is run, although they could be over-protective of underperforming local hospitals. It remains to be seen how much power Ministers will really give up, especially on some of the difficult decision-making on failing and unsustainable NHS services and providers. If expenditure gets out of control in this more decentralised NHS, then DH Ministers may find it difficult to resist taking over the controls. As I discuss further in Chapter 16 the challenge is still about real competition within the NHS and real political and clinical appetite for replacing failing services and organisations.

15

Assessing Labour's NHS stewardship

The NHS is Labour's creation. Now over 60 years old it is, with good reason, a popular national icon and part of the fabric of British society. The public popularity of the NHS has forced the Conservatives to revise their attitude to it. Before the 2010 Election they reassured the public that they would protect NHS frontline services in a difficult public expenditure climate, cut management costs and targets and devolve more power to clinicians and the local level. Since the Election the Coalition Government has promised a more radical set of changes in its "Liberating the NHS" White Paper that will both alter some Labour reforms and accelerate others. NHS resilience will be tested by these further changes and inevitable budgetary constraints, in part because Labour's reforms ran out of steam as Ministerial appetite for reform weakened substantially after 2007.

On the whole the NHS provides reasonable quality healthcare universally to the UK population at a price which is the envy of many other countries. Compared with the US healthcare system the NHS is superior both in terms of population coverage and what the population gets for the money spent. Despite the increased investment in the NHS under Labour, the UK still spends less of its national wealth on healthcare compared with many advanced countries but that is not necessarily a bad thing. The question remains – have the huge sums pumped into the NHS by Labour produced the major transformation that might have been expected? This chapter assesses the successes and failures of Labour's stewardship of the NHS in the 13 years it was in charge.

Investment, asset use and financial management

In 1997 Labour inherited an NHS in a parlous state in terms of funding, buildings, equipment and services. It looked like an NHS that had only 6% of GDP spent on it. People were understandably discontented with the long waiting times for access to services, the unnecessary deaths from killer diseases and the decrepit buildings and lack of modern equipment. The NHS was a 1940s service at the end of the 20th Century. More money needed to be invested so that more staff could be recruited and better buildings and equipment provided. But instead of starting this investment process soon after it was elected with a massive majority, Labour waited too long before doing so. Gordon Brown, with the self-image of an Iron Chancellor, kept to the Conservative spending plans for two years when

Conservative Ministers themselves like Ken Clarke acknowledged that they would not have done so.

It was to be 2000 before Labour produced a new plan for the NHS. This delay in increasing investment was the first mistake. The result of this delay was that the extra investment needed was then made too quickly. Giving a starving man foie-gras and champagne is probably not the wisest thing to do. The extra investment should have been made in a more measured way and through a more robust planning and financial management system. It took Health Ministers a long time to recognise fully how poor the NHS financial management systems were once the money had left Richmond House. Only with the 2005/6 financial meltdown described in Chapter 9 was this fully revealed. Much of the NHS simply lacked the financial expertise and control mechanisms to handle the scale of the extra resources provided between 2000 and 2010. It did not have the planning, performance management and financial control machinery and expertise to cope with six successive years of 7% real terms growth. In very simple terms Ministers and DH top management could not triangulate whether expenditure, levels of NHS activity and recruitment of personnel were consistent with each other; nor could they assess adequately whether the expenditure represented good value for money. Too much was paid for the delivery of improved access to services and shorter waits. Expansion of staff numbers was seen as almost an end in itself; and the generosity of new contracts for some personnel inflated staff costs further (as Chapter 6 illustrates).

There is little doubt in my mind, as earlier chapters demonstrate, that the NHS has failed to use well much of the extra money it has been provided with, despite delivering better performance overall. Both Conservative and Labour governments can reflect on periods of failure over NHS financing – one pursuing a policy of slow starvation and the other too rich a diet of financial excess. Neither has cracked a major problem which continues to bedevil much of the NHS – weak financial management and cost control and poor use of assets. Although matters have improved since the 2005/6 financial meltdown described in Chapter 9, NHS financial management and cost control is nothing like good enough for such a large £100billion a year business that the NHS is today. Continuing concerns about NHS financial management have been expressed by the NHS's own chief executive. Buried in the Operating Framework for 2010/11 issued by Sir David Nicholson is a passage on page 31 that states "there is a large number of PCTs and NHS trusts that have only ever met minimum acceptable standards....... This cannot continue, as it presents a risk to the sustainable financial health of these organisations as the NHS goes forward."[1]

PCTs are ultimately responsible for most of the spend in the NHS but none are rated 'excellent' for the management of resources and far too many are still rated 'fair' or 'weak' – as are many acute hospital trusts. Half acute hospital trusts are still not in a fit financial and business planning state to become FTs seven years after the legislation was passed. This state of affairs has been greatly contributed to by the weak financial control exercised over them by PCTs. Under Labour PCTs have been allowed to continue mismanaging demand to permit acute hospitals to 'over trade', especially in the areas of elective surgery and emergency admissions. CHKS (an independent health intelligence provider) recently revealed that between 2007/8 and 2008/9 only 15 PCTs (i.e. 10%) cut emergency admissions; and the rest of PCTs recorded an average increase in emergency admissions of 5% in a single year. During the same period elective admissions rose by 6% in a single year as trusts scrambled to meet the 18 week target.[2] Increases of this kind in acute hospital activity will bankrupt the NHS if they are allowed to continue. PCT commissioners as a whole have failed to cut significantly the tariff income of acute hospital trusts when they 'over-trade' by dropping the tariff price to marginal cost or less if they do more work than has been agreed with them for a particular financial year. Without changing reimbursement there is no financial incentive for hospitals to change behaviour. Only belatedly has the DH started to intervene by saying in the operating framework for 2010/11 that any emergency activity above 2008/9 will be paid only at 30% of the tariff price – even that level may be too generous a price.

If we want the NHS to improve and provide better value for money in a period of tight public expenditure, Ministers and the NHS will have to tackle with greater consistency than under Labour how resources are used and controlled locally. Without much greater cost-consciousness and better financial management systems it is difficult to be confident about the future of the NHS in its present form. The wasteful way extra resources have been used in some places in the past decade is an indictment of the financial expertise and management leadership in far too many local areas, alongside inadequate performance management by some SHAs.

This poor demand management and financial control by PCTs has been given a strange twist by the DH decision in 2008 to announce a new funding formula for PCTs that changed their target allocations from that used in my Ministerial time. Under the old system the distances from PCT targets in 2008/9 ranged from 3.7% under target to 13% over target; but under the new system that range changed to 6.2% below target to 23.4% over target. Yet the Health Secretary decided that all but one PCT should receive increased cash budgets for 2009/10 and 2010/11 irrespective of target allocations. As the King's Fund said there "appears to be little correlation between the percentage increases PCTs should expect under the new formula assessment of their needs and the increases in their allocations".[3] With the tough financial climate coming in 2011 the NHS has now been landed with a major source of confusion and disgruntlement over allocations alongside their local financial management problems. Labour's failure to take the NHS resource allocation system out of politics was a mistake that now needs to be rectified.

On the plus side, Labour can take great credit for the replacement of many unsatisfactory buildings, especially hospitals and primary care facilities and the huge increase in modern equipment, particularly diagnostic and imaging equipment. Nobody could deny that in 1997 the NHS required a massive injection of capital and much of this new investment has been put to good effect. There was nothing wrong in principle with the Private Finance Initiative to provide local areas with long-overdue modernised hospitals. Without PFI many communities would have been left waiting much longer than necessary for their new hospitals. LIFT and other schemes have provided better GP and community facilities and there have been a significant improvement in many GP premises even though some are still poor or far too small.

However despite these successes, too often the NHS has overdosed on the scale of particular hospital schemes built; and some trusts are now struggling to meet the long-term revenue consequences of their over-ambitious schemes with inflexible contracts. Some schemes have reflected the hospitals of the past more than the medicine of the future, with inflexible new buildings that assume a usage and presence on a site that is likely to prove unrealistic. History may well show that in the past decade the NHS has built too many expensive Taj Mahals when shorter-life more flexible, industrial buildings would have been more appropriate and better value. If I had not reduced the scale of the PFI programme (see Chapter 9) I suspect we would have had even more costly healthcare monuments. Labour Ministers cannot escape some responsibility for allowing some of the excesses of the PFI programme.

Many NHS staff managing these major new building projects learned on the job and rarely moved on to manage another one. People rarely challenged the UK's attachment to hospital wards and bays rather than more single rooms which would have assisted infection control. Although I managed in 2004 to establish a target of 50% single rooms in new buildings this was probably too low and came too late for many of the new NHS hospitals. Despite this major building programme the NHS still has not rid itself of mixed sex wards and the lack of privacy and dignity that this brings. The continued survival of mixed sex wards shows the obstinacy of the NHS at its worst and its ability to thwart Ministers committed to securing change that directly benefits patients.

In this major rebuilding programme some hospital trusts have made good use of their surplus land and buildings to finance new facilities.

University College Hospital in London is a good example where a whole hospital – the Middlesex Hospital – was sold to help finance new hospital development and has now been demolished. Across the NHS as a whole though there remains a major problem of underutilised and vacant buildings and surplus land. The NHS owns too much land, puts too small a building footprint on it and fails to use buildings and capital equipment as intensively as it could. In crude terms it doesn't sweat its assets very well. Although hospital trusts are supposed to declare surplus assets many continue not to do so. Some do not even know the extent of their spare assets. This has been a much neglected area by Ministers and top NHS management. The unsatisfactory management of many NHS fixed assets is a deep-seated problem and extends back well beyond Labour's NHS stewardship although Labour could have done more to tackle it. In about 50% of hospital trusts the assets are now in the control of independent FTs which makes it even more difficult now to ensure their efficient utilisation. As the NHS faces an increasingly challenging financial climate – especially around capital investment - this neglect of how fixed assets are used becomes more significant.

Labour has produced plenty of new and refurbished community facilities but many are not large enough to deliver new models of care outside a hospital. Yet it is a Labour Minister, Lord Darzi, who has produced the only major UK idea in a generation for a new model of care delivery – polyclinics providing integrated services for populations of 50,000 or more closer to home than district general hospitals. If the NHS is to rebalance its service delivery away from large acute hospitals to services closer to home it will require a new model of this kind and a major programme of rebuilding and adaptation to its existing property estate. Little work was done under Labour on a fundamentally different approach to the use of NHS fixed assets that is required and how local NHS estate personnel could be retrained to achieve the kind of major change of approach to capital development needed. In major cities like London where land is in short supply and expensive, it is often the NHS which has the biggest land bank, even if the local NHS does not realise it. More productive use of NHS fixed assets remains a serious challenge for the new Coalition Government, with the need to acquire more external expertise.

Targets and performance measurement

Labour Ministers relied heavily on centrally determined and driven targets to hold the NHS to account for the extra investment. These targets have been delivered through a system of 'command and control' down the NHS Chief Executive's management line. This has often disempowered local trust boards and many clinicians who often did not see themselves as part of the delivery mechanism or the 'owners' of the targets. These centrally-driven targets were not a complete solution for delivering improvements but they did secure improved NHS performance and significant benefits for patients. Targets have limitations but they are not the villains described by many NHS staff and Conservative and Lib Dem politicians. The much-maligned central targets made a significant contribution to improving patient access to services and speed of service delivery, as shown in Chapter 2. These improvements saved and lengthened thousands of lives, notably in the areas of the killer diseases – cancer, coronary heart disease and stroke. Targets have cut waiting times for services and improved access to GPs and to hospital Accident and Emergency services. They have also helped to improve performance on healthcare acquired infections as shown in Chapter 11. Although there is still much to be done, relentless focus on HCAIs through targets has made hospitals safer for patients despite some bad cases in particular hospitals. By the end of 2008/9 MRSA bloodstream infections were 62% below the base line that I had helped establish in 2003/4: this was better than the target of halving these infections by the end of 2008. Clostridium difficile infection rates were also reduced in that year by three times the targeted rate.

Targets alone have not produced all the NHS improvements made under Labour. However used appropriately and sparingly, centrally determined targets, with committed performance management and publicity for adverse performance, have shown that they can deliver real change. A 2009 study published by the Nuffield Trust shows that when targets are combined with 'naming and shaming' through public reporting of performance - as happens in England - they produce much better performance than where they are not – in Scotland, Wales and Northern Ireland. The report compares Scotland and North East England which have similar-sized populations, income, deprivation and health status. Scotland spent 6% more per head in 2006 than North East England but the latter delivered 18% more outpatient attendances, 40% more day cases and over 50% more in-patient admissions on much lower levels of staff per head. As one of the authors of this report said, these English policies "may have been deeply unpopular but they appear to have worked".[4]

Whatever the unpopularity of Labour's NHS targets the evidence suggests that they are an important item in the Ministerial and managerial toolboxes for producing improved performance across the NHS as a whole, which is important for national consistency and public satisfaction. What gets measured gets done, especially if failure to deliver is broadcast to a wider world. It would be perverse now, having shown that targets can be effective, to abandon them entirely as a policy tool for NHS improvement. Placing obligations through targets on local NHS management to show that taxpayers' money is being used to deliver measurable change for the public is important for securing both public support for a tax-funded NHS and greater geographical consistency in what is supposed to be a national service. Speed of access to healthcare is clinically relevant, especially with killer diseases like cancer. Delays can mean more deaths and disabling conditions, considerations often overlooked by the critics of targets. Totally abandoning targets that produce both patient benefits and convenience would in my view be politically irresponsible and deserving of electorate punishment.

If it makes elected politicians feel more comfortable and it appeases NHS staff to call targets something else – such as entitlements, guarantees, quality indicators, so be it. However let us not delude ourselves. The past decade under Labour has demonstrated that if we want a higher performing tax-funded NHS across the country as a whole we need a manageable number of key clinically-relevant targets, independently audited and published, as part of the armoury for demonstrating Parliamentary and public accountability. Without these national measures of performance we will not be able to identify which parts of the NHS are letting down patients; and the NHS will not be able to fulfil one of its founding principles - equality of access to equivalent services wherever you live.

Targets have been most effective where they have been applied to things that NHS providers have control over and which clearly benefit patients. They have been less effective in those areas where individual behaviour by the public has been the crucial ingredient of change, such as teenage pregnancies and sexually transmitted infections. But in all areas of NHS performance, service access is a major consideration for the public and a guarantor of equity, so a set of measurable service access guarantees will continue to be an important way of reassuring the public that they are being treated fairly under the NHS, compared with other areas.

What has been lacking with targets is a clearer linkage to the cost of delivering them. Throughout the NHS there is little relationship between performance measurement and budgetary control. This is because too few clinical services and decision makers know the cost of a unit of production – a day in a hospital bed, a specialist outpatient consultation, an A and E treatment, an ambulance collection, a GP consultation or out-of-hours visit or a pharmaceutical prescription. The result is that the service improvements delivered under Labour have been delivered largely irrespective of cost and certainly largely in staff ignorance of the unit costs of doing so. The result has been that too few managers or clinicians can easily assess whether there are more cost-effective ways of delivering improvements. At the core of these problems are commissioners, their financial and performance systems, their approaches and the way their performances are monitored.

Commissioning health and social care

Where Labour ended up with PCT commissioners is a muddle over the validity of PCTs allocations; continuing weakness in managing demand in the acute sector; an absence of linkages between performance measurement and costs; failure to use the tariff to both reinforce demand management and incentivise more cost effective treatment approaches; and an inability to commission sufficient effective community-based services. Without reform of these areas - and quickly – the NHS is guaranteed to have a surge of financial failures – both PCTs and acute trusts – that will undermine public confidence in the way the NHS manages its financial affairs. At the heart of these problems has been an inability to separate commissioning from provision and to develop a commissioning capability that safeguards the extra investment made.

Labour has emulated the Conservatives in failing both to deliver a proper purchaser/provider split and to create an adequate commissioning capability. Labour's first attempt at establishing commissioners in the 2002 organisation was a costly disaster. It was never going to be possible to produce over 300 competent PCT commissioning organisations. Although I managed to halve that number in 2005 we lacked the political will to face down union interests and reduce the number of commissioners much further - to one where it was more likely that we could find, group and develop the analytical capability and management talent to do the commissioning job properly. This political inability to impose an effective purchaser/ provider split also made it very difficult to apply the discipline of competition to the inefficient PCT community services.

More recently Labour put some effort into improving the know-how and competence of PCT commissioners but insufficient change has taken place to prepare the NHS for the harsher financial climate ahead. There are far too many PCT commissioners, many of whom are unable to control the expenditure of acute hospitals who continue to expand their activities and expenditure much as they wish. PCTs remain conflicted by hanging on to their community service provider arms and applying little rigour to performance managing them. For the most part PCTs have been nervous about dealing with failure in hospitals, GP services or community services and have avoided seeking public and political support for change. Many PCTs have thwarted the advance of GP commissioning. Too many SHAs have lacked the will to galvanise PCTs into change, preferring to play a waiting game to see which way the political wind blows.

Labour's unwillingness to resolve these various issues satisfactorily during a time of plenty means that the job of reshaping commissioning now needs to be done much more rapidly and more radically than was under consideration in my time as a Minister. This is particularly the case in London which has far too many underperforming PCT commissioners and community-based services. However simply replacing PCT commissioners without the know-how and the will to commission effectively with GP commissioners in the same situation will only make a bad situation worse. Some commissioning expertise has been developed under Labour in general practice, PCTs and SHA as well as the private sector. This now needs to be carefully harnessed and linked to private sector expertise and local government, as I discuss in the next chapter.

Labour cannot be criticised for financial neglect of community-based services. Between 1997/98 and 2008/9 the expenditure on GP medical services increased from about £4billion to £8billion in real terms. Indeed it had risen to nearly £8.5billion in 2005/6 until I began securing better value for money from the new GP contract, as described in Chapter 7. Similarly in community health services expenditure increased dramatically in real terms in the same period from about £2.8billion to over £7billion. If one adds in the increasing expenditure on community pharmaceutical and dental services nobody could accuse Labour of neglecting NHS service outside hospitals. What Labour can be criticised for is pumping extra money into community and primary care services without requiring a more rigorous performance management regime to be put in place that could clearly identify both the benefits produced by the extra money and the underperforming service providers. At least there is now financial and performance data that reveals the weak acute hospital performers but this is not the case with community-based services.

Work done in particular areas such as London and Yorkshire reveals that performance by PCT community services is highly variable and some are downright poor. If the weakest were brought up to the performance of the best there is scope for at least a 20% improvement in productivity. Yet there are still no systematic arrangements among PCTs for comparing performance across either community health or GP primary care services, apart from information on GP patient access and the patient satisfaction surveys for GPs that I introduced. Commissioners have developed virtually no systems for assessing the value for money of the services outside hospitals that they pay for. Following the Darzi Next Stage Review the DH has admitted finally that community health services lack robust data, tariffs or metrics.

There is little point in having a fully-fledged purchaser/provider split if the commissioners of services are not required to have in place an effective performance regime for services outside hospital that covers at least unit costs and levels of activity and that enables them to challenge and replace under-performing providers. It is the absence of such a regime that represents a major problem over using commissioners to drive efficiency and value for money in NHS community services. In mental health services for example we spend nearly £8billion a year - more than double the amount in real terms spent in 1997/98 – but we have virtually no performance metrics for either hospital or the community services. If we add this to expenditure on GP, community services and public health large sums of public money – approaching £25billion a year – are being spent on public services that commissioners, government and the public know little about in terms of the efficient use of resources or value for money. It is largely an article of faith that these non-acute hospital services are doing a "good job" – and we know some aren't. Neither Labour nor Conservative governments or DH and NHS management have tackled this performance measurement gap through effective commissioning. Monitoring the performance of these services presents a real challenge to the Coalition Government's ideas on GP commissioning consortia.

Many of the consumers of healthcare also need social care yet the integration of these services is still poorly developed and a continuing source of public complaint. Joint commissioning of health and social care advanced little under Labour, despite continuing rhetoric on the subject. In some localities the gulf between the free at the point of use NHS and the means-tested local authority adult social care services is likely to have widened under Labour because of the funding differential practised between the two services. Adult social care has been treated far less generously than the highly visible NHS, with social care budget increases over the last 3 years averaging little more than 1% a year, compared with increases of 5 or 6 times that being provided to PCTs for the NHS. As we live longer and have more people with degenerative diseases the pressure on adult social care is building up rapidly; but with less generous budget settlements local authorities consistently tighten their eligibility criteria for services. Over time this increases demands on the NHS. There has been little political encouragement of the well-funded NHS to reach across the boundary to further their own interests by helping their poorer neighbours. There have been a few local initiatives to integrate health and social care commissioning and service provision but little by way of widespread change.

Labour's Royal Commission on long-term care of the elderly reported in 1999 recommended moving to free social care for the elderly but a minority report cast considerable doubt on the affordability of this recommendation. The Government sided with the minority report and made few changes. After devolution however Scotland introduced in 2002 a version of free care for over 65s which has run into increasing financial difficulty, as foreseen by the Royal Commission minority report. In the 4 years between 2003/4 and 2007/8 costs doubled, with the numbers claiming increasing by 36% in that period. In England ten years after the Royal Commission report Labour cautiously produced a Green Paper on reforming adult social care that exposed the difficult political and policy issues involved in paying for this care as our population ages but the working population shrinks. To its credit this 2009 Green Paper, "Shaping the Future of Care Together" made clear that the extra money social care needed could not all come from the taxpayer and that in the future service users and their families would have to pay more, possibly using some new forms of insurance to help. Unfortunately Labour then rushed out a pre-Election 2010 White Paper promising a National Care Service, following Gordon Brown's ill-conceived and unaffordable Personal Care at Home Bill to provide free personal homecare.

This late Labour flurry of activity on social care may have been unsatisfactory but it was more ambitious than either Conservative or Liberal Democrat thinking. The political controversy it engendered did at least ensure that the issue of sustainable funding for adult social care and support was placed higher on the public and political agenda. The Coalition Government has now set up a 3-person Commission on Funding Care and Support – of which I am a member – to come up with ideas for a future funding settlement. Greater integration of health and social care commissioning and provision of services will continue to remain much needed but is likely to stay a second order issue until a way is found of increasing the overall funding base for adult social care. In summary, progress on NHS commissioning and joint commissioning with social care has been disappointing under Labour, given the extra money invested.

Competition and choice

The improvement that NHS commissioning needs should go hand-in-hand with re-energising the work started by Labour in 2003 on creating a more diverse NHS market of service providers. The NHS has never followed adult social care which has had a mixed economy of providers for more than two decades, strengthened by the Conservative's community care reforms of the early 1990s. Labour's progress on bringing in independent sector providers to the NHS faltered with the departure of Tony Blair as Labour sought to appease union interests. Much of the momentum built up in earlier years on bringing in new providers for elective surgery and diagnostics has been lost as private sector providers became disillusioned and disinclined to risk capital investment without clearer political support. Disbanding the DH's Commercial Directorate that drove much of the competition agenda between 2003 and 2007 was a mistake that reflected the political loss of appetite for keeping the independent sector enthused and interested in the NHS as a market.

The NHS default position of local public monopoly is well established in far too many areas and this inhibits its ability to deal with failing in-house providers or to expand patient choice. Theoretically the NHS has retained until recently a position of PCTs being able to choose the service providers most suitable for their population's needs, irrespective of whether they come from the public, private or voluntary sectors. The reality since the departure of Tony Blair has been that in most areas the NHS has been the preferred provider; and Andy Burnham made that position explicit in September 2009. The NHS badly needs a return to a more active competition policy of any willing service provider that began under Blair because it is these alternative providers who can act as a challenge mechanism to NHS monopolies, bring in innovation and provide wider choice to patients and commissioners. Matters looked more promising in 2004. Then John Reid gave his estimate of the level of private competition that the NHS needed that so upset the unions by proposing a level of private participation of up to 15%. Back then this relatively modest amount of competition looked capable of changing NHS behaviour but now any such ceiling may need to be higher if real patient choice is to be provided and if we are to remedy the inevitable failure of many existing NHS services as the financial screw tightens.

There continue to be real barriers of entry to the NHS market for new providers and significant difficulties for successful NHS providers taking over underperforming organisations. Even in community services where the costs of market entry are less it has proved difficult to achieve competition. Where the barriers to NHS entry are higher, in acute hospital services, the lack of political will to overcome them has made competition virtually impossible. This means that the NHS can far too easily stick to its monopoly default position, reinforced by the convoluted and costly tendering and contracting processes experienced by new service providers who attempt to enter the NHS market. The Burnham "NHS preferred provider" policy has made it very difficult to market-test inefficient PCT community services as they become separate provider arms within PCTs. Even when the policy was challenged by ACEVO and Care UK (see Chapter 14) and hastily rewritten, DH Ministers declined to give a clear message on the desirability of open competition. Instead, with SHA collusion, PCTs have been seeking mergers amongst themselves or vertical integration with acute hospital trusts. The NHS likes to keep things in the NHS family and will do so if Coalition Ministers let them, as Labour Ministers have done latterly.

Initially Labour made a much better fist of introducing more choice of hospital and GP services and deserves credit for this. However extending choice needs more competition and diversity of providers and the loss of competition momentum means that the choice initiatives begun under Blair have themselves lost momentum. Too many SHAs and PCTs have lacked the appetite and political support to bring in the new providers needed to extend choice and deal with the underperforming hospitals and community services. Failing NHS services are given too many chances to improve and the financial subsidies to survive, with the result that populations – often the poorest – do not receive the quality of services they should and taxpayers fail to obtain value for money. A politically-driven NHS preferred provider policy remains an open invitation to inadequate and costly service performance that does patients and taxpayers no favours. It is an overt encouragement to staff to under-perform, as the recent Nuffield Trust Study indicated.

The one area where Labour has continued to generate some competition is that of primary care, as indicated in Chapter 7. The new Alternative Provider Medical Services (APMS) contracts creatively introduced by some PCTs under Labour have enabled local contracts for GP services to be bid for by a wider range of service providers – public, private and voluntary. This has enabled new providers to gain entry to NHS, often in poorer areas where there was serious under-provision. By 2009 35% of the 173 GP practices holding APMS contracts were administered by private companies. This is hardly a major break through given that there are over 8000 practices but it represents some modest progress on competition. To his credit Alan Johnson launched a longer-term programme of 100-150 GP-led health centres in areas with the greatest shortage of GPs and some of these are likely to involve the private sector.

As Chapter 4 indicates there is a public appetite for exercising choice in healthcare if the necessary information is made available but all too often relevant information is not readily available so patients find it easier to go to the existing local service. Only with more readily available relevant information and a wider choice of service providers will more NHS users have the kind of choice that started to be envisaged under Labour. More choice and competition have considerable implications for the NHS's workforce and their unions and as a result some Labour Ministers have found these issues difficult to pursue, especially if they are union-sponsored.

Workforce and productivity

Most of the extra money Labour pumped into the NHS has gone on a rapidly expanding workforce. Undoubtedly some of this expansion was needed to improve performance and deliver more stretching service targets; but as with the extra money, this workforce expansion was too rapid. NHS staffing increased by about 300,000 people under Labour, or an average of some 2.5% a year. The rate of increase between 2002 and 2005 was even greater. Much of the increase was in higher paid groups of staff. This together with generous new contracts, use of agency staff and the inherent wage drift in the NHS has meant a rapidly rising pay bill. Understandably Labour has been proud of the huge increase in NHS staff and the better terms and conditions of service provided but this has been accompanied by a cost and poor productivity legacy that will now have to be dealt with as the period of growth ends.

The increased pay bill would not have caused problems if it had been matched by increased productivity. Quality of service has improved to some extent but on the only measure available to us – that of the Office of National Statistics – NHS productivity in Labour's period in office has declined significantly. As Chapter 6 shows healthcare inputs went up nearly 60% between 1997 and 2007 but outputs went down by about 4%. About two-thirds of these inputs were accounted for by the pay bill. In no year under Labour have outputs exceeded inputs. The recent Nuffield Trust Study could be said not to show that England's NHS staff have been super efficient but rather that they are less inefficient than their counterparts in other parts of the UK. With a staff sickness rate of nearly 11 days a year, the NHS is a day a year higher than the public sector average and 4 days a year higher than the private sector average. This is hardly a sign of a well-motivated, well-managed and productive workforce.

This does not mean that none of the NHS workforce is talented, committed or hardworking but it does mean that they may well be working in an inefficient environment, are sometimes poorly managed and are unable to give of their best. Whatever the underlying problems, the need to repair the public finances means that we cannot support over the next decade the kind of burgeoning NHS staff numbers and pay bill of the past 10 years. There has to be a significant improvement in productivity/efficiency if even the current staff numbers are to be maintained. Politicians keep promising to protect frontline staff but most of the staff appointed under Labour regards themselves as 'frontline.' If the NHS is to live within its means and become more efficient then frontline, as well as back office staff, have to improve their productivity.

What the Labour years suggest is that some aspects of the NHS pay bill that have been regarded as 'givens' will need to be examined more critically in a world of straitened public finances. The NHS has considerable pay drift which means that true wage costs are higher than headline annual increases. Employer pension contributions are much more generous than in equivalent private sector schemes. GP partners are small businessmen with NHS contracts, not NHS employees, but they still have one of the most generous public sector pension schemes. Pensions have been pushing up NHS costs faster than the rate of inflation.

In the past public sector pay has been settled by reference to private sector pay but if that pay is dropping or standing still to preserve jobs, the same logic could be said to apply to the public sector. Agency staff and fees have grown under Labour and need to be cut even more significantly than I was able to achieve. National pay bargaining inflates the NHS pay bill unnecessarily in regional labour markets where the cost of living is lower; and removes incentives from local employers to curb cost increases. These are all contentious issues for NHS staff, unions and Ministers, but as money becomes tighter moving away from inflationary pay bargaining systems should not be ignored, no matter how difficult changing them may seem. The NHS pay bill has to become better related to productivity and efficiency than it has been since 2000. My own Ministerial experience shows that it is possible – but unpopular – to drive harder bargains with NHS staff representatives than has often been the case in recent years. The best way to protect frontline jobs is improved productivity and more realistic pay bargaining systems. However the greater efficiency that the NHS requires may mean major changes to the way services are delivered, something that has not happened fast enough under Labour.

Changing service delivery

The acute hospital is a major NHS icon. These hospitals account for approaching 40% of the NHS revenue spend and most of its capital investment. Before 1997 many of these hospitals had fallen into serious disrepair and lacked important modern equipment. A major re-building and re-equipment of NHS hospitals has been undertaken by Labour using the Private Finance Initiative. This was much needed. However re-building and replacing many of these hospitals through PFI schemes means that the NHS will need to meet the bills for them for another quarter of a century. This has proved and will continue to prove a serious financial challenge for some acute trusts. The majority of NHS clinical staff work in hospitals and these institutions are prized by local communities. But as Chapter 11 demonstrates some of these hospitals have become expensive underperformers, sometimes with dangerous levels of HCAIs that damage and kill patients. Nearly 50% of acute hospitals are still not organised appropriately or managed sufficiently well to become FTs. Over 40 acute hospital trusts have historic debts and many of these do not generate income surpluses to pay them back – which effectively means that other parts of the NHS have to do so.

Labour's 2006 White Paper and the Darzi Next Stage Review suggested that more of the services the public needs could be provided outside hospitals - with their high overheads - and much closer to home. Too many NHS resources go into treating ill-health and not enough into preventing disease and health promotion. Yet PCTs have been allowed to go on spending money on costly but failing acute hospitals that cannot pay their way and whose quality is in decline. The regulators have shown the problem places but still the NHS Leviathan is reluctant to change direction. In part this is because there has been miniscule Ministerial or political appetite for tackling the problem of excess and underperforming capacity in acute hospitals and the waste of taxpayers' money that this involves. As Labour has been in government during this period of NHS plenty it must take responsibility for this political inaction.

The situation can only get worse and not just in the 80 or so acute trusts that have failed to become FTs but also in some of the weaker FTs whose future income may reduce. The NHS is now close to a tipping point on the future of some acute hospitals and the use that is made of their sites. The future public expenditure prospects facing the NHS mean that running the same number of acute hospitals with the same or similar configurations of services will be impossible to sustain. Bailing out loss-making hospitals can only be done when there is the money to do it. When the Coalition Government abolishes PCTs and SHAs it will fall to new commissioners and Ministers to tackle the entrenched problem of excessive and wrongly configured acute hospital capacity.

The weakest part of Labour's legacy is the failure to bring clearly before the public the importance of reconfiguring and reducing the work done in acute hospitals if the NHS is to be able to cope with the inevitability of an ageing and less fit population, medical advances and reduced public expenditure. It has been clear for some time that hospital departments treating too few patients to cover their costs were bound to compromise service quality. We have known for example that many maternity and paediatric units are in this position and need to merge. Some Accident and Emergency Departments need to stop pretending that they can really offer their populations anything more than an Urgent Care Service, with serious cases needing to go elsewhere. Some District General Hospitals will need to be downgraded to local hospitals or even community hospitals or polyclinics, possibly after merger with other trusts. Whatever the local political discomfort over these changes they cannot be put off for ever as many politicians across the political spectrum seem to envisage. The resources poured into acute hospitals have unbalanced the NHS, especially in the way the 17million people with long-term chronic conditions are treated and has reduced the investment and improvement needed in public health and health promotion.

Labour has invested very large sums of money in NHS services outside acute hospitals but it has done so without much in the way of a performance regime that tells us much about their outputs, benefits or efficiency. At least in the acute sector we can identify more clearly where things are going wrong even if the political will is lacking to take appropriate remedial action. This information deficit in community-based services and the scale of failing acute hospitals represents now a challenge for the regulatory system and the new Coalition Government. Both will need to be more courageous over underperforming and failing services than Labour has been and be willing to tackle the contentious issue of service reconfigurations.

Regulation, performance and failure

When Labour came to office in 1997 the NHS approached the Millennium desperately needing extra investment after years of Conservative neglect. Large sums of money were then tipped into an NHS system that was virtually free of any systemic regulation or performance regime – apart from the regulation of individual NHS professionals. The belief since the beginning of the NHS seems to have been that provided you audited the books, checked on the qualifications of health professionals and dealt with gross professional misconduct by individuals that was all the regulation the NHS needed. Because the private healthcare sector made profits this meant it required regulation to protect patients but NHS patients were not thought to require this regulatory protection. It was the Blair Government that rightly changed that perspective and moved to treat public and private healthcare provision on a more even-handed regulatory basis. It also injected NHS hospitals with a much heavier dose of performance measurement and monitoring.

Labour has established a performance management system for the acute hospital sector, including public comparisons, which is effectively naming and shaming. It has incentivised better performance with freedoms from central control for higher performers who could become Foundation Trusts. It brought in star ratings for hospitals that were published so that the public could see who were the poorly performing hospitals and could choose between them. A National Patient Safety Agency was established to collect and publish data on healthcare errors. Many in the NHS disliked the targets and the spotlight on poor – sometime dangerous – organisational performance. Pioneers like Sir Bruce Keogh even started comparing individual doctors' performance and showing how this can reduce death rates by improving medical practice. The Keogh worldview has grown amongst doctors in the past decade. Labour has encouraged measurement, performance review, inspection, regulation and public access to information about NHS performance. These are all major advances of great public benefit for which Labour deserves credit even if their introduction was sometimes piecemeal and uncoordinated.

Independent inspectorates were established to oversee star ratings and to examine NHS organisational practices and performance. I helped draft and introduce the first coherent set of national standards in 2004. We were in new territory for the NHS and the introduction of changes was sometimes clumsy. The Commission for Healthcare Improvement quickly gave way to the Healthcare Commission which in turn was merged with the adult social care Inspectorate (CSCI) into the new Care Quality Commission. I plead guilty as charged on this last merger. An independent regulator for Foundation Trusts, Monitor, was established in 2004. More recently the Labour Government, somewhat quixotically, established a Competition and Collaboration Panel – a contradiction in terms, particularly as the Brown government had little interest in pursuing NHS competition.

The NHS has moved in 10 years from little regulation to a crowded and sometimes confusing field. Alongside regulators we have had Strategic Health Authorities – soon to be abolished – and DH performance management of the NHS, albeit with little by way of metrics for community services. Surprisingly however there is no convincing system for overseeing the performance of commissioners who commit most of the NHS budget. Health professional regulation has expanded with a Council for Health Professional Excellence overseeing the individual professional regulatory bodies like the General Medical Council who have begun to tackle the complex issue of professional revalidation and to sharpen up their disciplinary procedures. Uncertainty still exists between the roles of commissioning, performance management, inspection and regulation (registration and licensing). Nowhere is this more apparent than over the replacement of failing service providers. There are still important regulatory shortcomings, especially the appropriate division between quality and economic regulation and Labour's failure to guarantee easier entry for new service providers to local NHS markets. Although the performance management record of SHAs has been mixed their abolition will leave a serious management gap at the regional level where governments since 1948 have found it useful to have a management presence.

Labour's ferment of NHS regulatory and performance activity has made good some of the deficiencies of the past but has not produced a stable regime or credible system for dealing with repeated poor performance and unsustainable and failing organisations. Looking at the past two decades it is difficult to see that DH/NHS top management and Ministers have been willing to commit to a robust and speedy system for replacing poorly performing and failing NHS providers, especially in the acute hospital sector. The system published in 2008 and enacted in the 2009 Health Act (see Chapter 14) is very cumbersome. It is difficult to see its lasting value, unless it is streamlined and supplemented by a more transparent system of competition and market-testing that deals with performance failure at an earlier stage.

Better performance data, more regulation and reduced financial growth rates will inevitably expose more NHS failure. Choice and competition make that failure more difficult to cover up - which is part of their purpose. Under Labour there has continued to be a lack of political will to ask the public to face up to the fact that NHS services can and do fail and an effective regime for dealing with that failure is necessary for an effective NHS to flourish. Weak commissioning, eliminating competition, reducing choice and unenforced regulation can all mask failure but they also waste a lot of what will be increasingly in short supply – taxpayers' money.

In the past decade the NHS has been protected from dealing effectively with poor performance and failure by Labour's massive injection of extra money. This has enabled poor performers to be bailed out so that Ministers could avoid many of the difficult and controversial decisions around failing and uneconomic hospital services. Local communities have been able to indulge their fantasies about what acute services they can have on tap locally. Services in the community have been put under too little pressure to improve their performance and value for money. The Blair government's pressures of competition and choice never achieved full maturity and were then subsequently relaxed by his successor. As the public money dries up the absence of strong commissioning, competition and an effective failure regime in the NHS – for hospitals and non-hospital services – will cause problems. Let us hope that the Treasury is now more alert to this issue through becoming the managers of the newest failing public services – banks. Now that "too big to fail" has joined the political lexicon it could be applied equally well to some of the large and over ambitious PFI schemes which lock the NHS into lengthy and expensive payback arrangements that in turn may well cause other service providers to fail. Ministers, DH and NHS management will need to show more innovation and creativity than has often been exhibited in the NHS.

Innovation, technology and research

The NHS has a mixed record on innovation and adopting new technology. However despite the implementation difficulties with the Connecting for Health programme the NHS has come a long way since 1997 on embracing IT. Labour deserves the credit for pushing on with change in this area, often against considerable political opposition. There have been major advances with digital imaging, electronic prescribing, Choose and Book systems and many other local IT programmes. A national spine through which information can be transferred by the English NHS is a major achievement, with high reliability. Patient records can now be transferred electronically when people change GP. The NHS has a secure email system where it had none 5 or 6 years ago.

The acute hospital trust sector has performed much less well in replacing its often antiquated patient administration systems while money was more plentiful. Main contractors and software suppliers have too often let down the NHS; but there have also been many weak contributions by the NHS through failing to put the management effort and resources into changing their antiquated systems. Too often medical leadership, inside and outside DH, has been lacking although clinical champions within the Connecting for Health programme itself have done a sterling job. What should have been - and may still be the NPfIT's jewel in its crown – a networked electronic patient record – is still too far away from completion. If patient safety, clinical quality and NHS efficiency are to be improved, completing NHS implementation of electronic patient records and a national network of modern patient administration systems is now critical to success in the NHS. The job would have been nearer completion by now if NHS and programme management had been more effective and a wider range of local systems and choice had been encouraged and implemented through main contractors. Abandoning support for completing this programme speedily would be a major political and managerial error that would leave a 21st century healthcare system without the ready access to clinical and operational data it needs to become more efficient and effective.

The NHS reputation for innovation in areas like telehealth, telecare, medical devices and new drugs is not a particularly good one within the industries selling into the healthcare market. Too often the UK is seen as a country that invents things, develops them for human use but then fails to adopt them extensively in NHS clinical practice. This is bad for patients and for UK plc in economic terms. A lot of effort has been made under Labour to improve matters, as earlier chapters have shown. The HITF exercise, the 2003 Genetics White Paper, closer working with the pharmaceutical industry and Lord Darzi's Next Stage Review changes on innovation all exemplify political commitment to working with industry to improve NHS innovation take up. But bringing research from the laboratory to the bedside still has a long way to go.

Labour has a good track record of backing expansion of publicly funded R and D in the medical and biosciences areas; and did try to improve the focus on translation of discoveries into cures. The difficulty so far has been that, in the jargon, innovation has not been operationalised into the NHS clinical and management cultures. Innovation is often still a fringe activity with lots of local champions and central initiatives that fail to go to scale. What the past decade has shown is the need to make the take-up of innovation more widespread and mainstream. This may require new approaches to the way funding streams, particularly capital, are used. We have not yet found a compelling way of incentivising innovation and take up of new technology across the NHS. Despite the efforts and improvements of the past decade it is still easier if you work in the NHS not to change or to change rather slowly. DH has not used the NHS annual operating framework to build a bridge for R and D work into the NHS's day-to-day operational work. This is an area that needs much more attention by the Coalition Government which may find what needs to be done difficult to reconcile with localism.

Balancing the scorecard

Overall the NHS has improved enormously over the past decade. After decades of underinvestment Labour was right to undertake a period of sustained investment; and in the absence of other measures it was reasonable to use centrally-driven targets to show national and local improvements flowing from the extra money. Independent evidence suggests the targets have produced improvements in access and waiting times and have helped reduce deaths from killer diseases. It is not too much to suggest that the NHS could not have survived many more years of the Conservatives' neglect. The middle classes would simply have gone private and the social contract underpinning the NHS would have been broken.

There is much for Labour to be proud of and even political opponents acknowledge the NHS improvements and advances that have been made. Public satisfaction with the NHS has improved significantly under Labour and stands at 75%-80% of people satisfied with it, depending precisely on which questions are asked. At the time of the 1997 election, the NHS was usually one of the public's top concerns in most opinion surveys but at the 2010 election it was down at fourth or fifth position – below the economy, unemployment, crime/law and order and immigration. The public usually sees the NHS as having improved more than education under Labour. However the NHS is consistently rated higher by those who use it than by those who rely on the media for their view of the NHS.

Labour can claim legitimately that its stewardship has improved the NHS, brought it much closer to the best performers in Europe and has pleased the public. However there is evidence to suggest that the public considers the NHS could be more efficient. The public does not like its high rates of healthcare acquired infections or NHS bureaucracy. There would have been something seriously wrong with both the NHS and the Labour Government if significant NHS improvements could not be achieved with the huge sums of taxpayer money injected since 1997. If you pose a different question - "Has the extra money been used well and prepared the NHS for a harsher public expenditure climate?" - objective observers might be far less satisfied than some of the public satisfaction surveys.

The NHS picture I see and have tried to describe is more mixed than either Labour or Conservative politicians claim. Alongside the many improvements and higher public satisfaction ratings there have been some serious mistakes. These include the 2002 reorganisation; the DH/NHS loss of financial control in 2005/6; a stop-start-stop approach to competition and choice; a failure to make commissioning effective and to separate it from service provision; an over large workforce with an excess of bureaucracy and poor productivity; and the lack of an effective failure regime for replacing seriously underperforming and unsustainable NHS providers.

The lack of policy and financial attention paid to adult social care compared to the NHS has been a misjudgement and unhelpful to the NHS as well. So has the inability to finish the job on Connecting for Health which Labour courageously started. Some of these mistakes were political in nature; while others were down to poor management in DH and the NHS. The rapid expansion in resources made available to the NHS exposed how badly equipped Ministers, the DH and the NHS were organisationally and managerially to cope with this extra taxpayer largesse.

Labour's reluctance to consistently confront vested staff and management interests over the need for more reform and rapid change has proved a political weakness. As a supporter I consider that the NHS could be so much better; more efficient, without any loss of quality; and more responsive to the country's health needs. The large extra sums of money have not been as well spent by the NHS as they could have been. If any government increases a public service's share of the national wealth from about 6% to nearly 9% in a decade then its performance should have improved much more than the NHS has achieved. For me this means that the NHS still has plenty of capacity to improve with the resources now at its disposal, providing the right policy, political and managerial decisions are made. Central to continuing improvement is strengthening financial management and control both within DH and across the NHS because unreliability in this area remains both part of Labour's legacy and a threat to the NHS's future.

The NHS is now completing its final year of very generous funding and has to adjust to more straitened circumstances. The NHS Chief Executive encouraged the NHS to build up a surplus of £1billion for the tough times ahead and told it in mid-2009 that from 2011 to 2014 the NHS would need to make efficiency gains of £15billion-£20billion over the 3 years. This would mean the NHS running on an annual basis at £20billion a year less in cash terms after 3 years and sustaining those savings and gains over time. The reality now is that the NHS has to do something it has never done – increase efficiency by about 4% a year – but also do this for 4 successive years.

In the parsimonious years of the Conservatives, when presented with savings requirements the NHS's traditional response was to ration service access by waiting lists. Many expect the old sheet music to be dusted off so these tunes can be played again to an anxious public and political cadre. Labour's investment legacy does make it possible for the NHS to rise to this financial challenge, providing we expect a lot more of the NHS than a Labour government often did. The time has come for the elected political class to ask more of the NHS for the extra taxpayer's money invested in it. Treating the NHS like some fragile child that has to be overprotected from the harsher public expenditure climate the UK now faces, demeans the NHS and the people who work in it. This national icon could and should do better. There are many clinicians, managers and staff who would like to be let off the leash to show what they can do. Political leadership needs to be more robust about what is expected of the NHS and more honest with the public about what needs to change. The NHS agenda needs to be reset, as discussed in the final chapter.

16

Feast to famine – resetting the NHS agenda

Why change is needed

This book has been written while the world is changing dramatically around the NHS. Under its feet the financial tectonic plates have shifted with increasing rapidity. The combined effect of a global recession and massive bank bailouts mean that the public debt has increased to unacceptable levels. Reducing this debt is a top political and economic priority and will mean a lengthy period of restraint in public expenditure. Some believe that the State has grown too big. If this is the prevailing public and political mood, this will impose its own longer-term constraints on NHS growth. Whatever transpires politically the NHS will not see again for a long time, if ever, a decade of annual real terms growth of 5-6%. Despite election-fuelled promises about protecting the NHS and the frontline, healthcare will have to share in the public services pain and the reduced state proportion of national wealth. The 2010 comprehensive spending review announced that the NHS would receive 0.4% real terms growth over the next years – 0.1% a year. This is the lowest 4 years increase for the NHS since the early 1950s. The Spending Review also allocated £1billion of NHS spending to social care which means that there will actually be a real-terms reduction in NHS funding over the next 4 years. The prospect of higher inflation and VAT and NI contributions can only make matters worse.

The NHS can hardly complain about this change of circumstances after its generous treatment for over a decade by Labour. It is better prepared than ever to identify the efficiencies that will now be required; and has only itself to blame for not preparing better for a period of more meagre rations. It is clear now that such a period will last for at least this Parliament and possibly longer. Yet the harsher financial climate will not stop demography providing an increasing number of older people requiring health and social care services; or scientific and medical advances producing new treatments; and rising public expectations over access to and quality of services. All these pressures – which all advanced healthcare systems will face – produce their own cost challenges. The NHS Chief Executive told the NHS in 2009 that it faced a funding gap of £15-20 billion in England by the end of 2013-14, so doctors and managers have had plenty of warning. This means that for the next 4 years the NHS has to make sustained efficiency improvements of 4%, as already indicated.

The history of the NHS does not encourage an optimistic view of it meeting this challenge. Although it has improved services with Labour's extra investment its productivity improvement has continued to be extremely modest relative to the scale of the extra investment. Many within the NHS have resisted reform, especially more competition; and the BMA and other unions continue to oppose more competition. Labour started reform too late and under Gordon Brown took its foot off the reform accelerator. As the financial screw is inevitably turned it is vital that we return to a serious programme of NHS reform, irrespective of who is in government. The Coalition Government has accepted this but Labour still seems reluctant to embrace radical NHS reform and remains in denial about NHS underperformance during its time in government. This reform now has to come quickly because of the urgency of delivering real terms cash savings. Making structural reforms to the NHS at the same time as delivering big efficiency gains will be extremely risky and difficult to achieve; but taking some risks is now inevitable because of the delay in tackling the NHS efficiency agenda.

Resetting the NHS agenda will not be easy politically, managerially or clinically. Further change will be unpopular with many staff and puzzling to the public, neither of whom has been well prepared for what lies ahead. Previous delays in reform areas like commissioning, competition and reconfiguring acute hospital services mean that the action to be taken now will have to be more radical and to take place faster. Some of the savings will have to come from the paybill and it is inevitable that organisational structures will have to change and become more streamlined. The Coalition Government's plans have plenty of risks, financial and otherwise, in terms of both their substance and the speed of implementation. However they are right to be considering radical change, particularly as it builds on the reforms started in Tony Blair's premiership.

There are many ways for the NHS to do things differently in order to achieve better value for money and to improve services to patients, so it should not be all gloom. However to bring about necessary change requires elected politicians to be much more honest with the public about the NHS's shortcomings as well as its strengths. They need help in this from clinicians, more of whom need to climb out of their comfort zones and show some leadership, especially over change in acute hospitals. Many more elected politicians and clinical leaders need to support continuing reform and improvement in the NHS rather than regarding it as somehow disloyal to a national treasure or politically inconvenient to expect much better from their local NHS services. MPs constituents' interest would be much better served by a more 'critical friend' approach to improving the performance of local NHS service providers and being less afraid to replace persistently failing or unsustainable services much more speedily.

Simply blaming bureaucracy, managers or targets for all NHS ills may be politically convenient but it is an inadequate response to a serious problem.

Equally we should not pretend that GPs are 'super-heroes' who with a dose of patient empowerment can put the NHS world to rights. Reducing bureaucracy, inappropriate targets and high overheads together with GP and patient empowerment are all worthwhile. But they need to be part of wider system reform that changes the prevailing default cultural stance of the NHS which is introspective and anti-competition. There also needs to be a willingness to realign the share of the available resources so that more goes to ill-health prevention, community services, long-term conditions and social care rather than to acute healthcare. A wider vision is required from many NHS decision-makers if the NHS is to retain public confidence and popularity in the difficult economic period that lies ahead.

There is no 'silver bullet' to put the NHS to rights. There is a range of systemic changes that offer the prospect that the UK could retain a tax-funded NHS with minimal co-payments and universal coverage whilst keeping the total health budget within a reasonable proportion of GDP. These changes would have to be more financially harder-edged than those in the Darzi Next Stage Review, however laudable its proposals were. If the NHS is not reformed in a more robust way financially and culturally then it is inevitable that the total cost will continue to rise faster than UK inflation and economic growth at a time when public expenditure is overstretched. This in turn means that the proportion of GDP spent on health services and long-term care will rise well past 10% of national income (as it has in the US, Germany and France). This would mean healthcare funding increasing either from taxation or co-payments (or both). Significant extra expenditure on the NHS would almost certainly mean cuts in other public services, as is happening now with the current relative protection of the NHS. Rapid rises in taxation to fund the NHS will damage economic growth and the prospects of a balanced economy – again as has happened and will continue to happen in the US. The alternative to taxation for funding rapidly rising healthcare expenditure would be to cap the public costs of the NHS at some level and use other rationing devices such as co-payments and longer waiting times – with expansion of private insurance to fill the funding gap.

Faced with these unattractive options more radical reform of the NHS should begin to look more appealing politically and to a reluctant NHS. In the hope that the collective mindset – political, managerial, clinical and public – is willing to contemplate more radical reform I am setting out some ideas for resetting the NHS agenda. These proposals are not intended to be a complete blueprint for change in the NHS. Instead they are intended to help construct a more coherent and robust financial and accountability framework for using the resources made available from taxation to run the NHS and reduce political interference. It is the absence of such a framework that still bedevils an NHS which continues to waste resources, deals inadequately with failure and poor performance and lacks the challenge mechanisms to drive change and productivity.

It is however an insufficient response for the challenges the NHS faces to simply hand over the purse strings to clinicians, replace access targets with outcome measures (likely to be longer term in impact) and somewhat randomly cut swathes of managers. These changes, together with more competition and choice, are required in some measure and within realistic timescales. However if they are pursued without a stronger operating architecture for the NHS they will fail and could well damage the NHS irretrievably. The NHS needs a radical overhaul of its operating framework and further organisational streamlining; but to retain the title of a 'National Health Service' it also has to retain a set of national requirements/entitlements that are met by local commissioners and providers. These requirements must be monitored and enforced on behalf of the public with published performance data and independent inspection and regulation. Simply devolving more decision-making to local clinicians and local authorities without adequate financial controls and accountability structures linking local and national levels will damage the national social contract that underpins the NHS and the risk-pooling it ensures for rich and poor alike.

The Coalition Government is showing a refreshing boldness of approach to NHS reform in contrast to the stuttering uncertainty of the Brown years in No. 10. Its flow of consultation documents on commissioning, choice and information are encouraging in their breadth of thinking and ambition and should not be glibly dismissed by professional and political opponents. However these proposals are incomplete in their thinking – unsurprisingly given their speed of production – and suggest an excessive optimism over the benefits of rapid devolution and the ability of GPs and the public to engineer beneficial and cost-control led change. For these changes to be implemented successfully, a more robust framework of governance, accountability and financial control than has so far been revealed needs to be put in place. The NHS will always need some central direction and control if it is to remain a tax-funded and national service. It would be naïve politically to believe otherwise. The more effective are the local challenge mechanisms of patient choice and service competition, the easier it is to devolve more autonomy. But these mechanisms are still relatively weak drivers of change. The financial control and performance framework surrounding the current Government's changes needs strengthening, together with some adaptation of those changes if some of the long-standing endemic weaknesses of the NHS are to be rectified and structural changes are not to lead to financial implosion. A more credible transition and implementation plan than has so far been revealed will be required also if the NHS is not to descend into financial and service chaos.

The legacy and its shortcomings

Let me start with a brief statement of the legacy the current Government inherits. To some extent these are statements of the obvious from earlier chapters but nevertheless they bear brief repetition.

Funding. The NHS has received a massive and necessary extra investment of resources and increased staff under Labour but has not used this extra money as well as it should have done. Its productivity improvement has been negligible or non-existent – depending on how you choose to measure it – across the hospital and community spectrum. By contrast social care has been funded far less well, given the demographic challenges it faces and will continue to face. Endless tightening of its eligibility criteria and the inadequate funding of social care can only increase NHS expenditure in the medium term.

Acute hospitals have consumed a disproportionate amount of the increased resources at the expense of public health and preventing ill-health and moving care closer to home. Some acute hospitals are serial underperformers with long-term deficits and bailouts from other parts of the NHS. They have little prospect of achieving sustainability with their current configuration of services and will continue to suck in resources inappropriately from other parts of the NHS. Scientific and technological advances make it necessary to concentrate more highly specialist health services in fewer hospital centres; but also to deliver more routine procedures closer to home with lower overheads. Political and clinical leadership has been lacking to drive the necessary reconfiguration of hospital services, especially in London and the big cities.

Targets have improved patient access to services under Labour which has been both clinically beneficial and good for public satisfaction with the NHS. Removing access targets is likely to increase waiting times across the NHS and is unlikely to benefit patients however much it pleases some NHS staff. Outcome measures are desirable but can be difficult to define and only show change over the long term: better output measures may be a more achievable objective in the near future but access targets should be retained.

Commissioning has not been separated from service provision which has produced conflicts of interest, much poor quality commissioning and an inability to replace unsatisfactory providers. Too many bodies have been involved in commissioning with too many small commissioners lacking adequate analytical capacity. PCTs have thwarted the greater involvement of GP commissioning. GP practices average less than 7,000 patients each and can only commission effectively in much larger consortia with proper incentives and adequate data and analytical capability. SHA performance management of commissioning has been poor in many places; and PCT capacity to manage demand has been weak in many areas. The PbR tariff has not been developed or used sufficiently to drive efficiency gains in both the hospital and community sectors.

Choice and competition remain weak drivers of change in an NHS with a strong preference for local monopoly and 'keeping it in the family.' The NHS prefers elected politicians to prop up its failures rather than replace them or encourage a diversity of providers under a sustained policy of 'any willing provider' from the public, private or voluntary/social enterprise sectors. Public monopolies no more serve the public interest than private monopolies; and an extension of regular market-testing is long overdue in the NHS as the basis for producing service improvement, as well as extending patient choice. Some FTs have not been as entrepreneurial as expected.

Information on NHS use and activity has improved considerably under Labour through targets, performance management measures and improved inspection and regulation. But there is still a very long way to go before public access to information is sufficiently good to drive choice and competition and improve patient self-care and challenge of professionals. NHS informatics and IT remain under-funded in a service where data is inadequately linked to finance; and too much data is hidden from public view or is only available in a difficult to use format. The failure to complete implementation of an electronic patient record has hampered improvement of clinical care, patients' control of their health data and research activity.

Management capability and professional skills in back office services remain a major weakness and impediment to a more efficient NHS. Overall the management cadre have not handled the extra investment provided that well, especially in relation to financial control. Financial management, human resources/organisational development, purchasing, IT services and facilities management are all areas of significant weakness in the NHS. The available management talent is spread over too many small organisations and with insufficient outsourcing to improve NHS expertise and reduce costs. The top general management cadre has insufficient clinician managers and a diminishing pool of talent for the needs of an expanded NHS. Without better ways of developing in-house management talent or importing more talent from outside, the NHS management capability could be a significant constraint on radical change and improvement in efficiency.

Research and innovation have been encouraged and promoted by Labour but all too often new discoveries and technological breakthroughs remain distant from day-to-day operations in a parallel research universe. The annual operating framework contains virtually nothing about using new technologies to improve performance; and has been little used to advance IT and informatics in an NHS slow to implement the full NPfIT or achieve the 4% of annual NHS expenditure on IT recommended over half a decade ago by Sir Derek Wanless.

The capital infrastructure of the NHS in terms of buildings and equipment has been improved enormously by Labour but in some cases unaffordably. The real estate footprint of the NHS is far too large for the buildings on it and the use made of them. There are virtually no consequences for using public assets badly in the NHS and few incentives to use them well. This is a major area of waste, ripe for fundamental change through external professional intervention and new financial rules. The NHS could sweat its assets far more and use surplus assets either to generate more income or produce the capital resources for new developments.

The NHS workforce has grown far too fast under Labour for the job it actually does and should either shrink or improve its productivity substantially. Redesign of services to use NHS labour more effectively is still in its infancy; and there is a reluctance to challenge established ways of delivering services – both clinically and administratively. National pay schemes and pay bargaining inhibit local initiatives on linking pay to productivity and local accountability for pay bills. Political mantras about how many doctors, nurses and other NHS staff have been employed tell the public little about how or whether the NHS has improved.

Recognising the reality of this inheritance across the political parties would be a good starting point for what needs to be put right, together with an acceptance that Labour started to make many desirable system improvements. However too many changes were piecemeal, too many had false starts – the excessive numbers of PCTs and SHAs, multiple reorganisations of inspection and regulation are examples – and too many were not driven hard enough – competition, choice, the PbR tariff and IT changes. The cross-party local political bidding to save failing and unsustainable acute hospital services is a long-standing problem and remains so, with the Coalition Government showing little appetite for tackling it. The consequences of this failure are an inadequate redistribution of resources and effort to community services, public health and social care.

The anti-managerialism of many elected politicians across the parties seems to blind the political class to the lack of professional skills and talent in many of the non-clinical services on which the NHS will always depend. A healthcare system cannot be run just by doctors and nurses. Restricting the pay for new managerial talent to a perverse interpretation of the Prime Minister's salary package – it could be said to be over £500,000 if in kind benefits are included - will only make matters worse, both in the NHS and across the public sector. Cheap political point-scoring on public sector senior manager pay could prove very expensive for taxpayers in the long run. The introspective, monopolistic culture of the NHS that rejects competition and learning from outside its boundaries is deep-seated and requires political challenge not political over-protectiveness and reinforcement of failure.

What needs to change?

Over the years the NHS has had a variety of changes imposed upon it by different governments. Many of these have concentrated on organisational change but often with inadequate functional analysis and too few of the accompanying process and systems changes required to ensure the new organisations perform better. The Coalition Government are in danger of repeating this experience. For most of its history the NHS and politicians have argued about whether it has enough money to do its job but with scant attention to whether it uses well the resources it does have. 'We need more money, more staff' has been the traditional mantra of those working in the NHS. Because the NHS has grown into such a self-absorbed organisation most of its staff are reluctant to look outside it for ways of doing things differently. For the most part it doesn't see itself as a business which needs to run its affairs efficiently and with a high level of professional expertise in the way it uses assets – buildings, equipment, people and cash. Many of the efficiency gains produced by the private sector and indeed some parts of the public sector have for the most part passed the NHS by. Importing skills, lessons and people from the outside world is not something that the NHS likes to do. Better to keep it in the family.

When attempts are made to bring about significant cultural change as happened under the Blair government, the Empire Strikes Back. Introducing choice, new providers and competition, improved regulation, paying for what you do through a tariff, targets, commercial purchasing, a purchaser/provider split all caused the NHS hackles to rise and resistance to set in. Bringing about NHS change becomes like a First World War battle, capturing a few yards at a time – often with casualties – and then along comes a new general who beats a retreat. As the Coalition Government tries to take the Blair reforms to their logical conclusion, history suggests they may have the same experience. The warning signs are already there from a bolshy BMA and other public sector unions. To make reforms stick the Coalition Government will have to be very determined and persistent and move quickly before another election comes along.

To avoid financial trouble for the reforms a new framework for the way resources are distributed, used and accounted for needs to be introduced, backed by legislation and within which the NHS is required to work. It is a framework that should provide the necessary glue to retain the 'N' in 'NHS' but with a lot of local and clinical freedom of operation within a more businesslike framework. The new edifice needs to be designed and described as a package, even if some of it takes longer to construct. Its purpose is to provide a stronger emphasis on the way assets and resources are used; strengthen substantially the challenge mechanisms within the NHS; let in more participation from outside; and reduce the role of elected politicians in the decision-making processes for dealing with service failure. Ministers should shift their role to overseeing the working of the machinery; setting priorities and modifying them as circumstances change; and deciding the broad patterns of expenditure and its distribution. Having shown the leadership to introduce new machinery and explain its purposes to the public, elected Ministers should try to abandon the habits of a lifetime and restrain their urges to keep taking over the plane's controls. Trying to capture those controls for party political advantage or personal advancement is generally bad for the nation's health.

In the hope that there is some interest in a less partisan and more technical/managerial approach to reshaping the NHS as we move into a more austere public expenditure era I have crafted an outline framework that I believe would improve many of the NHS shortcomings that I have identified and increase the prospects of success for a reform-minded government. Adoption of these changes should get the NHS past a biblical life expectancy of three score years and ten and retain the public's affection for it, despite some short term pain. This framework tries to improve the integration of the NHS with social care whose impact on the NHS has been so little recognised in the higher echelons of the Department of Health over the years. The NHS needs a lot less high flown rhetoric and much more effective management within a more robust financial and performance framework.

The new framework has 7 key elements:

(i) Controlling and allocating the Department of Health global sum

(ii) Strengthening financial and asset management

(iii) Improving commissioning functioning, organisation and accountability

(iv) Integrating standards, monitoring and enforcement

(v) Improving competition, choice, pricing and regulation

(vi) Increasing productivity and reshaping service delivery

(vii) Making better use of research and innovation

Controlling and allocating the DH global sum

As Labour left office the annual budget of the Department of Health was £116billion. This was larger than the combined budgets of the Ministry of Defence and the Department of Children, Families and Schools and was exceeded only by the Department of Work and Pensions. Of the DH budget, £100billion was NHS expenditure. By comparison expenditure on adult social care was about £13.5billion from a mix of central government grants and locally raised revenues. In Labour's last year the NHS budget grew by 7% and the adult social care budget flat-lined in real terms.

The Office of Budget Responsibility's projections for expenditure for these two service areas show health going up from 8% of GDP now to 10% in 2040; and long-term care rising from 1.2% of GDP to 1.9% in 2040. Combined they hit the 10% of GDP mark around 2020 and continue their relentless rise thereafter. As the population ages OBR project that by 2050, 20% of our GDP goes on health, long-term care and state pensions – virtually all of which are largely funded by the then shrinking working population from tax revenues. This situation poses problems for any government, especially the relentless rise of health and long-term care expenditure as a proportion of the national wealth. As the main users of health and long-term care services are older people there is an increasing burden for the shrinking working population. It means also that other public services get squeezed out unless taxes rise or more co-payments are introduced.

The good news is that the UK has not allowed health and long-term care expenditure to take such a large part of its GDP as countries like the US (well over 15%) or France and Germany (heading towards 15%). In all these countries insurance systems – social and private – have done a poor job of containing provider or transaction costs so we should beware siren voices trying to persuade us to move to an insurance-funded system. Nevertheless as a country we face some difficult questions. Do we want to accept a relentless rise in the proportion of our national wealth consumed by health and social care? Do we want to slow or cap it? Or do we wish to shift the balance between tax-funded and co-payments?

The political debate has focussed little on these questions. Instead more recently there has been much political bravado about 'protecting the NHS' or 'protecting the frontline.' As the size of the public sector shrinks back nearer to its norm of 40% of GDP the large proportion of that going to health and long-term care seems to me a matter for wider public debate. Rather than sliding, almost accidentally, into a situation where more and more of our national wealth and tax revenues are taken up by the NHS and long-term care I believe that the case is growing for the government of the day being required to announce to Parliament the percentage of GDP they are proposing to spend on the NHS (including staff pensions) and adult social care each year, possibly with their projections for three years ahead. This would enable the issue to be kept in the public eye and debated by those in work who will be picking up the increasing tab. Some might even think we should place a statutory cap on a tax-funded NHS to help impose more financial discipline in the way services are run.

Without going this far, identifying and ringfencing particular parts of the NHS/social care budget would help to impose greater financial discipline on those parts of the NHS's budget that have shown a propensity to grow at the expense of other services that might well be more in the wider public interest. As I have tried to show it has been acute hospitals that have consumed much of Labour's growth often at the expense of public health and social care. The Coalition Government have shown an appetite for ringfencing public health expenditure – an approach that we in Labour failed to pursue at the time of the 2006 White Paper on services outside hospitals. This political appetite for ringfencing public health could be extended to other areas.

I would like to see the DH Department Expenditure Limit (DEL) clearly subdivided between NHS, public health (with a broad definition) and adult social care, with an annual percentage rise identified (in cash and real terms) for each category. Within the NHS figure it would be for the Health Secretary to provide published guidelines to the new NHS Commissioning Board on the balance between say acute hospitals, mental health services and primary/community services. If situations occurred that made it necessary to amend those guidelines mid-year – for example a winter hospital crisis – then the Health Secretary should be free to do so, provided the decisions were made public and could be modified in a new financial year. To ensure that the relatively small and historically vulnerable public health/ill health prevention budgets were protected from raiding parties the ringfencing could be enshrined in statutory instruments so that a Health Secretary had to explain to Parliament why changes were being made.

An approach of this kind would require clear definitions of the categories, some road-testing and inevitably some boundary disputes. The civil service mandarins will no doubt argue that the definitions are difficult to formulate and will restrict Ministerial flexibility, exactly as they did in 2006. They would of course be right – especially about reducing flexibility – but that is the whole purpose of changes of this kind. They are intended to prevent acute hospitals gobbling up all the growth in the NHS and give new community-based models of care delivery like polyclinics a chance to develop. So there has to be some inflexibility if we wish important but more vulnerable and less glamorous services to develop and flourish.

If this sharper categorisation of the global sum made available to a Health Secretary is to be successful it needs to be closely integrated with two other components of the NHS financial system – resource allocation and the PbR tariff. Both are at present under the control of the Health Secretary and the tariff is still a work in progress that badly needs extension and completion. Both are vulnerable to the charge of political manipulation for party advantage. Both need to be made independent of the Health Secretary. The Coalition Government has said that the new NHS Commissioning Board will be responsible for allocating resources to commissioners and will manage the overall NHS commissioning revenue limit. This is an important advance. However it has decided that the Board and Monitor will share responsibility for settling NHS tariff prices. This seems to me to need further consideration because tariff-setting has to be not only independent of Ministers but consistent with the demand management and revenue control responsibilities of the Commissioning Board who ought to have the final say in this area.

What is needed now is a speedy independent review of the resource allocation system to ensure that it is in fact based on a realistic assessment of the resources likely to be available to commissioners over the next 3 – 5 years. This means eliminating the situation that exists now in which many PCT areas are either well over or well under their target allocation systems with no credible way of achieving the target allocation. This ensures that those commissioners below target allocations have a ready excuse to overspend. There is also an outstanding problem of some areas having large accumulated debts which it would be both unfair and unrealistic simply to pass on to new GP commissioning consortia, thereby setting them up to fail.

However it seems to me unlikely that the new Commissioning Board could easily construct a fair allocation system based on the burden of disease and disability for geographical areas as small as seems envisaged for some GP consortia, especially if there are to be some 400 of them. Many of the current PCT areas are already too small to measure easily both disease burden and the labour and other costs of coping with it. Doing this for even smaller areas is likely to be problematic. Whilst it is right to pass revenue resource allocation to the new Commissioning Board a lot more work seems required to create a workable and fair revenue allocation system. The Board is likely to need to operate a loans and banking system to enable it to move from the existing set of allocations, deficits and loans to a new and fair set of funding arrangements. This is particularly so if the Board is to operate without an intermediate tier like SHAs who have traditionally smoothed out local under and overspends to balance the NHS books overall.

The Coalition Government is right to want to accelerate the development of best-practice tariffs and to introduce an increasing number each year. This will mean moving rapidly from crude average pricing. But it will be critical to NHS financial health for many more of these tariffs to be based on delivering procedures outside hospitals at much lower prices and for more marginal cost payments (or lower) to be used by commissioners to control over-trading and uncooperative service providers. This tariff work is highly complex and technical and requires road-testing before the introduction of new tariffs. For some while it is likely that commissioners will have to use more broadly-based performance-related contracts while the tariff is developed and refined further by the new Board.

Although an economic regulator will have much to contribute on this work the responsibility for determining tariffs and amending them should rest ultimately and clearly with the NHS Commissioning Board. It needs to be able to develop a tariff payment and contracting system that enables it to be held responsible fairly for bringing home the NHS revenue budget on target, as well as driving improved productivity across the NHS. It is the failure to force more hospital providers into marginal cost reimbursement (or less) when they overtrade that has caused so much trouble for NHS revenue budgets in recent years. This issue will remain a major challenge for the new Commissioning Board rather than the new economic regulator.

What is being suggested here is that within about three years we have a new transparent system for sharing the annual division of DH spoils between the NHS, public health and adult social care and the proposed growth trajectories for each. Within that there should be provision for ringfencing, possibly reinforced in secondary legislation, those areas likely to be damaged by the NHS acute hospital juggernaut. Within the agreed global sum allocations it should be for the new NHS Commissioning

Board to oversee the construction and operation of a revised resource allocation system for commissioners that is based primarily on need - as defined by geographical disease and disability burden. Alongside this the Board would need a banking and loans system; and should have the lead responsibility for developing and operating a more refined tariff payment system for service providers based on clinical best-practice. This should have a strong element of marginal pricing to deter overtrading by acute hospitals and to drive NHS productivity improvement. While the tariff is being improved, performance-based contracting should be used. This approach would remove resource allocation and tariff-setting from political control and these responsibilities and provisions should be enshrined in statute on passage of the new Health and Social Care Bill to avoid political and bureaucratic backsliding.

Strengthening financial and asset management

These macro-level changes would in no way remove the need for a massive improvement in financial management and control systems at the local level and much better use and management of NHS fixed assets. First, the issue of financial management. There is an almost touching belief in many NHS and political circles that if you pump more money into the NHS then improved patient services will come out the other end. I have tried to show in this book that there is little evidence to demonstrate a clear correlation between particular amounts of money and particular levels of improvement. On productivity there is no reliable evidence of significant improvement for the extra workforce investment. There is evidence that targets produced much better service access but sometimes at disproportionate cost, particularly when achieving the last portion of the target.

The fundamental problem is that the NHS lacks credible local financial management systems that link in a meaningful way monies spent, workforce used and activity delivered. The result is that nearly all NHS organisations cannot show what has been achieved year by year in a standardised way for the money spent. Most NHS trusts and services do not have a detailed costing system that shows the service line costs in each of their service departments. Only in a relatively few FTs is there a functioning service line accounting system that enables trusts to know the costs of their services so they can begin the process of establishing which are paying their way and which are losing money. Outside hospitals, primary care and community services provide little financial information to show whether their activities represent value for money.

This absence of good financial management building blocks at the local level makes it extremely difficult to present a coherent picture nationally of what the NHS has delivered for the money invested, accounting period by accounting period. Instead Ministers are reduced to bragging about extra inputs provided – more doctors, more nurses, more equipment, new buildings – and targets achieved, most of which relate to acute hospitals and access to services. There continues to be no particular relationship between resource inputs and the targets or other outputs. For services outside hospitals it is almost impossible to describe with any precision, locally or nationally, what particular benefits the public has received in relation to the extra money spent on them. If the Coalition Government succeeds in replacing targets by outcome measures – which is by no means certain – it will still face the same problem of relating these outcomes to expenditure and showing that they have been achieved at a reasonable cost and represent value for public money.

It is the absence of a coherent set of standardised management accounts showing what has been produced at what cost, locally and nationally, for each accounting period that prevents effective NHS financial and performance management. This absence and the need to provide some accountability for spending a sizeable proportion of the nations' wealth each year has led to the current mish-mash of targets, elaborate national and regional performance management and inspection, together with a significant number of underperforming and failing organisations that no-one knows quite what to do with. Despite the so-called control systems that have been invented over the years, about 50% of our acute hospital trusts – with some big names amongst them – are unable to progress to FT status because they cannot demonstrate to the regulator their ability to plan and run their affairs autonomously. Alongside them are another 50% or so of PCT commissioners who are only 'fair' or 'weak' at handling their financial resources – many with large deficits – and who are largely unable to control the spending of their acute hospital trusts. This is not a reassuring inheritance for the new NHS Commissioning Board; and whether the new quality accounts will come to their aid is a moot point.

Yet need it be like this? Of course the NHS is a complex organisation with a diverse set of services. No-one wants to move to a situation where there are so many dials on the dashboard that they become conflicting and difficult to observe all at the same time. Nevertheless the Coalition Government, the NHS Commissioning Board and the new economic regulator would do well to consider, seriously and urgently, constructing a new financial management system for organisations providing NHS services so that costs are properly understood and expenditure is more directly linked to the income it produces and a clearer set of desired activities and outputs. If this can produce a move to quality and outcome measures so much the better; but the journey to that managerial nirvana is likely to be longer and to require reliable costing and output stepping stones along the way. A starting point would be to require all NHS service providers contractually to use an agreed service line accounting system that provides the necessary information on costs to commissioners and the public. This would enable the NHS to begin building a financial management system from the bottom up using IT, rather than doing what the DH and the NHS do so well – requiring huge volumes of central returns.

To make a change of this kind requires a clear understanding about what it is essential and practical to measure in terms of outputs, outcomes, quality and prices and in ways that are compatible with each other, using wherever possible common local data sets. To produce a technical specification that meets a range of needs and implement it will take some time and money; but the current range of unsatisfactory performance measurements are both expensive and morale-sapping for many in the NHS, without producing much by way of good results for managing services. The creation of a new infrastructure for managing the NHS and a period of austerity requiring the securing of greater value for money, makes it timely to undertake a fundamental review of the current systems for measuring cost and performance in the NHS. This should cover the tariff, annual financial accounts, quality accounts and the needs of inspectorates and regulators. Synthesising these needs into a simpler and more coherent financial management system is likely to take several years and changes would need to be introduced in stages. However a start could be made with the universal application of service line accounting within 2 years that was enforced contractually so that those who did not meet the Commissioning Board's requirements in an agreed timescale suffered financial penalties that reduced their income.

The Health Secretary should take the lead in creating a standing mechanism for undertaking this work with strong accounting representation from outside the NHS, a clear remit and key outputs and milestones, together with the involvement of the NAO. An interested Minister should oversee progress on this work to ensure momentum and to deal with the inevitable bureaucratic infighting and delaying tactics by the various enthusiasts for the status quo. I would like to see a Financial Management Standards Board established, possibly within the NHS Commissioning Board, with a clear remit and a lifespan of no more than 5 years and with a reporting line to the Health Secretary and with an expert Director with accounting and statistical skills from outside the NHS. As the work progresses it will be essential to ensure that it is applied across the NHS at the local level through the activities of the Commissioning Board and the regulators and enforced contractually through financial penalties for non-compliance and qualified accounts.

Whilst there is much to commend in the Coalition Government's consultation document on 'An Information Revolution' it will repeat the mistakes of the past if information is not related to expenditure as part of a holistic performance regime that is enforced by commissioners on service providers. Maintaining parallel universes between expenditure and clinical activities will continue to make it difficult to measure value for money and truly compare performance among different NHS providers and commissioners and different geographical locations. If a new financial management system is not enforced, with serious consequences for non compliance, it will be difficult to devolve more autonomy locally without the risk of both financial control problems and serious geographical variations in performance and value for money.

Alongside work to improve NHS financial management systems it is essential to tackle the longstanding NHS problem of poor management of fixed assets. The NHS has a history of underutilised and vacant buildings and surplus land. Its footprint overall is larger than it needs to deliver the services it does. Facilities management is too often poor and a low NHS priority. It is only likely to improve with an injection of expertise from outside the NHS, probably through outsourcing. The major PFI hospital programme the NHS is completing will bring its own challenges of using the new assets as profitably as possible in order to meet the high unitary payments. Delivering more care outside hospitals will require new facilities at a time when public capital is in short supply and there is a reluctance to commit to long-term PFI payments. Freeing up and using existing fixed assets more intensively will assume greater importance. But the NHS lacks the expertise, will or incentives to tackle these problems.

A bright light needs to be shone on the poorly used fixed assets tucked away in the NHS. This can only be done by some more formal but manageable system of disclosure, measurement and valuation. Unless organisations are required to disclose information about the utilisation of their fixed assets and to justify their holdings in relation to their service levels and forward business plans little will change. Without this kind of disclosure it is difficult to create an effective system of capital charging that incentivises good use and penalises poor use of fixed assets. If all hospitals become FTs under current legislation without any change of approach it will become even more difficult to place new obligations on them in relation to fixed assets. In practice the surplus buildings and land are unevenly distributed so some hospitals that become FTs become unfairly advantaged by the present system of transferring assets to them – the land-holdings of the Royal Brompton on the Fulham Road being a good example.

As described in Chapter 11 attempts were made in London to grapple with this issue. These revealed that in non-FT sites only some 18% of NHS-owned land was built upon and within that figure another 18% was underutilised. About 25% of the buildings were functionally unsuitable and there was about £1billion maintenance backlog which means more buildings falling into disrepair. Little has changed as a result of this exercise because there are no serious consequences for NHS and DH inaction. Only where the assets are required for a major redevelopment are trusts galvanised into action. Again with expensive diagnostic kit the assets are not used as intensively or efficiently as they could be because there are few if any consequences for not doing so.

For significant change to take place in the way fixed assets are used and managed across the NHS a centrally-orchestrated programme of change would be needed. This does not mean reverting to 'command and control.' It does mean a standardised system of operating across the NHS that discloses the scale, usage and maintenance of fixed assets in a straightforward way linked to the published annual accounts and their auditing. Placing this information on a standardised basis in the public arena would provide the basis for levying capital charges in a way that disincentivised poor usage. It would also be desirable to create some kind of pooling levy on disposal or development of assets to even out the randomness of asset distribution and to create an NHS capital pool from which people could borrow. It would be necessary for such a system to be applied to FTs in the future and possibly to consider some form of retrospective levy where major capital gains had been made in say the last 5 years. In addition consideration might be given to the Exchequer securing for the NHS a proportion of the profit when equity stakes in PFI schemes are sold on by the original lender.

It is a matter of choice as to whom the unpopular job should be given for devising such a system. It is difficult to see it operating well without the approval and support of the Health Secretary who is likely to need to give such a system some form of statutory underpinning if compliance is to be assured. HM Treasury will also have an interest, as will Monitor. It might well be best for the Health Secretary to establish an expert group to design a new system for better management of NHS fixed assets and how this should be implemented in a timetabled way and managed over the longer term. A good deal of external investment and estates management expertise would be required for this to be done successfully. However it will be the political will to make a lethargic NHS behave differently in this area that will be the most essential ingredient for change.

Improving commissioning functioning, organisation and accountability

The changes proposed above for financial and asset management would make easier the job of commissioning which is one of the great disappointments of Labour's reform programme. PCT commissioners have had the best part of a decade to show their mettle. Even allowing for the reorganisation of some 4/5 years ago (which only affected about 50% of PCTs in any case) PCT commissioners overall have simply not delivered – as the all-Party Health Select Committee so trenchantly declared just before the 2010 election. Some improvement has been made as a result of Mark Britnell's World Class Commissioning initiative but far too many PCTs lack the analytical capability and organisational muscle to effectively manage demand, drive productivity and replace underperforming providers, whether GPs or acute hospital services.

Labour's failure to secure a purchaser-provider split in 2005 is a partial excuse for inadequate commissioning; but even on provision of community services PCT performance has been less than remarkable. The plain truth is that we have far too many PCT commissioners and relatively few who can secure meaningful change in the pattern of service delivery within the resources available or effectively replace unsustainable, underperforming and downright failing providers. Inadequate performance management by too many SHAs has simply allowed this situation to continue. The PCT commissioning model has been given its chance but has failed to deliver the commissioning-led NHS we need. It is no surprise that the Coalition Government has lost patience and intends to abolish the PCTs. However whether they have yet found an alternative and effective commissioning solution seems to me more doubtful.

The Government's White Paper of July 2010 has some of the ingredients for a more effective NHS commissioning system. A greater involvement of clinicians in commissioning and more integration of health and social care in commissioning are important advances. It is right to replace a system of PCT commissioning that is not working after being given plenty of time to do so. Establishing an independent national board to select local commissioning organisations, oversee their performance and to determine resource allocation and payment tariffs usefully takes these matters out of the hands of Ministers. If delivered the improvements in access to information promised in 'An Information Revolution' will greatly help better commissioning. All these changes properly implemented are likely to produce improvements in NHS performance.

However there are some important missing ingredients from the Coalition Government's recipe for commissioning. What is to be the resource allocation system within which commissioning will operate? How will the competence of commissioners be ensured and failing ones replaced speedily? Will consortia have the will and capacity to challenge and control the spending of powerful acute hospitals? What will happen to services currently commissioned regionally and nationally that are likely to be unsuitable for GP consortia commissioning? Can one really run commissioning nationally without some form of intermediate tier between a national board and local commissioning bodies? (No government has managed to operate without some form of intermediate tier since the start of the NHS.) How will GP consortia be linked to the work of Health and Wellbeing Boards and social care commissioning? How will GP consortia be held to account for the expenditure of the large sums of public money entrusted to them? As incumbent service providers can a consortia of GPs really be trusted to foster competition from 'any willing provider'? Will the massive debts and deficits of some PCTs simply be handed to GP consortia to deal with? These are only some of the questions that need convincing answers before Parliament approves new legislation.

At present the Coalition's commissioning framework looks insufficiently robust to bear the financial weight that is to be loaded onto it and leaves too many of the current commissioning weaknesses unresolved. This could well lead to gross failures of demand management and financial meltdown in a fairly short order, with major consequences for patients and the reputations of GPs. Many PCTs failed as commissioners because they were both too small, too involved in provision of services and lacked the expertise to commission effectively. What should have happened in 2005 was the creation of fewer, larger PCTs – around 40-50 – for the whole of England – with greater analytical and financial capability, with a strong GP capacity for commissioning more local services through consortia and the hiving off of PCT provider services. This did not happen but the lessons from this Labour failure – and indeed from the Conservative GP fund-holding failed experiment – need to be learned for any new commissioning system to have a reasonable chance of success with the minimal risk of failure.

There is a strong case for pressing on with GP commissioning consortia providing there are sufficient willing participants, they are sufficiently large, they have clearly defined budgets and roles and they are required to demonstrate access to the financial analytical and IT capability to do the job they are taking on. Individual consortia should not be responsible for commissioning the regional and national specialised services. For these there needs to be a system at least as good as that defined by Sir David Carter's 2006 report. GP consortia need to be required by statute to promote competition and choice through accepting any willing provider when an incumbent is unsatisfactory. Their ability to do this has been called into question by the publicly expressed views of the BMA leadership, notably its Chairman and the Chairman of the GPs Committee. The Government has also seemed reluctant to use market-testing in the transfer of PCT provider arms. A robust statutory system for preventing GP conflicts of interest and collusive local behaviour between GPs and hospital services will need to be put in place – with appropriate sanctions for misbehaviour - if there is to be true competition within the NHS.

I support the idea of giving the NHS Commissioning Board the job of defining what GP consortia can and cannot do and that I think means effectively licensing consortia for particular geographical areas. The Board needs to be able to replace consortia when there is repeated failure of performance or adherence to Board guidelines and they should review these arrangements periodically – say every 3 years. It follows that the Board should be able to appoint alternative commissioning entities when there are no willing or suitable local GP participants using competitive processes to do this. This is essential if recalcitrant GPs are not to hold the NHS locally to ransom. For a period of time it would be wise to allow the Board to retain some effective PCT commissioners if suitable GP consortia are not available in some areas.

For GP consortia to work effectively they will require better analytical capability, financial management skills and IT than many existing PCTs have had. The probable scale for producing this capability cost effectively is likely to be much larger areas than that covered by many GP consortia or even many existing PCTs. This in my view means creating and licensing/accrediting an appropriate number of expert commissioning hubs to help service consortia. I see little point in creating such hubs unless they are capable of servicing populations of at least a million people and they can work for a number of GP consortia. The scale and complexity of London is likely to require some bespoke commissioning arrangements, particularly for its many highly specialised services and research capability, as well as to deal with the much-needed rationalisation of acute hospital services. The Coalition Government needs to give more thought to arrangements in London than has so far been revealed.

If GP consortia are to work successfully it will require the Commissioning Board to ensure that they have access to and use accredited commissioning support hubs which can come from the private sector, public sector (ex-PCT or SHA staff) or partnerships of the two. This to my mind is likely to require the Board to run an open competition against agreed specifications to secure a sufficient volume of accredited or licensed analytical hubs to meet the needs of GP consortia. Simply leaving a large number of different consortia to do the due diligence and quality assurance on these support capabilities is likely to be a costly mistake that dooms a lot of first-time consortia to failure. The new Commissioning Board is going to have little financial room for manoeuvre and can ill-afford too many financially failing commissioning consortia. It will therefore require a reporting and monitoring system for consortia to enable it to intervene early or where there are signs of financial distress. Such a system is likely to rely heavily on the quality of the consortia's support hubs which is why there is a need for an accreditation/licensing system after a proper competitive process.

No doubt some will see an approach of this kind as unduly bureaucratic and fussy but the Government must learn from the experience of PCTs, particularly as some £20billion needs to be taken out of the NHS cost base by 2014/15 and there are already big deficits in some areas that are likely to be inherited in some form by the newcomers. PCTs are required to be demand managers and to balance their books annually but too many failed both tests, particularly the smaller ones with big powerful acute hospitals in their territories. GP consortia could easily suffer the same fate particularly if they show undue favour towards inefficient existing local providers. On present plans there will not be 10 SHAs to practice financial black arts to bail out consortia by arm-twisting the financially strong to compensate the financially weak. The new NHS Commissioning Board will need an effective banking and loan system also to enable it to produce an annual balanced budget but it will also need to be a lot more effective than some SHAs have been at replacing failing commissioners. Most of the debate on NHS competition so far has related to service providers but the new model of GP consortia commissioning lends itself to more competition among commissioners if there is the political will to use competition in this area.

The Commissioning Board must be able to enforce demand management and financial control duties on all commissioning entities and to do this without political interference if they are to be truly accountable for £80billion of public money. The Board's ability to intervene and replace commissioners failing in their financial responsibilities should be incorporated in legislation to avoid doubt. That will mean that the service reconfigurations to secure balanced and sustainable budgets through more cost-effective service delivery can be enforced by the Board. Many PCTs and SHAs have failed to do this or been prevented politically from doing so. A major argument for commissioning through GP-led consortia is that they will be able to persuade the public to accept service reshaping and replacement. GP consortia may need to be helped in that task by knowing that the Commissioning Board has a legal power to require them to do so and can replace them. What is clear is that if GP consortia and the NHS Commissioning Board cannot act speedily to replace inappropriate and failing services this whole reorganisation will have been in vain. Where GP consortia, CQC and Monitor evidence points to service reconfiguration then the Commissioning Board must have the authority to act after timetabled public consultation and without a political veto. It is in the public interest to convey that authority unambiguously in primary legislation.

The Government's proposal for giving a right of appeal against reconfigurations to the Health and Wellbeing Boards (and then to Health

Secretary) well undermine the accountability of GP consortia and the Commissioning Board unless the Health and Wellbeing Boards are more integrated into the whole commissioning process than currently seems to be envisaged. At present these Boards have important joint planning and partnership functions but lack much in the way of budgetary responsibility. However it would be possible to view these Boards – which might well operate on a larger geographical area than GP consortia – as a form of intermediate tier between the NHS Commissioning Board and GP consortia. The Government sees them as operating at the upper tier of local government which would mean counties and large cities, with populations around at least 1 to 1.5 million people. They might well be a suitable scale for regional planning and specialised service commissioning and could provide a scope for improving strategic integration of health and social care commissioning, as well as providing some democratic involvement in commissioning. This scale of operation might well be a more appropriate population size for NHS resource allocation than many GP consortia.

Abolition of PCTs will require the Coalition Government to establish a new geographical basis for NHS resource allocation that effectively pools risk on the basis of disease and demographic health burden. Many PCT areas were not only too small for commissioning effectively but for resource allocation as well. Many GP consortia may well have the same shortcomings and will certainly be too small for commissioning more specialised services on a regional basis. Having some 40 or so Health and Wellbeing Boards co-terminus with upper tier local government could form a more satisfactory basis for resource allocation and for working with GP consortia than the Coalition Government has so far envisaged. They would also be about the right geographical size for accredited commissioning hubs to support effective GP consortia commissioning. Moves in these directions would require a change of heart by the Government and different accountability and governance arrangements but such a change of approach seems to me worth considering, providing new accountability arrangements can be designed that do not undermine those of GP consortia and the NHS Commissioning Board.

For the Commissioning Board to do its job properly it must be able to rely on the governance arrangements within which GP consortia operate and this still remains an area of uncertainty. Consortia should have a clear corporate identity with an accountable chief officer and board of directors operating within similar terms to company law (including the inability to trade insolvently). This would mean adherence to Commissioning Board guidelines on their practices, producing independently audited annual accounts in a timely fashion and publishing minimum performance data on what they have achieved in accordance with the Commissioning Board's requirements so that comparisons could be made with other consortia. With these arrangements in place it would be possible for the Commissioning Board to allocate budgets direct to consortia and have them accountable for those budgets direct to the Board. Providing the Health and Wellbeing Boards were properly constituted under statute and produced independently audited accounts they could become the commissioners of designated specialised services within allocations made by the Commissioning Board, as well as taking responsibility for securing public consultation on service reconfigurations but still with the final decision resting with the Commissioning Board. They could also be required to increase joint commissioning between health and social care and to advise on weak GP consortia. I would like to see further consideration being given to the allocation of functions and the inter-relationship between Health and Wellbeing Boards and GP consortia in order to strengthen the commissioning processes and reduce financial risks but under the overall direction of the new NHS Commissioning Board.

The technical organisational and governance issue discussed here need more work before the Coalition Government's commissioning changes are implemented if the mistakes of the past are not to be repeated. Simply moving the organisational furniture around or expecting groups of GPs to do financial heavy lifting beyond their capability will not improve NHS commissioning or create financial stability. But other changes are also needed.

Improving standards, monitoring and enforcement

A key part of commissioning is setting standards for service providers and enforcing them. For much of this system commissioners in the past have been dependent on others. For a decade or so Ministers and the NHS have wrestled with different arrangements for setting national standards and indicators/targets that give some national guarantees about what the public can expect from a the NHS, irrespective of where they live. It is clear from this experience that the public are not just interested in clinical standards and indicators but they value access/convenience and the way that they are treated just as highly as clinical excellence. So the setting of standards cannot simply be left to clinicians, although they should have a considerable say in them. It is fair to say also that without lay and political involvement the improvements in access to services and dignity of treatment would not have been delivered by clinicians left to their own devices. Nor would action on clinical failure such as healthcare acquired infections and medical and surgical errors. It has taken political and lay interventions in these areas to energise the NHS to tackle these problem areas more vigorously. 'Leaving it all to the doctors' does not necessarily work for the benefit of patients, even if one doesn't accept the view of George Bernard Shaw in The Devil's Disciple that 'all professions are conspiracies against the laity'.

Performance monitoring and management has relied heavily on central controls from DH and their SHA agents, especially through the use of national targets. More latterly independent inspectorates/regulators – the Healthcare Commission, Monitor and the Care Quality Commission – have played a bigger role in informing commissioners and the public about the performance of providers especially acute hospital trusts. This has exposed a growing divide between the best performers and the worst, together with the weaknesses of PCTs in taking remedial action with poor performers. With the exception of Monitor the other inspectorates/regulators and most SHAs have been better at exposing shortcomings than actually securing change and improvement.

The Coalition Government is keen to reduce bureaucracy and targets but they are in danger of removing a credible system of national standards by which the NHS can be held to account. In my view there are 3 primary components of standards that need to be retained:

- Best clinical practice standards and guidelines.
- Organisational standards and requirements.
- Patient entitlements in terms of service choice and access and the way patients are treated.

A system of national standards should not be so overwhelming that they leave little room for local discretion. It is however essential glue for a national service and making clear to the public what they can expect from the NHS, irrespective of where they live. These standards also place some obligations on staff throughout the NHS which need to be clearly understood and acted upon. Of course a fair degree of devolution is required in precisely how these standards are met; and areas need to be able to learn to meet standards with different approaches. But if there is no clear underpinning set of national standards that the public can expect and check they are receiving then the case for a universal tax-funded NHS, largely free at the point of use, starts to become less strong. We know that the public object strongly to postcode lotteries in the provision of services (especially life-saving treatments). Without a national set of standards we end up instead with a variety of local interpretations of what kind of NHS is satisfactory, all in the name of devolution and localism but with little clarity of public expectations and an inevitable diminution in equity of treatment. If we are to have an NHS Constitution – and the Coalition Government wishes to continue with Labour's innovation – then it makes no sense not to have some clear national requirements in the three areas described above.

Each of these three primary components need someone responsible for keeping them up-to-date, a robust and acceptable information underpinning and a monitoring and enforcement capability. One of the weakest parts of the NHS in my experience is the lack of serious consequences for persistent and gross failure. We have improved enormously our ability to establish where things are going wrong but not at acting effectively to put things right and stopping repetition of the same mistakes. My heart tends to sink when I watch a public sector spokesman saying on television that no individual was to blame, it was system failure, we have learned the lessons and it will never happen again. Usually at least three of those four statements are untrue, both within the NHS or elsewhere in the public service.

NICE has been identified as the architect of clinically-approved quality standards that the new NHS Commissioning Board would use in setting commissioning guidelines. This is a welcome clarity of responsibility. It is important that NICE retains a strong focus on cost-effectiveness, especially in relation to new drugs, so that the NHS retains some relationship between clinical standards and resource availability in a service that will always be cash limited. If the NICE system for approving new drug treatments is weakened and more lobbying of politicians by drug companies and patients replaces it, equity and value for money will suffer. In monitoring adherence to standards I would like to see more use of published standardised mortality rates for individual hospital services and departments and survival rates for particular conditions, especially cancers. More publicly-accessible data on the performance of individual clinicians within a stronger system of clinician peer review is desirable and could be linked to professional revalidation. The use of peer review to drive up clinical standards is less well established in the UK than in for example the USA; and needs a push from clinician-led commissioning.

The pricing mechanisms for reimbursing hospitals and pharmaceutical companies should be more closely linked to clinical benefit. The tariff for paying hospitals (or other services) needs to be expanded and to be more closely related to best clinical practice, as the Government seems to intend and as is discussed further below. The research-based pharmaceutical industry needs to be moved to a reimbursement system that is more based on value-pricing than the nearly 50 years-old PPRS. Weaning 'Big Pharma' away from 'me too' drugs and the search for the next blockbuster as we move to an era of personalised medicine is now overdue. However until an effective system of 'value pricing' is in place for pharmaceuticals it would be unwise and probably financially damaging to remove NICE's system of technology appraisals for evaluating the cost-effectiveness of new drugs. Whether value pricing can be developed as quickly as the Government intends, remains to be seen.

Not all the standards the public expects from the NHS and that it should be judged by are clinical. That is why a set of organisational standards are required as well which are independently audited and inspected against. This is where I detect a weakening of resolve on the part of the Coalition Government. These performance measures should be integrated wherever possible with the financial accounting system, as already discussed. This would make it easier for the public to see if they are getting value for money. We already have many organisational standards and targets that provide an indication of organisational performance. These need to be brought together, and probably reduced in number, to give an indication of organisational performance on an annual basis. They should cover areas like patient choice, cross-infection rates, patient satisfaction with food and cleanliness, survival and readmission rates, waiting times for appointments and operations/treatment, management costs as a percentage of turnover, proportion of professional staff who are locums or agency staff, extent of mixed wards and toilet/bathing facilities and numbers of complaints. Any competent NHS manager needs information of this kind to judge the responsiveness of their organisation to the public, so collecting this information and publishing it should not be seen as a bureaucratic chore but a feature of good and accountable public sector management.

If we are to have a registration and quality assurance system using the CQC, as the Coalition Government propose, it seems to me that this needs to be backed by an organisational requirements system that the CQC monitors and inspects against. Its role should not be confined simply to clinical standards, but overseeing a comprehensive annual assessment of providers that is published within 6 months of the end of the financial year and feeds into an annual assessment of the NHS as a whole. This assessment process should not be limited to acute hospitals but applied to different classes of providers. The measures in that process would need to be built up over time in conjunction with the NHS Commissioning Board and Monitor. It should be designed to give strong clues about underperforming organisations so that remedial action can be taken. The public would do well to look at any weakening of resolve by the Coalition Government on setting and monitoring organisational standards for NHS providers because any such weakening can only work against the interests of patients and taxpayers.

The third component of a standards system is patient entitlements. The Coalition Government's commitment to the NHS Constitution needs to be reinforced by more specific requirements in the areas of service access, choice, dignity and patient records. Possibly the most significant of these is access standards. However much some in the NHS dislike access targets, they have stopped the NHS reverting to its traditional posture of deciding when to deal with patients, often with adverse clinical consequences. Any significant diminution in access targets and their enforcement will damage patients clinically and will damage the NHS's reputation. Abolishing clear national standards on waiting times and access would be a massively retrograde step for patients. Access standards now need refining not weakening and should be enshrined in a cluster of measurable patient entitlements that embrace hospital, GP and community services. There is little point in having a new patient watchdog in the form of Healthwatch if they do not have some measurable items to look out for.

The Coalition Government have committed themselves to a wide range of choices that patients are going to be given in terms of their providers and services accessed. These need to be converted into measurable performance standards that patients can expect and providers can be measured against. There have to be some consequences for providers who repeatedly breach their obligations on choice – for example not showing consultants slots in the Choose and Book system - starting with financial penalties after due warning. Similarly in two other area of guarantees that are important to patients – dignity and access to patient records.

To put together a set of enforceable standards covering all three of the areas proposed is an ambitious project but key to improving commissioning and patient outcomes and satisfaction. They need to be integrated into annual assessments of provider used by commissioners and placed in the public arena. Advances in these areas are only likely if the NHS chooses or is required to use IT more effectively. We are still only in the foothills of providing the public with the information they need both to manage their own health and make meaningful choices about how, where and when they access services. Technology provides huge opportunities now to collate, synthesise and disseminate more widely meaningful data and information. The Government has set out an ambitious programme on information in the NHS and stated that the NHS Commissioning Board will be the prime authority for setting the standards on information and implementing them through the commissioning framework. This is the right approach but it will be a major challenge in terms of finishing the implementation of the National Programme for IT, especially the electronic patient record; ensuring that the needs of different information users are met; and securing take-up and exploitation of IT across the NHS.

Major issues of procurement and programme management will have to be tackled to deliver the ambitious 'information revolution' envisaged. This will require the Commissioning Board to be able to acquire the necessary technical capability to do the job and exert the necessary pressure through commissioning guidelines to ensure better compliance on IT innovation from NHS service providers than has been demonstrated so far. Increasing the proportion of NHS spend on informatics and IT will be necessary and this may require the kind of centralised purchasing and oversight that is less consistent with the prevailing mood of localism sweeping through public services. Local specification of information needs and technology requirements is undoubtedly necessary but so are national arrangements for architectural compatibility and securing value for money. Based on previous experience it is highly unlikely that undirected local procurement of IT goods and services will secure the best value for public money. The work of the Information Centre should be more strongly focussed on the commissioning needs of the new Board and local commissioners, the work of regulators and the needs of patient-decision making. Much of the progress on commissioning, choice and competition that is sought is likely to turn on the improvements in information, informatics and IT that the NHS Commissioning Board can secure. What is not in doubt is that major change in the NHS provider market is also badly needed.

Improving competition, choice, pricing and regulation

Labour started late and finished early on choice and competition. After accelerating in both areas between 2003 and 2007 the Brown Government then lost momentum. It retained a somewhat fictional policy of PCTs using 'any willing provider' to best meet the needs of their population, only for Andy Burnham to give the game away in 2009 and formally bury this policy by stating that the NHS was the 'preferred provider'. The failure to push on with the removal of the service provider arms from PCTs in 2005 only made it easier to limit choice and competition – as well as weaken commissioning. The loss of momentum on competition effectively meant that the range of choices for patient remained much more limited than it need have been. Many providers in the private, voluntary and social enterprise sectors lost heart and interest in NHS contracts. Securing those contracts often proved an expensive and ultimately frustrating exercise. Labour Ministers have allowed the NHS closed-shop mentality to flourish and for the default-setting of the NHS to be local monopoly and 'keeping it in the family'. They have been reinforced in their behaviour by the BMA and other NHS unions, not to mention a fair number of managers and clinicians in underperforming hospitals. Accelerating choice and competition will only accelerate judgement day in those trusts and the painful service reconfiguration decisions needed.

If private sector clinical regimes were utilised in the NHS then clinicians would need to work as productively in the NHS as they do in their private practice activity. This would be good news for patients and taxpayers but not for the revenue base of many NHS acute hospitals.

It is refreshing therefore to see the Coalition Government's commitment in their July 2010 White Paper to extending choice and competition which they have reinforced in their December 2010 response to consultations. The major expansion of patient choice and of any willing provider should drive competition significantly providing the NHS culture does not thwart it and Ministerial actions match their rhetoric. The proposals for extending choice in maternity services, diagnostics, long-term conditions, mental health and end of life care all ought to expand the range of providers offering NHS services. However for competition to become a reality it will be essential for commissioners to allow a more diverse range of providers into the game, for information about their offerings to be widely available to patients and for the Choose and Book system to be adapted significantly.

Aspiration to extend choice and competition will need to be backed by detailed processes, not least periodical market-testing of services so that new providers can enter local markets on equal terms with existing providers. The NHS has an impressive track record of preventing this happening, both locally and nationally. Without imposing some national and legally-based requirements that change local behaviour the NHS will see off another set of good Ministerial intentions, playing on public fears about losing local services and bogus arguments about the quality of non-NHS providers. Many if not most of the doctors offering services in private hospitals are the very same doctors treating NHS patients in NHS hospitals. Historically a misplaced sense of loyalty to the NHS family has thwarted competition from outside. Cosy restrictive practices have suited local providers and commissioners alike. Life was more comfortable without new kids on the block, whether or not they came from the NHS or the independent sector. People seem to forget that in most other countries the state does not provide all the hospital services.

The NHS has already conformed to type with the separation of the so-called Autonomous Provider Organisations (APOs) from PCTs. In many cases this has and is being done without any market-testing. Vertical integration of community services with local acute hospitals looks likely being the option of choice for 'keeping it in the family'. Twenty or so APOs have or are seeking to become NHS trusts as a preliminary to applying to Monitor to become Community Foundation Trusts. Fifteen or so braver spirits are seeking to become social enterprises. It is being left to PCTs locally how they decide to hive off their provider services before they themselves are abolished. The Coalition Government has done nothing to prevent this so non-NHS providers will not get much of a look in, whatever the rhetoric of new Ministers. The Office of Fair Trading

(OFT) will have no power to retrospectively review any completed mergers, although Monitor, as the new economic regulator, will have concurrent powers with OFT to carry out studies in the healthcare sector and refer concerns about restrictions on competition to the Competition Commission.

If the Coalition Government genuinely wants to secure the benefits of competition for NHS patients – lower costs, higher productivity and higher-quality innovative alternatives – they need to confront the reality of NHS behaviour and culture more head on than they have done so far. Closed-shop behaviour and restrictive practices should be seen for what they are – major disbenefits for patients and taxpayers alike. The reality of collusive behaviour between commissioners and providers must be tackled. New arrangements for commissioning through GP consortia will require much stronger safeguards against this behaviour than has existed in the past. The mechanisms for ensuring that 'any willing provider' can indeed compete to provide NHS services in different parts of the country will need to be formulated and enforced. The necessary mechanisms do not exist now and hitherto there has been virtually no cultural will for their enforcement even if they had been notionally in place. The conduct of the last Labour Health Secretary just before the 2010 election in preventing any market-testing of community health services in the East of England is eloquent testimony to the absence of political appetite for competition that has enabled the longstanding NHS culture to prevail. The Coalition Government will have to show that they have the appetite to move beyond the rhetoric of 'any willing provider' and put in place a commissioning and regulatory system that will make it more likely to become reality.

The lack of political, clinical and managerial support for competition within the NHS has had a highly damaging impact on commissioning, productivity, choice and price-setting. All these areas present problems alongside a regulatory system that does little to promote competition because it does not handle failure effectively. The NHS's almost obsessive unwillingness to confront and tackle provider failure – reinforced by the absence of political support for doing so –has bedevilled commissioning. At the heart of commissioning services there has to be a willingness and a system to replace service providers who consistently fail to deliver what is required at the price and within the timescales specified. This requires enforceable rules for doing so that also ensure the continuance of essential services. These rules must not be so convoluted, so biased and so time-consuming that they are never used. The new GP commissioning consortia are highly likely to favour incumbent providers and stick with them come what may unless new rules are introduced by the NHS Commissioning Board that break the NHS habits of a lifetime. This means that the nature of NHS standard contracts and the way they are let, monitored, reviewed and changed are key to introducing more competition. If incumbents are provided with loosely drafted contracts of lengthy duration and with no process for other providers to offer their services even when there is documented service failure, nothing much will change any time soon, especially in the acute hospital sector.

The NHS Commissioning Board will have to show that they mean business from the outset in establishing contracting challenge mechanisms to incumbency in the commissioning process for primary care, community services and acute hospital services. They cannot do everything at once but they should make clear early on that they intend there to be a thorough review of letting contracts to incumbents over a 5 year period and a willingness to intervene when poor practice is apparent. A start might be made initially by examining all new arrangements for community services since the date of the 2010 election that were not subjected to any market-testing; and a selected cluster of underperforming secondary care services where competition is thought likely to produce improvements for patients through a change of providers. Areas like maternity services, paediatrics, stroke, pathology and urgent care/out of hours services would probably head the list for such market-testing in a good few local areas around the NHS. Limiting the length of contracts and strengthening the independence of performance monitoring of compliance also needs attention. These are all areas where the legal framework within which commissioning operates requires attention. The Health and Social Care Bill presents an admirable opportunity to provide the NHS Commissioning Board with the necessary powers to enforce more competitive elements in the commissioning and contracting processes that are applied to NHS and non-NHS providers alike.

For the NHS to benefit more from competition more work needs to be done on the pricing and payment system in order to encourage greater productivity and avoid rewarding inefficient and costly provider behaviour. The PbR tariff system has both the potential to drive productivity and to incentivise more efficient and effective NHS provider behaviour. This potential is a long way from being exploited although the Coalition Government has recognised that potential. So far the over-emphasis in the tariff on the acute hospital sector and on average pricing for tariff items has proved both highly costly and a reinforcer of under-performing hospital services. At the heart of this problem is the absence of a more comprehensive tariff that incentivises use of cheaper effective clinical interventions and which would quickly enable commissioners to cut tariff rates to near marginal cost or lower when they see providers overtrading against agreed contract levels of activity. Speedier moves by the Commissioning Board to progress changes in these areas are highly desirable in the present state of the public finances. This area of tariff work needs to be taken out of the DH back rooms and given greater investment and prominence by the new Commissioning Board. If there are legal impediments to commissioners reducing tariff prices when required these need to be removed.

So far the argument has been made that NHS and non-NHS providers should compete on quality and not on price. Research suggests that there may be some case for this approach, especially when a degree of competition was just being introduced under Labour so that the NHS had some time to adapt its services to a new competitive environment. However two things have changed since then. The NHS has done a very effective job of preventing much competition; and the state of the public finances has deteriorated significantly. The absence of much competition means that the NHS can use restrictive practices to keep their average prices artificially high and not learn from new procedures that cut costs. It seems timely for this issue of no price competition to be revisited jointly by the NHS Commissioning Board and Monitor as the economic regulator, especially as the NHS badly needs mechanisms that can reliably drive productivity improvements of 3-4% a year over the longer term. If new providers can meet the licence and quality requirements for the NHS market and can offer reliable services below the NHS tariff price for a whole contract period it seems to me perverse to prevent them from doing so. It is also perverse to stop NHS providers offering services to more NHS patients within budget if they can do so by being reimbursed below tariff price.

Where this analysis leads is that NHS should begin a process for allowing providers to be able to compete on price as happens in most other fields of human endeavour where there is competition. With new commissioning and regulatory arrangements it would seem right to revisit the belief that competition within the NHS should be confined to quality and not price. Providing suitable standards are being met it should be possible for providers to compete on the basis of price and to offer new services at cheaper rates than existing providers as long as sustainability of supply can be guaranteed at the lower price. What is being suggested here is a major overhaul of the system of NHS pricing and provider competition in order to use the new commissioning system to drive up NHS productivity from its current lamentable levels, challenge provider incumbency through more competition from both NHS and non-NHS providers and increase patient choice of services through great diversity of providers of NHS services. The challenge of doing this is enormous given the deep-seated NHS cultural resistance to competition and political nervousness over confronting the NHS's closed-shop mentality. However public expenditure circumstances and a new Government's apparent willingness to challenge the way the NHS operates suggests the time might be right to have another go at injecting some price competition into the NHS.

To achieve change will require a level playing field to be created legally that enables effective competition to develop among a range of providers from within and outside the NHS. In doing this it is important to remember that the existing restrictive practices prevent efficient NHS providers moving to replace existing inefficient NHS providers. These changes are proposed not simply as a device to enable providers from outside the NHS to take over provision of more NHS services – the alleged privatisation of the NHS. It will mean that there is a regulatory set of rules and processes that are not controlled by DH Ministers or their civil service proxies. These rules and processes will need to be overseen by an NHS Commissioning Board whose commissioning and contractual guidelines are independently determined; a Care Quality Commission whose quality assurance and registration processes can be relied upon as independent and enforceable; and an economic regulator, Monitor, who will be entitled to examine and challenge restrictive practices and processes within the NHS and to use the licensing system to develop a speedier and effective way of dealing with underperformance, failure and unsustainability by using fines and licence suspension or revocation. None of this will be easy or quick.

When confronted with another public sector Leviathan that was a bastion of anti-competitive practices – British Telecoms – it has taken successive governments two decades to get to a point where the designated regulator felt able to reduce his regulatory powers. The OFTEL and OFCOM journey with British Telecoms has not been an easy or smooth one, with a number of setbacks and regroupings by the regulator. In telecommunications technological change through mobile phones and other means have fostered competition; and healthcare offers a similar technological prospect if competition is facilitated and institutionalised. Where this points to is a strong independent economic regulator backed by legislation being able to require NHS commissioners and service providers to change their practices. If Monitor, as an economic regulator for healthcare, is to drive change over time it will require the authority to secure information and change on a similar scale for that provided to OFCOM. Monitor will need to use its new regulatory powers to carry out market studies within the healthcare sector and refer concerns about restrictions on competition in both the hospital and community sectors to the Competition Commission.

The three legal pre-requisites for securing greater NHS competition seem to me to be:

- To establish Monitor as an independent economic regulator quickly with a clear duty to promote competition of service provision in the NHS and a range of powers similar to OFCOM.

336

- To empower the regulator to conduct an early review of NHS barriers to entry for service providers and to propose legal steps for their removal including identifying the circumstances in which market-testing was appropriate.
- To enable the regulator to propose a legal framework in secondary legislation for the speedy replacement of failing and unsustainable NHS services whilst protecting the public interest in terms of continuation of essential services.

This latter provision could be modelled on a shortened version of the convoluted existing arrangements by a new guide covering hospital, community and primary care services. The regulator should be able to appoint NHS trustee administrators to transition failing services into new arrangements that best met the public interest and safeguarded public assets but within a timescale set by the regulator. Alongside this the NHS Commissioning Board will need to keep after local commissioners to use competition to drive change and efficiency.

With changes of this kind there would be some greater prospect of the advantages of the competition being introduced into a competition-averse NHS, patients benefiting from much more service choice and the efficiency of the NHS increasing. It would take time to bring about and would involve a massive cultural shift by the NHS. However without a major cattle prod of this kind it will be extremely difficult to move the NHS along the paths of productivity improvement and service reshaping that are so badly needed.

Increasing productivity and reshaping service delivery

As already discussed in Chapter 6 the NHS's productivity improvement has been poor relative to the huge amount of money Labour has invested in it. Any business enterprise with such a performance would have had the shareholders clamouring for the replacement of the Board of Directors and takeover rumours would have been circulating. Yet the NHS sails on undisturbed and seems to bewitch elected politicians into believing that it needs special protection from harsh economic winds. This is a misguided world view. Healthcare is a consumption good much like any other such good. A nation consumes as much of it as it can afford. If the productivity and efficiency of the sector declines the nation suffers the consequences – it gets less of it for its money. As the efficiency screws are turned on the NHS's competitors for taxpayers' money so eventually more people will start to question the performance of the NHS – as some less timid souls are now starting to do.

A reshaped NHS needs as part of its architectural framework, better arrangements for driving productivity and reshaping services.

Implementation of many of the ideas in this chapter would themselves improve significantly the efficiency and productivity of the NHS and there is no need to go over this ground again. What is critical however is that for each operational year a clear statement should be made of the productivity improvement the NHS is expected to deliver and this should be clearly expressed in the annual tariff. The obvious candidate for determining this productivity figure in the light of the allocation to be provided to it is the new NHS Commissioning Board, after consultation with the Health Secretary and the economic regulator. I would suggest that the obligation to oversee and drive productivity ought to be part of the statutory functions of the Commissioning Board. However for any productivity target to have any true meaning and implementability it needs to be related to the whole area of NHS pay and pensions. The NHS is a labour-intensive industry; and most of Labour's extra money went on more staff but with a poor return in terms of productivity. The extra largesse did not even produce a happier workforce, only resentment when the flow of money slowed or reform was required. Perhaps a different approach should be tried.

National pay bargaining has been at the heart of the NHS since its inception and is not something the trades unions (including the BMA) will relinquish easily. The jobs of their central negotiators are at stake, apart from anything else. However it is already very clear that there are many local and regional labour markets in England and this is reflected in the market forces factor in the resource allocation system. Those different labour markets have very variable costs of living because the housing and transport costs in particular areas can vary considerably, as can the rate for the job for particular skills. The average cost of a house in London is twice the national average cost for example. Wage grade drift in the NHS is considerable as employers grapple with the consequences of national pay bargaining. Whilst there remains a strong case for retaining a national pension scheme with a common, tiered percentage employee contribution structure based on level of earnings, the system for settling pay, grading and conditions of service ought to move to one with much more local flexibility. If we are to ask NHS local employers to drive improved productivity it makes no sense whatsoever to impose unreasonable constraints on what they pay their staff – from cleaners to senior doctors and managers. This makes even less sense with greater localism and autonomy, more mutual organisations and a hospital sector full of autonomous organisations. These are all ingredients of the Coalition Government's vision for the NHS and any future Labour Government will find it difficult to put these particulars genies back in their bottles.

A major problem that the NHS faces is the rigidity of many staff contracts about their place of work. This makes it difficult to move staff away from a hospital base and hampers joint posts with local authorities. The national pay and grading system for the hospital sector is a significant impediment to reshaping the delivery of services away from hospitals to other locations. Employers need to be able to introduce more flexible contracts of employment and pay and grading systems that fit their local circumstances and patient needs. None of this means that they should be able to do this in an arbitrary manner and without proper discussion and negotiation with staff representatives. Instead however these discussions should take place locally and without the constraints of a rigid national pay structure. This greater local autonomy on the determination of pay would make it easier for the NHS to modernise working practices and service delivery and for staff to benefit from local team and individual incentive schemes aimed at greater efficiency and productivity.

I recognise that this approach will be seen as threatening to many staff and staff interests, as well as some in Whitehall who will think they are losing their ability to control public sector pay. However it would still be possible to have an annual guideline on the percentage increase in the overall NHS pay bill, alongside a productivity guideline (as described above) without seeking to micromanage local pay negotiations between employers and employees. If the NHS is to have more mutuals and social enterprises it will be difficult to achieve the benefits of those organisational models without a much more flexible pay and grading system based on more local employer/employee negotiations or groups of local employers and local employees. Union rights of representation can be perfectly well protected in such a decentralised scheme, providing they genuinely represent appropriate proportions of the workforce. After due notice local employers should be able to withdraw from national pay and grading arrangements.

Different employment contracts and accountabilities are often at the heart of the awkward boundary between health and social care that causes so much confusion and problems for patients with long-term conditions. Better integration of the commissioning and provision of means-tested social care and free at the point of use healthcare is much needed. One of the potential benefits of more localised commissioning by GP consortia and the existence of Health and Wellbeing Boards is the scope for blurring this boundary for the benefit of patients. The future disease and demography profiles will place huge pressure on social care budgets and finding sustainable and fair funding solutions is the job of the independent Commission on Care and Support appointed by the Coalition Government. My membership of that Commission makes it inappropriate for me to offer detailed thoughts on these funding issues before the Commission reports.

However it is clear that improved integration of service delivery to those with long-term conditions is critical; and that the NHS has to face up to a future in which it accepts a fuller responsibility for the care of those with underlying medical conditions that dominate the nature of their care needs. This would be better for patients and NHS budgets. We have to end the painful local tussles between NHS and local government over the funding of continuing care where local individual budget battles are fought out to the detriment of patients and their carers. Nowhere is this more apparent than in the area of dementia care where what is essentially a medical condition is treated differently from other medical conditions. The abiding principle in my view should be that where there is a diagnosed medical condition – as there is with dementia – and a patient's GP assesses that the condition is so serious that a family cannot be expected to care for someone at home because of the level of professional nursing supervision required then the NHS should pick up the tab for the necessary care, with the normal rules on loss of benefits applying as now whenever a person is admitted to hospital.

This approach would incentivise the NHS to do more to help support informal carers and care at home. This in turn would encourage more integrated service commissioning and jointly delivered care at home for people with long-term conditions. If more high cost care for the most dependent people was shifted from social care budgets to the NHS it would facilitate more preventative services being provided by social care that would postpone the need for NHS care – especially emergency admissions. A cultural shift of attitude by the NHS of this kind is needed for the sake of the NHS as well as for patients. Endlessly tightening social care eligibility criteria away from helping the less dependent as already stretched social care budgets shrink further can only damage the NHS finances in the medium-term. A better equilibrium is required between the NHS and local government in the area of long-term conditions if patient needs are to be better met. This might enable the NHS to reshape more of its care for ill or recovering people in medically supported nursing homes or community hospitals rather than the more expensive medical wards of acute hospitals.

More flexible and localised systems of services and of pay and grading will contribute to but not totally deliver the reshaping of services that the NHS requires without other changes. A more robust system of economic regulation as described above would also play its part as would a more comprehensive and coherently framed tariff and a move away from overpaying many acute hospitals through averaged-priced tariffs. However there is no substitute for well planned and well-executed sets of local service changes after appropriate public consultation. One of the dangers of a highly decentralised NHS could also be the implications for those services and buildings that need to be planned, developed and funded on a regional basis. The NHS has suffered in recent years from over-ambitious PFI hospital schemes initiated by particular trusts without sufficient regard to the regional consequences. Medical advances themselves require many specialised services to be provided on a larger scale and in fewer centres whilst making it possible to provide more routine procedures closer to home. These technological and scientific changes mean a continuing process of reshaping the location of services, greater flexibility of use of buildings and a careful planning of services and the capital consequences of reshaping them. This agenda will pose a particular challenge for the NHS Commissioning Board who will inherit an NHS with service configurations that in many parts of England do not meet either clinical needs or the likely available resources (capital and revenue), together with an untried new localised commissioning structure. The sweeping away of SHAs – irrespective of their individual merits – will remove a regional capability that is likely to be missed and may well have to be reinvented. Before the Coalition Government gets too carried away with its quango-culling it would do well to dwell a little longer on the longstanding need for the NHS to have some form of intermediate/regional tier that planned and developed future service requirements and strategically directed professional (especially medical) education and training..

I did not align the new SHAs in 2006 on government regions by accident. There was a reason. It was to provide some overarching strategic view of services in a reasonably large and coherent geographical area and plan their future development as medicine, demography and other circumstances changed, as well as ensuring that budgets were balanced across sizeable geographical territories. The need for large-scale organisations alongside more local commissioning still remains. If SHAs are to go I would replace them by allowing the NHS Commissioning Board to bring together Health and Wellbeing Boards in larger groupings for particular planning and development functions as required. The precise nature of these higher-level planning entities seems to me a matter of political preference to a great extent but I am not in any doubt that something of this kind is needed. Further thought needs to be given on how best to achieve a suitable replacement for an intermediate tier before SHAs are shuffled off into the pages of history. This kind of regional planning presence also has a relationship to the final piece of the framework I believe the NHS of the future is likely to need which is the way the NHS uses research and innovation and translates ideas into clinical benefit for patients.

Making better use of research and innovation and the translation of ideas

As discussed in Chapter 13 quite a lot of patient benefit gets lost in the translation of new scientific discoveries into widespread day-to-day NHS clinical practice. The NHS has a reputation for being slow to take up new discoveries, even when they may have been made within the NHS itself. Industry often regards selling new products into the NHS as hard work. During Labour's time in office considerable improvements were made both in the investment in R & D and the proportion of that budget spent on translating ideas into safe clinical use. A new machinery of NIHR and OSCHR has worked hard to improve the effort put into translation. However there is still a way to travel in order to speed up the widespread use by patients of proven new products and procedures.

The NHS's policy and operational systems and processes still do not ensure that clinical practice changes faster and speeds up patient access to new technologies. The world of NIHR and OSCHR is still a long way from being integrated into the world of NHS operational decision-making. Despite the emphasis on new ways of working and the importance of innovation following the Darzi Review there was no reference to R & D in the 2009/10 Operating Framework issued by the NHS Chief Executive. Unlike most successful businesses the NHS's R & D effort has not been integrated systematically with the way the NHS operates on a day-to-day basis. R & D seems to operate in a parallel universe to the decision-making of most Board and executive management teams, relying heavily on local clinical champions to bring technological advances into practice. In an ideal world these technologies and their speedy adoption should be more influential in the commissioning and forward planning processes of the NHS. Nowhere will this be more critical than the advances in personalised medicine promised by genomic and epigenomic medicine.

The structural changes being proposed for the NHS provide the opportunity to revisit this whole area of integrating R & D and innovation into NHS operational decision-making processes. The starting place for such a change, as with so many other topics, is the new NHS Commissioning Board. If it is to control commissioning guidelines and a tariff these are mechanisms that can be used to foster the speedier take up of innovative procedures, especially where they represent better value for money. However this requires a level of horizon-scanning and monitoring for innovation that should secure speedier absorption into clinical practice. This is likely to mean a stronger role for NICE in relating R & D work to clinical standards and an R & D translation capability in the Board itself for picking up proven discoveries that the NHS needs to adopt more speedily. At present there is little organised briefing of senior decision-makers in commissioners or providers on the R & D work coming out of NIHR and OSCHR or the pharmaceutical and devices industries. Too many decision-makers lack the information to pursue these issues in their local processes. The Commissioning Board should consider how this knowledge gap can be filled and related better to the financial investment decision-making of commissioning and provider boards. This approach might be reinforced by an annual research briefing for local boards that identified the high-impact changes coming out of translation R & D that they should be thinking about in terms of local implementation.

These concerns about the translation of R & D discoveries into the mindsets of NHS decision makers echo the problems of NHS investment in information technology and informatics. Although Labour's investment in IT was hugely better than what went before and improved NHS IT capacity considerably, progress was thwarted on both the NPfIT and the pursuit of telecare. NHS use of information both for better management and patient benefit and choice is some way from what is required. Investment in informatics is both unsystematic and inadequate. The Coalition promises 'An Information Revolution' but this will not take place without much greater investment in both technology and skilled people. Exhorting and hoping for the best locally will not deliver rapid change if the past is anything to go by. Essential as local buy-in is to successful IT change so is knowledge, incentives and contracting skills. It is far from clear how the information revolution is to be delivered without some grouping of the limited skills and money and some drive from the centre to ensure that those with the skills to implement new IT systems can be secured for the benefit of the NHS.

This looks like another 'to do' for the new Commissioning Board, aided by a more dynamic Information Centre. At the heart of the problem of faster take-up of IT in the NHS has been access to knowhow, an investment-funding stream and the managerial and clinical will to convert antique local systems to something suitable for a 21st century health and healthcare system that links into local authority IT systems as well. It is difficult to see change happening fast without financial incentives and an affordable way of securing the knowhow locally to purchase and implement new systems.

A central capital development fund operated, at least in part, on a loan basis seems to me likely to be needed. Some central assessment and part-procurement of approved implementers to help local organisations choose and implement systems also seems to me necessary if the NHS is to get the skills they need at an affordable price. This approach would not foist on local people software systems that do not fit their needs or are unproven. If an electronic patient record and more rapid use of telecare is to happen mechanisms of this kind are going to be required. They will almost certainly require some form of financial top slicing centrally and a system of repayable loans to secure local commitment and a degree of recycling of central funds. The natural resting place for hosting such arrangements is likely eventually to be the NHS Commissioning Board, although the DH could handle some of this work in the shorter-term.

A summing up

Labour saved the NHS but did not secure it for the future. The advances under Labour should not be forgotten – higher investment, more skilled people, more modern equipment and many better buildings. Waiting times and waiting lists dropped significantly and overall access to hospitals and GPs improved. Deaths from killer diseases fell considerably but the UK still lags behind the best performers in Europe in areas like early diagnosis of cancers. A tariff for paying hospitals replaced the inefficient block grant system and patient choice was established, in principle. Belated efforts were made to introduce some competition but efforts stuttered at the end. Foundation Trust were established and showed that hospitals could be run autonomously and could raise their game but the job was only half done with 50% of acute hospitals not making the grade.

Performance management and regulation improved but financial control and financial management still remains a major challenge for many commissioners and service providers. Commissioning has not progressed as it should have done and PCTs have been a huge disappointment as deliverers of change and as demand managers. Too much of the extra money has been gobbled up by acute hospitals, with political, managerial and clinical unwillingness to reconfigure hospital services more efficiently and bring many services closer to home. Productivity has been unsatisfactory given the levels of increased investment. The NHS remains a rather bureaucratic, inward-looking organisation resistant to competition and with a high propensity for 'keeping things in the NHS family'. There has been an unwillingness to rebalance the NHS adequately between the needs of public health and those of acute medicine in order to better reflect society's disease and demographic profiles. Compared with the NHS, social care has been treated far less generously under Labour.

As the UK faces a period of lengthy public expenditure austerity the NHS is better equipped in resource terms than virtually all other public services. Whether its mindset is adequately prepared for austerity is another matter. Many of its basic systems of financial management, asset use, IT, securing higher productivity and information-rich performance management are much weaker than they should be. Its challenge systems dealing with poor performers and replacing them are weak. It has become too used to central government giving it money with insufficient conditionality and backing off on reform and competition when vested interests raise their voices. This is the reality of the situation the Coalition

Government faces with its ambitious programme of reform. It is the situation and mindset that a Labour Government would face if it was suddenly catapulted into office.

This book tries to give a fair account and assessment of Labour's stewardship of the NHS, warts and all. I have drawn upon that experience in framing the ideas in this final chapter. The NHS badly needs a major overhaul of its business systems and processes if it is to use the resources provided to it much more effectively and efficiently. The way the NHS uses money, assets and people is often wasteful. Simply increasing the influence of clinicians without changing the way the NHS does its business will not deliver desired change. Without a more robust financial, economic and performance architecture greater devolution and clinician power could produce financial meltdown in the NHS, particularly with an inadequately planned and over-hastily implemented radical reorganisation which is itself likely to cost a lot of money. The Coalition Government needs a far better transition plan for its changes – many of which I support – than it has so far revealed and a set of financial controls that will guarantee to prevent financial and service implosion.

For many hardworking and committed professionals working in the NHS I recognise that my criticisms will seem unfair and my prescriptions unnecessary and over-managerialist. Some political colleagues will take the same view, especially those who have a low opinion of men and women in grey (or more likely black nowadays) suits. But it is better management – clinical and lay – that the NHS badly needs now and the business architecture to accompany it. I hope this book helps more of that architecture to be built in an institution that remains a national treasure but continues to need reform. As Ernest Rutherford, the eminent wartime physicist said – 'We haven't got the money, so we have to think.' That is the situation the NHS faces in 2011, as the risk of the money running out increases.

Notes

Preface – Scene setting

1. Lord Butler of Brockwell, profile in The House Magazine, 17 May 2010.

1 The NHS reform inheritance

1. Sir Roy Griffiths, letter to Norman (now Lord) Fowler, then Secretary of State for Social Services, 6 October 1983. This letter set out the findings of the NHS Management Inquiry set up in February 1983 and led by Sir Roy to give advice on the effective use and management of manpower and related resources in the NHS. Its main recommendation was the establishment of an NHS Management Board.
2. Margaret (now Baroness) Thatcher, speech as Prime Minister to the Conservative Party Conference, 8 October 1982.
3. Nicholas Timmins, *The Five Giants: A Biography of the Welfare State* (Harper Collins, 1995) p.465.
4. Ibid.
5. New Labour because Britain deserves better, 1997 Labour Party Election Manifesto.
6. The NHS Plan: a plan for investment, a plan for reform, Department of Health, July 2000.
7. Ibid.
8. Ambitions for Britain, 2001 Labour Party General Election Manifesto.

2 Investing in the NHS – money and targets

1. New Labour because Britain deserves better, 1997 Labour Party General Election Manifesto.
2. The NHS Plan: a plan for investment, a plan for reform, Department of Health, July 2000.
3. Ambitions for Britain, 2001 Labour Party General Election Manifesto.
4. Ibid.
5. Jennifer Rankin, *Public Expectations & the NHS*, Institute for Public Policy Research, September 2006.
6. The NHS Improvement Plan: Putting People at the Heart of Public Services, Department of Health, June 2004.
7. State of Healthcare 2008, Healthcare Commission, December 2008.
8. Ibid.

9. NHS performance ratings 2008/09, An overview of the performance of NHS trusts in England, Care Quality Commission, December 2009.

3 Creating an NHS market – foundation trusts, competition and tariffs

1. James Johnson, Privatisation by stealth is bad for your health Sunday Times, early 2006. (Article in capacity as Chairman of British Medical Association.)
2. NHS foundation trusts: report for year ended 31 March 2007, Monitor, June 2007.
3. The annual health check 2006/2007, Directory of performance ratings for NHS trusts, Healthcare Commission, late 2007, Table 3.
4. NHS Foundation Trusts – the story so far, Foundation Trust Network, July 2007.
5. NHS foundation trusts: review of six months to 30 September 2008, Monitor, December 2008, p.1.
6. NHS Foundation Trusts – the story so far, Foundation Trust Network, July 2007.
7. High Quality Care for All – NHS Next Stage Review Final Report, Department of Health, June 2008, p.61.
8. NHS foundation trusts: review of twelve months to 31 March 2009, Monitor, 24 June 2009.
9. State of Healthcare 2008, Healthcare Commission, December 2008.
10. Presentation by Monitor's Chief Operating Officer, February 2009.
11. NHS performance ratings 2008/09, An overview of the performance of NHS trusts in England, Care Quality Commission, December 2009.
12. Growing Capacity: Independent Sector Diagnosis and Treatment Centres, Department of Health, December 2002.
13. Independent Sector Treatment Centres, House of Commons Health Committee, Fourth Report of Session 2005-06, 25 July 2006, Volume 1, p.30 – para 73.
14. Ibid, p.17 – para 28
15. Ibid, p.30 – para 72.
16. Ibid, p.4 – first para.
17. Financial Times, 26 September 2007, p.2.
18. Nicholas Timmins, Financial Times, 6 February 2008.
19. Ibid.
20. Department of Health press notice, 15 November 2007.
21. Nicholas Timmins, Financial Times, 6 February 2008.
22. Department of Health press notice, 15 November 2007.

23. Personal papers.

24. High Quality Care for All – NHS Next Stage Review Final Report, Department of Health, June 2008, p.41 – footnote 76.

25. The right result? Payment by Results 2003-07, Audit Commission, February 2008.

4 Choice and commissioning

1. The NHS Plan: A plan for investment, A plan for reform, Department of Health, July 2000.

2. Building on the Best – Choice, Responsiveness and Equity in the NHS, Department of Health, December 2003.

3. Ibid, pages 3 and 4.

4. The NHS Improvement Plan: Putting People at the Heart of Public Services, Department of Health, June 2004.

5. Britain forward not back, 2005 Labour Party Election Manifesto, pages 63 and 64.

6. Patient choice – how patients choose and how providers respond, King's Fund, June 2010.

7. MORI survey for Department of Health, April 2005.

8. *A review of the effectiveness of primary care-led commissioning and its place in the NHS*, Martin Smith, Nicholas Mays, Jennifer Dixon, Nick Goodwin, Richard Lewis, Siobham McClelland, Hugh Mcleod, Sally Wyke, The Health Foundation, October 2004.

9. Practice-based commissioning: achieving universal coverage, Department of Health, January 2006.

10. Ibid, p.10 – para. 47.

11. Health reform in England: update and commissioning framework, Department of Health, 13 July 2006, p.14.

12. Health reform in England: update and commissioning framework, annex – the commissioning framework, Department of Health, 13 July 2006, p.4.

13. Putting commissioning into practice – implementing practice-based commissioning through good financial management, Audit Commission, November 20007, p.2.

14. GP News, 26 September 2008.

15. *Practice-based Commissioning: Reinvigorate, Replace or Abandon?*, King's Fund, November 2008.

16. Lords Hansard, 8 July 2009, Col. WA156.

17. Health reform in England: update and next steps, Department of Health, 21 December 2005.

18. Health reform in England: update and commissioning framework, annex - the commissioning framework, Department of Health. 13 July 2006, p.29, para. 3.5.

19. John Carvel, The Guardian, 30 June 2006, front page.

20. Review of Commissioning Arrangements for Specialised Services, Department of Health, May 2006.

21. The NHS in England: the operating framework for 2007/08, Department of Health, 11 December 2006, p.21.

22. The NHS in England: the operating framework for 2008/09, Department of Health, 13 December 2007, p27, para. 3.11.

23. The NHS in England: the operating framework for 2007/08, Department of Health, 11 December 2006, p.17, para. 3.13.

24. Mark Britnell, Public Servant, March 2009, p.24.

25. NHS performance ratings 2008/09, An overview of the performance of NHS trusts in England, Care Quality Commission, December 2009, pages 112-115.

26. NHS Next Stage Review, House of Commons Health Committee, First Report of Sessions 2008-09, Volume 1, p.61, para. 3, January 2009.

5 Cutting bureaucracy and streamlining the NHS

1. Review of NHS data collections 2005: report for the Department of Health and the NHS Health and Social Care Information Centre, Department of Health, July 2006.

2. Department of Health press notice, 20 May 2004. Written House of Commons statement by John Reid on same day.

3. Reconfiguring the Department of Health's Arm's Length Bodies, Department of Health, 22 July 2004.

4. An Implementation Framework for Reconfiguring the DH Arm's Length Bodies, Department of Health, 30 November 2004.

5. Lords Hansard, 15 July 2009, Col. WA219.

6. The James Committee on Taxpayer Value. Proposals on NHS released by Conservative Party during second half of 2004.

7. Britain forward not back, 2005 Labour Party Election Manifesto, p.61.

8. Taking healthcare to the patient: transforming NHS ambulance services, Department of Health, 30 June 2005.

9. Commissioning a patient-led NHS, Letter to NHS and local authority chief executives, directors of social services and PEC chairs from NHS Chief Executive, Department of Health, 28 July 2005.

10. Ibid p.9, para. 35.

11. Niall Dickson, Health Service Journal, 12 July 2007, pages 14 and 15.

12. Patricia Hewitt, Speech to NHS Chairs, 20 September 2005.

13. Configuration of NHS ambulance trusts in England: a consultation, Department of Health, 14 December 2005.

14. New architecture of local NHS, Department of Health press release, 12 April 2006.

15. Review of the NHS financial year 2006/07, Audit Commission, October 2007.

6 A people business – or where the money went

1. Office of National Statistics Labour Force Survey 1997-2006.

2. NHS Health and Community Health Services and General Practice Workforce 1996-2006, The Information Centre. Figures for all years are as at 30 September each year.

3. Ibid.

4. Ibid.

5. Ibid.

6. Ibid.

7. Ibid.

8. Information from Income Data Services incorporated in article by Nicholas Timmins in the Financial Times of 20 March 2006, p.3.

9. Letter from author to all MPs, July 2006.

10. Letter from author to all MPs, 30 October 2006.

11. Ibid.

12. Lords Hansard, 15 July 2009.

13. Office of National Statistics UK Centre for the Measurement of Government Activity: Total Public Service Output and Productivity, June 2009. This covers the period 1997-2007.

14. Lords Hansard, 16 July 2009, Col. WA259.

15. *Aspiring to Excellence*, Final report of the Independent Inquiry into modernising medical careers led by Professor Sir John Tooke, January 2007.

16. Workforce Planning, House of Commons Health Committee, Fourth Report of Session 2006-07, Volume 1, March 2007.

17. Modernising Medical Careers, House of Commons Health Committee, Third Report of Session 2007-08, Volume 1, May 2008.

18. High Quality Care for All – NHS Next Stage review Final Report, Department of Health, June 2008.

19. NHS Next Stage Review, House of Commons Health Committee, First Report Session 2008-09, Volume 1, p.59, para.175, January 2009.

7 GPs – gatekeepers or change agents?

1. The Provision of Out-of-Hours Care in England, National Audit Office, 5 May 2006.

2. NHS Pay Modernisation: New Contracts for General practice, Forty-first Report, Public Accounts Committee, 9 October 2008.

3. Ibid.

4. GP Earnings and Expenses Enquiry (EEQ) 2005-06, Final Report, The Information Centre, 2008.

5. GP magazine, 26 October 2007, front page.

6. Alan Johnson speaking at NHS Alliance conference, October 2008.

7. NHS Pay Modernisation: New Contract for General Practice, Forty-first Report, Public Accounts Committee, 9 October 2008.

8. General and Personal Medical Services England 1999-2009, The Information Centre, 25 March 2010.

9. Ibid.

10. Ibid.

11. Ibid.

12. Ibid.

13. Ibid.

14. Lords Hansard, 21 January 2010, Col. WA279.

15. General and Personal Medical Services England 1999-2009, The Information Centre, 25 March 2010.

16. GP Patient Survey 2008/09, Ipsos/MORI, 30 June 2009.

17. Lords Hansard, 21 January 2010, Col. WA279.

18. Unpublished report by consultants on London's community health services, 2009.

19. DH estimate of community services inefficiency after Darzi final report.

20. Author's information on Autonomous Provider Organisations.

21. Lords Hansard, 9 March 2010, Column 136.

22. What the Doctor Ordered: Study of GP fundholders in England and Wales, Audit Commission, 1996; Giving GPs budgets for commissioning: what needs to be done, Nuffield Trust, 23 June 2010.

23. Commissioning, House of Commons Health Committee, Fourth Report of Session 2009-10, Volume 1, March 2010.

24. Equity and excellence: Liberating the NHS, The Stationery Office, 12 July 2010.

8 Computer games – connecting for health

1. National Strategy for Local Implementation, Department of Health, 1998.

2. Delivering 21st Century IT for the NHS, Department of Health, 2002.

3. John Oughton giving evidence to the Public Accounts Committee, 2005.

4. Ben Verwaayen, interview in Sunday Times (Business), p.9, 14 May 2006.

5. Supporting Transformation, National Programme for IT in the NHS, Benefits Statement 2006/07, Department of Health, late 2008.

6. Michael Cross, The Guardian, 19 October 2006, p.7.

7. Supporting Transformation, National Programme for IT in the NHS, Benefits Statement 2006/07, Department of Health, late 2008.

8. Department of Health: The National Programme for IT in the NHS, National Audit Office, 16 June 2006.

9. Nicholas Timmins, Financial Times, 30 May 2006.

10. Supporting Transformation, National Programme for IT in the NHS, Benefits Statement 2006.07, Department of Health, late 2008.

11. David Nicholson communication on NPfIT Local Ownership Programme, August 2006.

12. House of Lords Debate on Public Sector IT Projects, Official Report, 21 June 2007, Columns 376-377.

13. Jonathan B. Perlin, *Transformation of the US Veteran Health Administration, Health Economics, Policy and Law (2006)*, Vol.1, pages 99-105.

14. John Carvel, The Guardian, 19 December 2006.

15. The National Programme for IT in the NHS: Progress since 2006, National Audit Office, 16 May 2008.

16. Lords Hansard, 6 January 2010, Col. WA108.

9 Financial meltdown and recovery

1. Author's list of NHS Counter Fraud Management Service achievements prepared for 2005 Election.

2. Author's personal papers.

3. Ibid.

4. Ibid.

5. Ibid.

6. Audit Commission review of the NHS financial management and accounting regime – a report to the Secretary of State for Health, Audit Commission, July 2006.

7. Review of the NHS financial year 2006/07, Audit Commission, October 2007.

8. Written Ministerial statement to the House of Commons by Alan Johnson, 29 November 2007.

9. Review of the NHS financial year 2006/07, Audit Commission, October 2007.

10. NHS performance ratings 2008/9, An overview of the performance of NHS trusts in England, Care Quality Commission, December 2009.

11. Lords Hansard, 14 July 2009, Col. WA207.

10 Keep taking the tablets – pharmaceuticals and the NHS

1. Safeguarding public health, MHRA Corporate Plan 2004-05 to 2009-10, MHRA, April 2004.

2. Heart drug available without a prescription, Department of Health press notice, 12 May 2004.

3. Report of an Independent Review of Access to the Yellow Card Scheme, The Stationery Office, 5 May 2004.

4. Department of Health, press notice, 17 January 2005.

5. Richard Brook, Daily Mail, 23 March 2004.

6. (a) Committee on Safety of Medicines's Expert Working Group Report on SSRIs, MHRA, 6 December 2004; (b) National Institute for Clinical Excellence guidelines on the treatment and care of people with depression and anxiety, NICE, 6 December 2004.

7. GSK investigation concludes, MHRA press release, 6 March 2008.

8. The Influence of the Pharmaceutical Industry, House of Commons Health Committee, Fourth Report of Session 2004-05, Volume II, EV372, 3 February 2005.

9. Better healthcare through partnership: a programme for action, report of Healthcare Industries Taskforce, Department of Health, 17 November 2004.

10. Serious Organised Crime and Police Act, 2005.

11. Ian Sample, The Guardian, 21 July 2009.

12. The British National Formulary for Children, first published 2005 and now updated at 2010-2011.
13. 1999-2009 – A decade of excellence, National Institute for Health and Clinical Excellence, July 2009, p.10.
14. Ibid, p.7.
15. Ibid. p.7.
16. High Quality Care for All – NHS Next Stage Review Final report, Department of Health, June 2008.

11 Acute hospitals – cathedrals of cures or expensive luxuries?

1. NHS Performance ratings 2008/09, An overview of the performance of NHS trusts in England, Care Quality Commission, December 2009.
2. Investigation into outbreaks of Clostridium difficile at Maidstone and Tunbridge Wells NHS Trust, Healthcare Commission, October 2007.
3. Investigation into Mid Staffordshire NHS Foundation Trust, Healthcare Commission, March 2009.
4. *The Hospital Guide*, Dr Foster, November 2009.
5. High Quality Care for All – NHS Next Stage Review Final Report, Department of Health, June 2008.
6. National performance ratings 2008/09, An overview of the performance of NHS trusts in England, Care Quality Commission, December 2009.
7. Deaths in Acute Hospitals, National Confidential Enquiry into Patient Outcome and Death, 2009.
8. Winning ways: working together to reduce healthcare associated infection in England, Report of Chief Medical Officer, Department of Health, 5 December 2003.
9. Improving patient care by reducing the risk of hospital acquired infection: a progress report, National Audit Office, July 2004.
10. High Quality Care for All – NHS Next Stage Review Final Report, Department of health, June 2008.
11. Health Act, 2009 and The Code of Practice for the Prevention and Control of Healthcare Associated Infections, 2006.
12. Statement by Healthcare Commission, 16 June 2008.
13. State of Healthcare 2008, Healthcare Commission, December 2008.
14. Private briefing provided to author.
15. Lords Hansard, 14 July 2009, Col. WA207.
16. NHS performance ratings, 2008/09, An overview of the performance of NHS trusts in England, Care Quality Commission, December 2009.

17. Ibid.
18. Ibid.
19. Unpublished consultants report to Queen Elizabeth Hospital Trust.
20. Lords Hansard, 20 July 2009, Col. WA286.
21. Lords Hansard, 16 July 2009, Col. WA261
22. High Quality Care for All – NHS Next Stage Review Final Report, Department of Health, June 2008.
23. Report of the Review of NHS Pathology Services in England, Department of Health, August 2006.
24. Report of the Second Phase of the Independent Review of NHS Pathology Services in England, Department of Health, December 2008.
25. Lords Hansard, 15 July 2009, Col. WA233.

12 Getting closer to home

1. A Framework for Action, report by Sir Ara Darzi for NHS London, 2007.
2. Ibid.
3. Independence, Well-being and Choice: Our Vision for the Future of Social Care for Adults in England, The Stationery Office, March 2005.
4. Saving Lives: Our Healthier Nation, Department of Health, June 1999.
5. Mortality target monitoring: update to include data for 2008, Department of Health electronic publication, 14 October 2009.
6. Choosing Health: making healthy choices easier, The Stationery Office, November 2004.
7. Health Survey for England 2004,Department of Health 2004.
8. Profiles of disease in 'Our health, our care, our say' White Paper, The Stationery Office, January 2006.
9. Information on carers in 2006 White paper.
10. EU comparisons in 2006 White Paper.
11. Responses to the consultation on adult social care in England: analysis of the feedback from the Green Paper, Department of Health, October 2005.
12. Our health, our care, our say: a new direction for community services, The Stationery Office, January 2006.
13. Ibid.
14. Ibid.

15. Ibid.

16. Our health, our care, our say: making it happen, Department of Health, 18 October 2006.

17. Ibid.

18. Our health, our care our say: investing in the future of community hospitals and services, Department of Health, July 2006.

19. Our NHS our future – NHS Next Stage Review Interim Report, Department of Health, October 2007.

20. A Framework for Action, report by Sir Ara Darzi for NHS London, 2007.

21. High Quality Care for All – NHS Next Stage Review Final Report and Regional Reports, Department of Health, June 2008.

13 Lost in translation – science, healthcare and politics

1. Our Inheritance, Our Future – Realising the potential of genetics in the NHS, The Stationery Office, 24 June 2003.

2. New Scientist editorial, November 2007.

3. *The Race to the Top: A Review of Government's Science and Innovation Policies*, Lord Sainsbury of Turville, 5 October 2007.

4. Public Attitudes to Science 2008, Research Councils UK, March 2008.

5. Public Attitudes to Stem Cell Research – establishing the UK stem cell bank, Medical Research Council, 2003.

6. Review of Human Fertilisation and Embryology Act: proposals for revised legislation (including establishment of Regulatory Authority for Tissue and Embryos), The Stationery Office, 14 December 2006.

7. Government proposals for the regulation of hybrid and chimera embryos, House of Commons Science and Technology Committee, Fifth Report of Session 2006/07, 5 April 2007.

8. House of Lords debates on Human Fertilisation and Embryology Act, 2008.

9. House of Lords Select Committee on Science and Technology's Report on Genomic Medicare, 7 July 2009.

10. John Carvel, The Guardian , 17 November 2008, front page.

11. Richard Thomas and Mark Walport, *Data Sharing Review*, Ministry of Justice, 11 July 2008.

12. Sir David Cooksey, *A Review of UK Health Research Funding*, December 2006.

13. The Review and Refresh of Bioscience 2015, a Report to Government by the Bioscience Innovation and Growth Team, Department for Business, Enterprise and Regulatory Reform, January 2009.

14. PHG evidence to House of Lords Science and Technology Committee's Inquiry into Genomic Medicine, quoted at paragraph 76 of Committee's final report.
15. House of Lords Select Committee on Science and Technology's Report on Genomic Medicine, 7 July 2009.
16. Medical Technology – Can we afford to miss out?, The Medical Technology Group, December 2009.
17. The operating framework for the NHS in England 2010/11, Department of Health, 16 December 2009.

14 Who's in charge? – accountability and regulation

1. The Future of Health and Adult Social Care Regulation, report of research into the impact of system reform on regulatory requirements, Department of Health, 23 November 2006.
2. Ibid.
3. Ibid.
4. The future regulation of health and adult social care in England, Department of Health, 27 November 2006.
5. Ibid.
6. The future regulation of health and adult social care in England: response to consultation, Department of Health, 24 October 2007.
7. Ibid.
8. High Quality Care for All – NHS Next Stage Review Final Report, Department of Health, June 2008.
9. Ibid.
10. Consultation on a regime for unsustainable NHS providers, Department of Health, 10 September 2008.
11. Ibid.
12. Ibid.
13. Framework for Managing Choice, Cooperation and Competition, Department of Health, 16 May 2008.
14. David Nicholson, 'Dear Colleague' letter launching Cooperation and Competition Panel, Department of Health, 28 January 2009.
15. Lords Hansard, 15 July 2009, Col. WA232.
16. Primary care trust procurement of guide for health services, Department of Health, 25 March 2010.
17. The Coalition: our programme for government, Cabinet Office, May 2010, p.25.

18. Equity and excellence: Liberating the NHS, The Stationery Office, 12 July 2010.

15 Assessing Labour's NHS Stewardship

1. The operating framework for the NHS in England 2010/11, Department of Health, 16 December 2009, p.31.
2. Growth in hospital admissions varies by 28 per cent, press release by CMKS, 3 March 2010 (and supporting report).
3. Sheelah Connolly, Nicholas Mays, Gwyn Bevan, *Funding and Performance of Healthcare Systems in the Four Countries of the UK Before and After Devolution*, Nuffield Trust, 20 January 2010.
4. Free Personal and Nursing Care, Scotland, 2007-08, National Statistics publication for Scotland, November 2009.
5. NHS Chief Executive's Annual Report for 2008/09, Department of Health, 31 May 2010.

Lightning Source UK Ltd.
Milton Keynes UK
10 March 2011

169052UK00001B/24/P